Translational Speech-Language Pathology and Audiology

Translational Speech-Language Pathology and Audiology

Essays in Honor of Dr. Sadanand Singh

Edited by
Robert Goldfarb

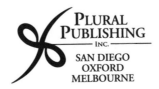

PLURAL PUBLISHING
— INC. —

SAN DIEGO
OXFORD
MELBOURNE

MW

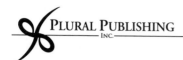

5521 Ruffin Road
San Diego, CA 92123

e-mail: info@pluralpublishing.com
Web site: http://www.pluralpublishing.com

49 Bath Street
Abingdon, Oxfordshire OX14 1EA
United Kingdom

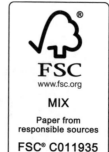

FSC
www.fsc.org

MIX
Paper from
responsible sources

FSC® C011935

Library of Congress Cataloging-in-Publication Data

Goldfarb, Robert (Robert M.)
 Translational speech-language pathology and audiology : essays in honor of Dr. Sadanand Singh /
Robert Goldfarb.
 p. ; cm.
 Includes bibliographical references and index.
 ISBN-13: 978-1-59756-445-8 (alk. paper)
 ISBN-10: 1-59756-445-1 (alk. paper)
 I. Singh, Sadanand. II. Title.
 [DNLM: 1. Speech Disorders—Festschrift. 2. Hearing Disorders—Festschrift. 3. Language
Disorders—Festschrift. 4. Translational Medical Research—Festschrift. WL 340.2]
 LC Classification not assigned
 616.85'5—dc23
 2012009023

4/2/14

❧ Contents ❧

Preface

There was a welcome message on the answering machine: "Robert, this is Singh. Call me back." He didn't call me Bob and I didn't call him Sadanand. Sometimes, the message included a South Asian–inflected addition: "It's ten o'clock. Call me back in an hour's time."

The purpose of the conversation was, not surprisingly, a book. I had met Singh occasionally over the years, and had used many College-Hill Press and Singular Publishing books professionally and as assignments to students, but we had never before exchanged more than pleasantries. Still, having arranged a symposium on ethics and looking for a publisher for the proceedings, I contacted only one. Who but Singh would have been open to a book whose focus was a 1939 master's thesis? He was planning to launch a new publishing company, Plural Publishing, and certainly wouldn't have been blamed if he passed on my proposal in favor of one likely to sell more briskly.

Singh published the book (Goldfarb, 2006), and it must have sold dozens of copies. Still, he wanted to use his influence as a publisher to advance the study of ethics in our professions, even if he didn't make any money doing it. Fortunately, the other two books I wrote for Plural sold quite a bit better. As a very successful businessman, Singh never stopped being a teacher, scholar, and mentor. A description of his legacy also should certainly include his constant and long-standing support and encouragement of new generations of clinicians and researchers.

As the reader will note in the essays that follow, Singh touched many of us in personal, professional, and profound ways. The authors of the essays in this volume include many of the boldface names in speech-language pathology and audiology from around the world. Some who, because of clerical errors, had not been invited in the first round of emails asked to join the project. These are people who do not need to pad their résumés, and include ASHA Fellows, Honorees, and named professors. That the essays reflect some of their most important work is a tribute to their esteem and affection for Singh. We have also included essays from burgeoning scholars, who are much newer to the professions. Singh always had time to listen to, and be interested in, the ideas of our younger colleagues.

The structure of the book raises two questions: Why are we using a translational model, and why have we written essays instead of chapters?

The following was sent to prospective contributors:

> *Translational SLP/A* will include investigations in the broad fields of laboratory, clinical, and public health research. Interdisciplinary and cross-disciplinary papers are encouraged. Aiming to expedite the translation of scientific discovery into new or improved standards of care, the book is intended to promote a wide-ranging exchange among basic, preclinical, clinical, epidemiologic, and health outcomes topics. Also encouraged will be essays describing public health research with potential for application to the clinic, disease prevention, or health care policy. Our professions are somewhat behind the curve, compared to medicine, in not addressing this issue directly, although there certainly have been efforts in this direction by individuals.

As we will see in Part II, discovery is a two-way street, with clinical findings informing scientific exploration, in addition to the "bench-to-bedside" approach to translational research.

The invitation to contribute included the understanding that all editor and author royalties will be donated to the San Diego Foundation/Dr. Sadanand Singh Fund. In a paragraph before the essays, authors discuss Dr. Singh's influence on their careers.

We have written mostly short essays of about 2,500 words with no more than 25 references. The 18th-century Scottish philosopher David Hume used the essay form to write about essay writing. A recent edition of *The New Yorker* features Princeton English literature Professor Jeff Nunokowa's thoughts on writing short pieces. "They are brief essays. That is to say, what Hume was getting at in the essay on essay writing: rendering the sphere of scholarship sociable" (Mead, 2011, p. 19). We hope the essay form will honor the memory of the most sociable of scholars, Sadanand Singh.

The book is divided into six topic areas.

Part I: In Memory of Dr. Sadanand Singh contains four essays. Jeffrey L. Danhauer's "Eulogy" includes a portion of the remarks delivered at the memorial ceremony for Dr. Singh on April 6, 2010. Thomas Murry wrote "In the Course of a Lifetime: A Multidimensional Relationship." In this essay, he acknowledged the 46 years of friendship with Dr. Singh, a relationship that began with the voice science work that they did while Singh was at the University of Texas and Murry was at the VA Medical Center in San Diego. The nature of speech analysis took a dynamic turn in the early 1970s with the use of multivariate statistics, and Dr. Singh was on the cutting edge of that scientific method of speech analysis. The work they did at that time helped to solidify a friendship that had developed in the speech science program at Ohio State University. John W. Oller Jr.'s essay, "Milestones and Cases Along the Way," includes reflections on Dr. Singh's influence on the book projects that became *Milestones* (2006) and *Cases* (2010).

The research cited in these books shows that organo-mercurials are also genotoxins that damage the genetics of plants, insects, lab animals, and humans. Jon K. Shallop remembers "My Personal Journey with a Good Friend and Scholar: My Tribute to Dr. Sadanand Singh." "It was a cool fall day in 1963 in Columbus, Ohio, when I met Sadanand. We were both new doctoral students in the OSU Speech and Hearing Sciences Program with Prof. John W. Black as our advisor. Dr. Black said, 'Shallop, you teach him English and he will teach you about Hindu philosophy.'" Indeed he did.

Part II: The Nature of Translational Research contains five essays. Ray D. Kent presents "Models and Concepts of Translational Research." He expands on the basic description of translational research as (T1) "bench-to-bedside" and (T2) "bedside-to-community." John C. Rosenbek discusses "The Science of Dissemination." Translation from laboratory to practice was hastened by Dr. Singh's dedication to publishing, but continues to be too slow and erratic, problems that Dr. Singh recognized and actively tried to solve. Audiology and speech-language pathology's dedication to a science of dissemination that moves the professions beyond publishing, continuing education courses, and yearly conventions may well help to finish what he began. Lauren K. Nelson is interested in "Promoting Resilience in Young Children: A Role in Prevention of Communication Disorders." Resilience is a term that refers to situations in which children overcome exposure to adversity to attain normal or above normal functioning in one or more developmental domains. Interventions focused on factors that promote resilience in young children might provide opportunities for speech-language pathologists to participate in primary prevention.

Wendy Papir-Bernstein presents the clinical perspective in "The Artistry of Practice-Based Evidence (PBE): One Practitioner's Path — Part I." This essay focuses on Types 3 and 4 of the translational research continuum (dissemination, diffusion, and evaluation), sometimes referred to as PBE. She correlates principals from the fields of information design and knowledge management. Karyn Lewis Searcy, Aubyn Stahmer, and Lauren Brookman-Frazee describe the "SoCal BRIDGE Collaborative: Across Treatment Disciplines." BRIDGE is a result of the collaboration among researchers, funding agencies, parents, and therapists to develop an early intervention treatment for children at risk for autism. Unique aspects include the research-to-clinical collaboration that expedites the process of implementing evidence-based practices and the recognition that parents need to directly collaborate in the treatment.

Part III: Public Health, Education, and Clinical Policy contains seven essays. Edie Hapner explores how the scope of practice for SLPs can include "Community and Office-Based Oral, Head, and Neck Cancer Screening and Education: Our Role and Responsibilities." By educating themselves on the risks, signs, and symptoms of this cancer, and by implementing simple visual oral examinations and adding case history questions that might identify the presence of concerning findings and the need for immediate otolaryngology follow up, speech-language pathologists have the opportunity to impact the survival rates from this cancer. Alison Behrman is interested in "Fostering Patient Compliance by Nurturing Clinical Expertise in Graduate School." The skills with which the therapist manages the problem of client adherence are those that comprise clinical expertise. She considers the neurological control of creativity, in part because she speculates that creativity plays a significant role in clinical expertise. Wendy Papir-Bernstein continues her view of "The Artistry of Practice-Based Evidence (PBE): One Practitioner's Path — Part II." She discusses the enhancement of program effectiveness for speech-language therapy programs in the practice-based educational arena, through the implementation of a reflective and self-directed approach to staff development and supervision.

Andrea F. Blau is both a practicing attorney and an SLP; she describes "The Interplay Between Legal Policy and Clinical Practice." She explores examples of how public policy, as expressed through our legal system, impacts our clinical practice, and how speech and hearing sciences in turn influences the practice of law. Joseph J. Montano reports on "Overdependence on Technology in the Management of Hearing Loss." He is concerned that oral rehabilitation may be neglected in clinical practice by both audiologists and speech-language pathologists. He recommends that services provided by audiologists be patient centered, not merely technocentric. Yula C. Serpanos and Abbey L. Berg reveal "Noise Exposure and the Potential Impact on Hearing in the Pediatric Population." The rise in societal exposure to environmental and recreational noise is associated with an increased incidence of high-frequency hearing loss in the pediatric and adolescent population. This essay reviews sources of noise exposure and presents recommendations to disseminate and make accessible information gleaned from research on noise-related hearing loss and its prevention to the profession and general population. Finally, Peter Flipsen Jr. advocates for "Off-Label Use of Norm-Referenced Tests in Speech Pathology: Insights Gained from Children with Hearing Impairment." The use of a procedure or treatment in a way for which it was not originally intended and particularly for which it was not specifically approved is often referred to as *off-label*. In the field of speech-language pathology one analog to such off-label use is the application of norm-referenced tests to populations for which they were not originally intended. As with off-label use by physicians, such uses in our field also rely heavily on the judgment of the speech-language pathologist.

Part IV: Communication Disorders and Movement Science contains five essays. Michelle Gray, Barbara Bennett Shadden, Melissa Powers, and Ro DiBrezzo recommend "Collaborating with Exercise Science: Helping Older Adults Maintain Cognition and Communication." Mental and physical exercises are widely praised as ways to forestall some of the less pleasant consequences of normal and pathologic aging. A particularly intriguing line of research and potential preventive intervention for speech-language pathologists is the effects of physical exercise (with and without cognitive exercise) on cognitive/linguistic functions. Fran Redstone explains "Movement Science for the SLP." Speech is perhaps the most refined and highly developed set of movement behaviors that humans produce. The speech-language pathologist's work begins when these systems are not fully integrated and affect the areas of swallowing or language. This often occurs in children with neuromotor disorders such as cerebral palsy. Carl W. Asp, Madeline Kline, and Kazunari J. Koike report on "Verbotonal Body Movements." Young children vocalize while moving their body. This movement develops motor and auditory memory through proprioceptive feedback to the brain. Body movements use the seven perceptual parameters to correct errors. Later, self-correction skills are developed and carryover is established for all communication problems, including second language learning.

Dana Battaglia applies "The Martial Arts of Communication." Training in martial arts parallels language intervention, and can therefore improve pragmatic skills, such as reciprocity; initiation, maintenance, and termination of conversation; and structure, including shaping, prompting, and fading. These skills are applied to clinical intervention with children who have autism-spectrum disorders. Susan Hendler Lederer recommends "Storybook Yoga: Integrating Shared Book Reading and Yoga to Nurture the Whole Child." Shared book reading can foster language skills such as vocabulary development and story comprehension, as well as emergent literacy skills such as phonological awareness and book concepts. By integrating shared book reading with yoga and music, we can foster development simultaneously in the cognitive, physical, emotional, and social domains.

Part V: Audiology and Hearing Science contains nine essays. David M. Baguley writes about "Reflections on Translational Research in Tinnitus and Hyperacusis." He asks some searching questions about the applicability of basic science to these symptoms, and about the insights that the clinical situation might give to the basic scientists. Significant treatment uncertainties exist, and research might seek to resolve these. Anthony T. Cacace and Robert F. Burkard ask, "What Is Auditory Neuropathy? Translational Studies That Distinguish Inner Hair Cell (IHC) from Auditory-Nerve (AN) Dysfunction." They discuss terminology and definitions, consider appropriate tests of measurement, and provide relevant examples to elaborate on this distinction. Anthony T. Cacace and Dennis J. McFarland show "Single and Double Dissociations as a Frame of Reference: Application to Auditory Processing Disorders (APDs)." The authors discuss psychometric factors as ways to improve this area of investigation. They include other options to help clarify some of the outstanding issues, including making a specific diagnosis and delineating processing specializations in the auditory and visual sensory modalities. In a third essay from this research group, Dennis J. McFarland and Anthony T. Cacace are interested in "Establishing the Construct Validity of the Auditory Processing Disorder (APD): Application of Psychometric Theory to Clinical Practice." There is a need to improve methods for assessment and diagnosis. The present essay discusses the application of psychometric methods that may facilitate this goal.

Marshall Chasin examines "Hearing Aid Settings for Different Languages." Using hearing aid fitting formulae designed specifically for English understandably has limitations. A discussion and study of various linguistic aspects of some non-English languages yields specific clinical information relative to hearing aid fittings. Frederick S. Berg provides materials for "Preparing Deaf Children for Regular School." Hearing and visual technologies, methods, and materials are described that help enable deaf children to learn spoken English and precise speech early in life, so they do not need special education or rehabilitation. Patricia M. Chute and Mary Ellen Nevins study Educating Children with Hearing Loss in the Technology Age." This essay explores the impact that cochlear implant technology has had on the student, the educational system, and the profession. James Jerger and Mary Reagor use data from the neuroscience laboratory in "Listening to Words: Event-Related Potentials Reveal Cognitive Complexity — Implications for Speech Audiometry." They ask whether electrophysiologic responses from the brain reveal a difference between (1) a simple repetition response to a heard word and (2) a decision based on a more complex listening task. This is one of two essays (the second is in Part VI) that uses the ERP paradigm. Part V concludes with Jeffrey L. Danhauer and Carole E. Johnson, who consider "Evidence-Based Practice in Audiology: Examples from Prevention and Treatment." One particularly effective methodology used in evidence-based practice (EBP) involves conducting systematic reviews (SRs) with meta-analysis on specialized topics. The authors have used SRs to promote EBP in audiology for the prevention, diagnosis, and treatment of hearing disorders.

Part VI: Speech-Language Science and Speech-Language Pathology contains sixteen essays. William Culbertson and Dennis C. Tanner begin with "Observations on Speech and Swallowing." Speech and deglutition

share certain neurologic pathways and anatomic structures. The essay is an interesting exercise in anatomic and physiologic analysis to contemplate similarities and differences in the two functions. Mary Pannbacker and Norman J. Lass raise some sparks in "Oral Motor Exercises: The Debate." Oral motor exercises are controversial among speech-language pathologists, with the view ranging from unconditional acceptance to total rejection. This essay describes the rationales for these views and their clinical implications. Sharynne McLeod considers "The Impact of Seeing Speech" in her essay. The production of consonants and vowels to generate speech is both an acoustic and articulatory event, mediated by cognitive decision making around the input and output of speech. William Culbertson considers "Phonological Processes and Traditional Phoneme Acquisition Norms." A traditional approach to speech articulation treatment purports that mastery of adoption of phonemes into a typical child's speech seems to develop first with articulations that are easier to produce and more visible. The emphasis has shifted to the rules for articulation of the entire syllable, rather than the simpler idea of perception and production of phonemes.

Estella P.-M. Ma and Edwin M.-L. Yiu describe "Voice Research in Hong Kong: Past, Present, and Future." This essay uses the Voice Research Laboratory at the University of Hong Kong as an exemplar to illustrate the development of voice research in Hong Kong over the past two decades. Reem Khamis-Dakwar uses event-related potentials for "Translational Display of Neurophysiologic Investigations in Communication Sciences and Disorders." Incorporating neurophysiologic methods in communication sciences and disorders (CSD) research enhances clinical practice. She presents clinically driven neurophysiologic studies conducted at the Neurophysiology of Speech and Language Pathology Lab. Lawrence J.

Raphael and I conduct "An Acoustic Analysis of a Case of Amusia." Presence or absence of aphasia or agnosia; site of lesion in the right or left hemisphere; and specific areas of damage in either or both hemispheres do not predict presence, type, or severity of amusia. The authors used acoustic analysis to examine effects of amusia on the pre- and poststroke piano recordings of James P. Johnson, composer of "The Charleston."

Leonard L. LaPointe, Frank Johnson, Malcolm R. McNeil, and Sheila Pratt examine "Birdsong and Human Speech and Language: What the Zebra Finch Uses, Loses, and Regains." The translational aspect of their preliminary research in this area is related to the potential use of acquisition, destabilization, and recovery of birdsong in the zebra finch as an animal model for investigation of intrinsic and extrinsic variables that might influence recovery. It may be possible to learn more about these recovery patterns of learned vocal behaviors and inform research on dissolution and recovery of speech and language in humans. Dennis C. Tanner reveals "Defense Mechanisms and Coping Styles in Aphasia." The essay examines the role defense mechanisms and coping styles play in the psychological adjustment to aphasia. Nonverbal coping styles and defense mechanisms, such as denial, displacement, and projection, remain available, whereas those requiring language, such as rationalization, intellectualization, and humor, are partially or completely compromised.

Cindy Geise Arroyo reviews "The Impact of Augmentative and Alternative Communication (AAC) Technology." Especially when inexpensive "apps" are available for electronic tablets, it is important to examine the use of AAC technology for individuals with complex communication needs. Mary Jo Santo Pietro and I propose "Using Set Theory in SLP Diagnosis and Treatment." A general theory of sets refers to what is known as the concept of the cardinal number, or the continuum problem, as well as the more familiar application of overlaps between two collections. The authors examine how set theory can apply to diagnosis and treatment in communication disorders associated with Alzheimer disease, aphasia, and disfluency. Carl W. Asp, Madeline Kline, and Kazunari J. Koike consider the global impact of verbotonal treatment in "Verbotonal Worldwide." Dr. Singh published two Verbotonal books, one in 1981 and one in 2006. He grasped the potential of this powerful strategy. His endorsement made Verbotonal a worldwide strategy for developing listening and spoken language for communication problems.

The recent burst of interest in minimal cognitive impairment is explicated by Kathryn Bayles in "Timing Is Everything: At Least for MCI." Neuroscience and medical science have shown that timing is crucial to learning, treatment, prevention of disability, and rehabilitation. This essay makes a case for early detection and treatment of minimal cognitive impairment (MCI) and a role for the speech-language pathologist. Brooke Hallowell explores another current topic in "Exploiting Eye-Mind Connections for Translation to Clinical Applications in Language Assessment." The eye-mind assumption is that where people look as they are viewing just about anything tells us something about what they are thinking. As anyone who has ever daydreamed or anyone who is blind knows, the assumption may be invalidated. Still, many scholars across a vast array of disciplines have developed clever ways to ensure and study close eye-mind relationships in a vast array of populations. There is tremendous potential in exploiting those relationships for translation of eyetracking methods into clinical use. The last essay, by Audrey L. Holland, is "Counseling Around the Edges of Traditional Treatment," which continues on a theme expressed in her 2007 book for Plural Publishing. Although most speech-language pathologists and audiologists recognize the value and need for counseling for children and adult clients and their families, it is extremely difficult, if not impossible, to find time to provide it. Dr. Holland outlines a stopgap way to meet counseling needs around the edges of our required interventions.

I am grateful to my fellow contributors, who gave freely of their time and expertise to produce a body of knowledge that is a tribute to Singh as well as a volume of which we can all be justifiably proud. Some of you are cherished friends, and others were kind enough to give me a peek into your lives during the course of our correspondence.

The thorough professionalism of the Plural family is, by now, familiar to most of the contributors, even though there have been some changes. The contributors and I mourn the passing of Sandy Doyle, who had guided production of our books for many years. We wish our former editor, Stephanie Meissner, success and happiness in her new ventures, and welcome Scott Barbour as a new editor. Tom Murry, who has been associated with Singh in publication ventures for more than four decades, and who is a contributing essayist, provided welcome and valuable advice at the onset of this project. Angie Singh has been a constant source of encouragement and enthusiasm in what we hope is a fitting tribute to the living memory of her husband.

My colleagues and administrators at Adelphi University have understood that editing and contributing to this book has been an intense undertaking. I am grateful for a timely sabbatical leave, research release time, and the excellent essays written by my friends in the Department of Communication Sciences and Disorders. Michelle Finik, my research assistant and a first-year graduate student, has been prompt and diligent in checking consistency of referencing in all of the essays, and assisted in the acoustic analysis for the essay on amusia.

Shelley Goldfarb has been a source of inspiration, love, and sanity since we were both teenagers. She is also to be commended here as an accomplished mathematician, helping to edit my essay on set theory. Finally, I'm sure that Singh would have joined me in a loving welcome to a new generation of scholars in the family, Elizabeth Goldfarb and Matt Simon.

REFERENCES

Goldfarb, R. (Ed.). (2006). *Ethics: A case study from fluency*. San Diego, CA: Plural.

Mead, R. (2011, July 4). "Earnest." *The New Yorker*, 19. Retrieved from http://www.newyorker.com/talk/2011/07/04/110704ta_talk_mead#ixzz1SMxQQdB2

❧ About the Editor ❧

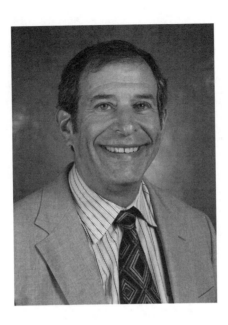

Robert Goldfarb, PhD, Fellow, ASHA, is Professor and Program Director of Communication Sciences and Disorders at Adelphi University and Emeritus Professor of Speech and Hearing Sciences at Lehman College and The Graduate Center, CUNY, where he was also Executive Officer. He has published extensively in the areas of adult aphasia, the language of dementia, and the language of schizophrenia, and is also coauthor of two tests: *The Stocker Probe for Fluency and Language* (1995) and *Time-Altered Word Association Tests (TAWAT,* 2013). He edited and contributed chapters to *Ethics: A Case Study From Fluency* (2006) and *Translational Speech-Language Pathology and Audiology* (2013), and is coauthor of *Techniques for Aphasia Rehabilitation Generating Effective Treatment (TARGET,* 1995), *Professional Writing in Speech-Language Pathology and Audiology* (2009), *Professional Writing in Speech-Language Pathology and Audiology Workbook* (2011), and *Language and Motor Speech Disorders in Adults, Third Edition* (2013).

Contributors

Cindy Geise Arroyo, DA, CCC-SLP
Department of Communication Sciences
  and Disorders
Adelphi University
Garden City, New York
Essay 40

Carl W. Asp, PhD
Director, Verbotonal Research Lab
Professor Emeritus
University of Tennessee
Knoxville, Tennessee
Essays 19 and 42

David M. Baguley, BSC, MSc, MBA, PhD
Director of Audiology
Cambridge University Hospitals
Visiting Professor
Anglia Ruskin University
Cambridge, England
Essay 22

Dana Battaglia, PhD, CCC-SLP
Assistant Professor
Adelphi University
Garden City, New York
Essay 20

Kathryn Bayles, PhD
Professor and Chair
Department of Communication Sciences
  and Disorders
University of Central Arkansas
Conway, Arkansas
Professor Emerita
Department of Speech-Language-Hearing
  Sciences
University of Arizona

Tucson, Arizona
Essay 43

Alison Behrman, PhD, CCC-SLP
Assistant Professor
Department of Speech Communication
  Studies
Iona College
New Rochelle, New York
Essay 11

Abbey L. Berg, PhD
Professor
Department of Biology and Health Sciences
Communication Sciences and Disorders
  Program
Pace University
Director of the Newborn Hearing Screening
  Program
The Morgan Stanley Children's Hospital of
  New York-Presbyterian
Adjunct Faculty
Departments of Otolaryngology—Head
  and Neck Surgery and Pediatrics
College of Physicians and Surgeons
Columbia University
New York, New York
Essay 15

Frederick S. Berg, PhD
Professor Emeritus
Department of Communicative Disorders
  and Deaf Education
Utah State University
Logan, Utah
Essay 27

Andrea F. Blau, Esquire, PhD, JD
Dr. Blau & Associates
Clinical and Legal Consultants

New York, NY
Essay 13

Lauren Brookman-Frazee, PhD
Assistant Professor
University of California, San Diego
Child and Adolescent Services Research
    Center
San Diego, CA
Essay 9

Robert F. Burkard, PhD, CCC-A
Professor and Chair
Rehabilitation Science
University at Buffalo
Buffalo, New York
Essay 23

Anthony T. Cacace, PhD
Professor
Communication Sciences and Disorders
Wayne State University
Detroit, Michigan
Essays 23, 24, and 25

Marshall Chasin, AuD, REg. CASLPO
Doctor of Audiology
Associate Professor
University of Western Ontario
Adjunct Professor
University of Toronto
Director of Research
Musicians' Clinics of Canada
Toronto, Ontario, Canada
Essay 26

Patricia M. Chute, EdD
Dean, School of Health Professions
New York Institute of Technology
Health Policy Fellow
Old Westbury, New York
Essay 28

William Culbertson, PhD
Professor of Health Sciences
Speech-Language Sciences and Technology
Northern Arizona University

Flagstaff, Arizona
Essays 31 and 34

Jeffrey L. Danhauer, PhD
Professor of Audiology
Chair, Department of Speech and Hearing
    Sciences
University of California, Santa Barbara
Acoustical Society of America
Fellow — American Speech, Language and
    Hearing Association
Fellow — American Academy of Audiology
Academy of Rehabilitative Audiology
California Speech and Hearing Association
American Auditory Society
Fellow and Founder — California Academy
    of Audiology
Santa Barbara, California
Essays 1 and 30

Ro DiBrezzo, PhD
Director
Human Performance Lab
University of Arkansas
Fayetteville, Arkansas
Essay 17

**Peter Flipsen Jr., PhD, S-LP(C),
CCC-CLP**
Professor of Speech-Language Pathology
Department of Communication Sciences
    and Disorders
ISU Meridian Health Sciences Center
Meridian, Idaho
Essay 16

Robert Goldfarb, PhD
Professor and Program Director
Communication Sciences and Disorders
Adelphi University
Garden City, NY
Emeritus Professor of Speech and Hearing
    Sciences
Lehman College and The Graduate Center
City University of New York (CUNY)
New York, NY
Essays 37 and 41

Michelle Gray, PhD
Assistant Professor, Exercise Science
University of Arkansas
Fayetteville, Arkansas
Essay 17

Brooke Hallowell, PhD
Professor, Communication Sciences and
   Disorders
Director, Neurolinguistics Laboratory
Ohio University
Athens, Ohio
Essay 44

Edie Hapner, PhD, CCC-SLP
Associate Professor
Department of Otolaryngology—Head and
   Neck Surgery
Emory University School of Medicine
Director of Speech-Language Pathology
Emory Voice Center
Atlanta, Georgia
Essay 10

Audrey L. Holland, PhD
Regents' Professor Emerita
Department of Speech and Hearing
   Sciences
University of Arizona
Tucson, Arizona
Essay 45

James Jerger, PhD
Distinguished Scholar-in-Residence
School of Behavioral and Brain Sciences
University of Texas at Dallas
Dallas, Texas
Essay 29

Carole E. Johnson, PhD, AuD
Professor
Department of Communication Disorders
Auburn University
Auburn, Alabama
Essay 30

Frank Johnson, PhD
Department of Psychology
Program in Neuroscience
Florida State University
Tallahassee, Florida
Essay 38

Ray D. Kent, PhD
Professor Emeritus
University of Wisconsin–Madison
Madison, Wisconsin
Essay 5

Reem Khamis-Dakwar, PhD
Assistant Professor
Director, Neurophysiology in Speech and
   Language Pathology (NSLP) Laboratory
Department of Communication Sciences
   and Disorders
Adelphi University
Garden City, New York
Essay 36

Madeline Kline, MS
Consultant, Verbotonal Research Lab
University of Tennessee
Knoxville, Tennessee
Essays 19 and 42

Kazunari J. Koike, PhD
Professor and Director of Audiology
Department of Otolaryngology—Head and
   Neck Surgery
West Virginia University Health Sciences
   Center
Morgantown, West Virginia
Essays 19 and 42

Leonard L. LaPointe, PhD
Francis Eppes Distinguished Professor
School of Communication Science and
   Disorders
Faculty, Program in Neuroscience
Faculty, College of Medicine
Florida State University
Tallahassee, Florida
Essay 38

Norman J. Lass, PhD
Professor, Department of Speech Pathology
    and Audiology
West Virginia University
Morgantown, West Virginia
Essay 32

Susan Hendler Lederer, PhD, CCC
Associate Professor
Department of Communication Sciences
    and Disorders
Adelphia University
Garden City, New York
Essay 21

Estella P.-M. Ma, PhD
Assistant Professor
Division of Speech and Hearing Sciences
Director
Voice Research Laboratory
University of Hong Kong
Pokfulam, Hong Kong
Essay 35

Dennis J. McFarland, PhD
Research Scientist
New York State Department of Health
Albany, New York
Essays 24 and 25

Sharynne McLeod, PhD, CPSP, FSPA
ASHA Fellow
Professor in Speech and Language
    Acquisition
Australian Research Council Future Fellow
Charles Sturt University, Australia
Bathurst, Australia
Essay 33

**Malcolm R. McNeil, PhD, CCC-SLP,
BC-NCD**
Distinguished Service Professor and Chair
Department of Communication Science ad
    Disorders
University of Pittsburgh

Research Career Scientist
VA Pittsburgh Healthcare System
Pittsburgh, Pennsylvania
Essay 38

Joseph J. Montano, EdD
Chief
Audiology and Speech-Language Pathology
New York Presbyterian Hospital-Weill
    Cornell Medical Center
New York, New York
Essay 14

Thomas Murry, PhD, CCC-SLP
Professor of Speech Pathology
Department of Otolaryngology — Head and
    Neck Surgery
Weill Cornell Medical College
Adjunct Professor
Department of Biobehavioral Sciences
Columbia University, Teachers College
New York, New York
Essay 2

Lauren K. Nelson, PhD
Department of Communication Sciences
    and Disorders
University of Northern Iowa
Cedar Falls, Iowa
Essay 7

Mary Ellen Nevins, EdD
Senior Strategist for Professional Learning
Oberkotter Foundation
Philadelphia, Pennsylvania
Essay 28

John W. Oller Jr., PhD
Doris B. Hawthorne Board of Regents
    Support Fund Professor IV
Department of Communicative Disorders
University of Louisiana at Lafayette
Lafayette, Louisiana
Essay 3

Mary Pannbacker, PhD
Professor
Program in Speech-Language Pathology
Louisiana State University Health Sciences
  Center
Shreveport, Louisiana
Essay 32

Wendy Papir-Bernstein, MS, CCC-SLP
Adjunct Assistant Professor
Lehman College, City University of New
  York
Speech Supervisor (Retired)
New York City Department of Education,
  D. 75
New York, New York
Essays 8 and 12

Melissa Powers, PhD
Assistant Professor
Department of Kinesiology and Health
  Studies
University of Central Oklahoma
Edmond, Oklahoma
Essay 17

Sheila Pratt, PhD
Associate Professor
Department of Communication Science and
  Disorders
University of Pittsburgh
Geriatric Research Education and Clinical
  Center
VA Pittsburgh Healthcare Center
Pittsburgh, Pennsylvania
Essay 38

Lawrence J. Raphael, PhD
Professor of Speech Science
Adelphi University
Coordinator of the Doctoral Program in
  Speech-Language Pathology
Professor Emeritus
The Graduate School of the City University
  of New York

Professor Emeritus
Lehman College of the City University of
  New York
Garden City, New York
Essay 37

Mary Reagor, MS
PhD candidate in Cognition and
  Neuroscience
University of Texas at Dallas
Dallas, Texas
Essay 29

Fran Redstone, PhD, CCC-SLP, NDT/C
Associate Professor
Adelphi University
Garden City, New York
Essay 18

John C. Rosenbek, PhD, BC-ANCDS
Professor
Department of Speech, Language, and
  Hearing Sciences
University of Florida
Gainesville, Florida
Essay 6

Mary Jo Santo Pietro, PhD, CCC-SLP
Professor
School of Communication Disorders and
  Deafness
Kean University
Director
Institute for Adults Living with
  Communication Disabilities
Center for Communication Disorders
Kean University
Union, NJ
Essay 41

Karyn Lewis Searcy, MA, CCC-SLP
Director
Crimson Center for Speech and Language
San Diego, California
Essay 9

Yula C. Serpanos, PhD
Professor
Department of Communication Sciences
    and Disorders
Adelphi University
Garden City, New York
Essay 15

Jon K. Shallop, PhD
Professor Emeritus
Mayo Clinic and College of Medicine
Rochester, Minnesota
Faculty Associate
University of Arizona
Tucson, Arizona
Essay 4

**Barbara Bennett Shadden, CCC-SLP,
BC-NCD**
University Professor
University of Arkansas
Fayetteville, Arkansas
Essay 17

Aubyn Stahmer, PhD, BCBA-D
Research Scientist
Child and Adolescent Research Center
Rady Children's Hospital
Department of Psychology
University of California, San Diego
Research Director
Autism Discovery Institute—Rady
    Children's Hospital
San Diego, California
Essay 9

Dennis C. Tanner, PhD
Professor of Health Sciences
Speech-Language Sciences and Technology
Northern Arizona University
Flagstaff, Arizona
Essays 31 and 39

Edwin M.-L. Yiu, PhD
Professor
Voice Research Laboratory and Swallowing
    Research Laboratory
Division of Speech and Hearing Sciences
University of Hong Kong
Pokfulam, Hong Kong
Essay 35

PART I

In Memory of
Dr. Sadanand Singh

ESSAY 1

❧ Eulogy ❧

A Portion of the Remarks Delivered at the Memorial Ceremony for Dr. Singh on April 6, 2010

Jeffrey L. Danhauer

The invitation to this event should have said, "Closed for Family Only," because if you ever met Singh, then you are part of his family.

I am Jeff Danhauer. I am Singh's best doctoral student, I am his best colleague, I am his best coauthor, I am his best business partner, I am his first and best son, I am his best friend, I am his father-in-law, I am his best confidant, I am the closest person in the world to him. Shocking you think? How can I stand here and say these things when each of you know in your hearts that you feel the same way and that you were his best . . . whatever?

Indeed, Singh had a way of making each one of us feel that way, like we were the most special and important person in the world to him. He did that to us from our very first meeting with him. Singh was special and made every one of us feel that we were too.

I remember one of our first doctoral classes with him at Ohio University. We only had about three or four students in the class, which was typical for doctoral seminars, and it was held in his office. I recall seeing this little brown man sitting on top of his desk with his legs all contorted into a lotus position and watching him pick at his bare toes while one of us was writing some of his fresh ideas on the blackboard. This was about as different as expectations for such a class could be, but the energy, enthusiasm, creativity, passion, and empowerment that he exuded was amazing. A lot of different adjectives could be applied to Singh, but punctual, conformist, prepared, planned, boring, and lazy are definitely not among them. Singh rarely prepared for his lectures. In fact, he never really lectured at all. His way of teaching was letting you right into the thick of whatever busy research he was conducting or article he was preparing at the time. We students learned by becoming immersed and active participants in his work and world. He was often late for class and we weren't always sure where class would be held on any given day, or just who would end up teaching it. We met in classrooms, offices, students' homes, and frequently at Singh's home on the farm. We worked hard and had great fun together. We literally worked, ate, slept, drank, played, raised our kids, and practically lived together in those days. None of us, including Singh, had much money then, but Singh found ways to introduce us to the best scholars in the field who all seemed to make their pilgrimages to the farm in Albany, Ohio to visit Singh, and ended up teaching us students as well. He was dynamic and a magnet for scholars. His casual, unorthodox style may not have been for everyone, but it certainly lit a fire in me that still burns today. He simply had an infectious magnetism that everyone had to feel at first meeting him.

Yes, we are here this evening to celebrate and memorialize the life of a great man, a man whose first name was difficult to manage for many. It was always funny to hear how people struggled with Singh's first name (is it "Sad—An—And Singh?" "Sad Man Singh?" or Singh's personal favorite "Sit—Down—And Singh?" Regardless of whether he was "Dr. Singh," "Daddy," "Gee," or just "Singh" he was a friend and family to us all.

Without going into great details, Singh was born in India in 1934, although the exact date was a source of debate for many years. He was born in a small farming village, but moved on to earn a PhD in aesthetics at Ranchi University; then came to the United States and earned another PhD in Speech Science at Ohio State University. From there, he went on to serve as Chair at Howard University until 1970 when he moved to Ohio University in Athens, Ohio, and then on to Chair the University of Texas at Houston, and finally came to California to Chair San Diego State University's program. He authored over 60 articles in scientific journals and several books, which firmly established his place in the Communication Sciences. His entrepreneurial side led him to create three outstanding publishing companies and an impressive Internet Search Engine and Database in ContentScan. It is from his teaching, publishing, promoting of

other people's works, and his endless philanthropy that Singh is most noted.

A little more historical perspective about how he got there. I recall that Singh and his second wife, Kala, came to Ohio University with all their belongings in an old light blue Ford sedan and only a couple hundred dollars to their name. Through hard work, willingness to take risks (some would have said foolishness), and a whole lot of luck, they created a great life together and produced two beautiful children in Kalpana and Samir to add to his three daughters (Meehna, Sheila, and Mooni) from his first marriage. Days on the farm would involve some academic work, usually writing articles, puttering around the barn playing with cows, trying to teach Singh how to ice skate on his pond in the winter, and painting and remodeling the house in the summers. At about the time that I finished my degree in 1974 and moved to teach at Bowling Green State University, Singh's entrepreneurial drives began to emerge and the family moved to Houston where we started College-Hill Press, which we ran out of their basement until we could no longer house the inventory, and then moved to a shared space with Kala's India Spice and Import Company. In those days, it was not uncommon for purchasers of our works to smell spices and shake rice grains from the pages as they read our books. We didn't charge extra for that, or the personal attention that Singh gave to each author. He used to say that helping an author complete a manuscript and converting it into a book was like delivering a child. Again, the reference to how Singh made each author feel like family, which is a major reason why both neophyte and seasoned authors alike came to our publishing companies over the years, which is still the case today.

Then after the Singhs moved to San Diego and his heart began to fail and we sold College-Hill, they traveled to India to regain their roots and an easier, more laid-back lifestyle. Unfortunately, following a beautiful sojourn to India, we all know what happened on the way home in Karachi and the terrorist attack. Singh, Kalpa, and Samir were severely wounded, but we all lost Kala. She was my age and was like a sister to me, but she was everything to Singh and I saw him dying by the day while trying to cope with his loss. How could he go on? How could he rebound? How could he nourish and raise those two young children alone? Some feared he would not pull through and it was like watching the end of a tragic love story. Nothing seemed to cheer him up.

Then one day, like a miracle, the family brought Angie from Washington, DC, and into all our lives. This young girl was like magic the way she took care of Singh and the kids, ran the household, and literally breathed new life into a dying man. After a while Singh and Angie fell in love and were married. The wedding ceremony was held in the same house they live in on the hill just across from where we are now. I am proud to say that my wife, Kim, and I served as Angie's surrogate father and mother and gave her to Singh in that ceremony. So, when I said earlier that she is my daughter and I am his father-in-law, you know what I meant.

Singh's strength recovered and we started an even bigger and better publishing company in Singular. Soon, they added two more beautiful children to the family in Sapna and Sanjay. Then, later, when Singh's health began to fail and they needed to slow things down again, we sold Singular and Singh re-entered retirement. Right! Nothing could retire the man's mind and creativity and soon his entrepreneurial juices began flowing again. It wasn't long until I received the calls that we were going to start a new venture, a glorified search engine and database initially focused on the Communication Sciences, but soon to expand to related disciplines. ContentScan was born

and this time nurtured by Samir and Jamie, who guided it on to bigger and better things.

However, Singh's true love and what he knew best was publishing and helping others promote their works. Within a couple years, he and Angie started Plural Publishing, which has already superseded College-Hill and Singular together. Again, I assure you present and future authors that your creative works and intellectual properties are in great hands with Angie Singh and her able team. Singh may be gone in body, but Angie sees that his spirit, soul, and memory go into every book.

El Gato, Lazarus, Superman. These are some of the names applied to Singh over the years as we have witnessed his amazing recoveries from near death on multiple occasions. It seemed as if he really was the cat with nine lives. Illnesses — pancreatitis, hepatitis, gout, quadruple heart bypass, repairs to his heart, the Karachi hijacking injuries, heart stents, heart pacemaker, and traumatic head injury from a fall two years ago — the list went on and on. They led to physical and emotional strains, but Singh never gave up. So, naturally, as he lay in bed at the hospital a few weeks ago, our hearts fully expected him to sit up and shake this one off too, but our brains knew that what our eyes were telling us was true. This was one he was not going to survive. The infection had just spread too fast and too far and the sepsis was taking over every organ in his body. But, I thought, why shouldn't Singh go out this way? For he was an infection.

Singh was an infection of the most communicable and contagious kind. From a first meeting with him, one was exposed, and it was too late and impossible to stop the spread. He infected my mind, and heart, and soul, and changed my life and ways of thinking and doing for as long as I breathe. I would never be the same again. He was an infection, a virus. Whether you are even aware of it yet, you are carriers of his infection as well.

Singh was known around the world to friends, family, and strangers alike. Even last summer on a vacation to Italy, the family attended a Papal Blessing at the Vatican. When Samir and Jamie pushed Singh's wheelchair to the front of the line, I am told that many people in the audience were heard to whisper to each other, "Who's that up there on the altar with Singh?" Well, maybe not, but if he's like the rest of us, then I'm sure the Pope got as much out of the encounter as Singh did. In spite of all his successes and accolades, which include the highest honors from ASHA and AAA and every major (and minor) state, national, and international societies of the communication disorders and medical-related communities, Singh was always a very simple man who never forgot his roots. I always had to laugh when Angie would dress him up in a fine suit and shirt and tie, only to look down at his feet and find him wearing sandals. They were what he felt most comfortable in and they fit his soul.

"Family" carries so much meaning, especially after spending time with Singh and his immediate family. And once you had, you were in their family. Singh helped me cope with the deaths of both of my parents. At Singh's death, I witnessed just how precious and respected life is. I have never seen such an uninhibited emotional outpouring of love and respect as that which I witnessed at that bedside with his family and children all huddled around him. Few men would ever be so lucky to have a wife like Angie who was never afraid to tell and show her husband and the world how dedicated and so in love with him she was, regardless of who was present.

Perhaps too often in our culture, we hurry the passage of a life and rush it to the point that it seems we don't want a loved one's passing to inconvenience us in any way from our daily routines. I must admit having felt that a bit in my own parents' passing. But with the Singh family, things are different. As Singh was passing, word spread quickly and almost all members of the family rushed to his bedside (even from India) to shower him with the love and respect of a king, or at least a valued patriarch. And even as he passed, after lying for almost two days in a coma, Singh found a way to let Angie and all the children know that he was fine and that they would be okay too. He had prepared them and already given them the strength, courage, and values to help them carry on and succeed with their important missions in life, just as he had. Then, for 13 days, the Singh households both in La Jolla and in his village in India mourned his death and celebrated his life with daily pujas and prayer ceremonies. On the 13th day, we had a ceremony on the pier over the La Jolla shore, just a few feet down the hill from where we are now. As about 80 of us family stood on the edge of the pier and watched as a small boat escorted by a dozen dolphins pulled up and the sons, Samir, Sanjay, and Jamie took out a small ziplock bag and cast his ashes into the sea. As they committed Singh's ashes to the water, the tide began dispersing them in what looked like a white shroud toward us on the pier, and they seemed to take on a human form as they spread. I felt like Singh was reaching out to us all for one last time, reassuring us that everything was okay. A portion of his ashes were held back, and the family will repeat this beautiful ceremony again this summer in Singh's village in India. They will commit the rest of his ashes to the Ganges as Hindi tradition requires, and as Singh wished. Surely, these ceremonies have held families together for ages and remind us that there is much more to life than just living.

I just left the AAA convention hall where no fewer than seven of my students and I presented papers a few minutes ago, which we dedicated to the honor and memory of Dr. Sadanand Singh, our academic father and grandfather. My students know that lineage. Actually, one of the papers is being delivered right now by a first-time presenter without me being present. I am sure that my students can handle it, because they are Singh's descendents, and I have passed on knowledge and confidence to them that he instilled in me long ago. I know he will see them through.

Few persons achieve a level of distinction in any field where they are instantly and distinguishingly recognized by just one name: Jesus, Elvis, Magic, Kobe, Einstein, Cher, Madonna. Even if people struggle with his first name, they know him by his last. Just Singh.

ESSAY 2

❦ In the Course of a Lifetime ❧

A Multidimensional Relationship

Thomas Murry

"The better part of one's life consists of his friendships"

A. Lincoln

This essay is a snapshot of my 46 years of friendship that developed between Dr. Singh and me and how that relationship expanded over those years from voice science to the world of publishing.

The nature of speech analysis took a dynamic turn in the early 1970s with the use of multivariate statistics, and Dr. Singh was on the cutting edge of that scientific method of speech analysis that ultimately turned into voice analysis. The work we did at that time helped to solidify a friendship that developed in the speech science program at Ohio State University.

INTRODUCTION

It is not difficult to review my remembrances of the times I shared with Sadanand Singh; it is only difficult to limit the number of remembrances of our times together. After all, they spanned 46 years and extended from coast to coast, north and south, from the voice science laboratory at Ohio State University to the study of voice through multidimensional scaling to publishing on a grand scale.

I met Sadanand in September, 1964, he a 30-year-old doctoral student and me a 20-year-old master's degree student at Ohio State University. He, along with Oscar Tosi and Yukio Takefutu, were doctoral students assigned to co-teach the speech science course with Dr. John Black. All three of them had been in the United States for only a short time. Sadanand and Yukio were my first exposure to Indian and Japanese natives speaking English. In our Saturday morning laboratory class at 8:00 AM, we began learning how to measure formants and scaling the differences in various speech parameters such as aspiration, plosiveness, and frication. Maybe it was because Sadanand was very different from other students I grew up with in high school and college that I enjoyed talking to him after classes. Maybe it was the fact that he knew so much more about speech science than I did, or maybe it was the fact that I was too shy to talk to any of the other students. Nonetheless, in those brief moments after the lab class on Saturday mornings, a lasting friendship began to develop. It would be several more years before we talked to each other on an almost daily basis. He moved to Washington, DC. I moved to Florida and then Connecticut but our paths seemed to cross in meetings of the Acoustical Society of America, and our friendship maintained.

Few people have known Sadanand for as long as I have and in so many circumstances. To some, he was their professor; to others, he was their publisher; and to others still, he was part of their family. To me he was all of those and more—a trusted friend. In fact, we were often referred to as brothers by our respective families. We shared good times and other times together. In the course of a day in Seabrook, Texas, we spent time at the Texas Institute of Rehabilitation Medical Center, returned to his home and stacked rocks along the back of his property to prevent the soil from washing away, and went out to the local Vietnamese market to select the freshest fish of the day for an evening family meal. And sitting at the round kitchen table with his brother, Vidyanand, a table at which we sat around many times over the years, we began to forge a small book company that became College-Hill Press. A long day for sure but that was the intensity of Sadanand, always energetic and always looking for ways to improve his profession. When he wanted something, he did not hesitate to search for a way to achieve his goal. He was spontaneous, energetic, and worked to show that "it" could get done. I'm not sure if anyone knew at the time we started College-Hill Press that many of the early books were stored in the back of the spice shop that his wife, Kala, operated in a Houston suburb. Maybe that was the sweet smell of success that took that company from one book to 32 books in its first year.

Sadanand was the kind of person one could talk to about anything. Whether there was a serious academic issue, a family matter, a decision to make, or just to enjoy an intellec-

tual interchange, Sadanand was there to listen. When my father died shortly after my mother's death, Sadanand talked with me about many problems people in India faced with poverty, disease, and especially the lack of education. His discussions helped get me through those difficult weeks following my return to California after the funeral. We often discussed the value of memories and the importance of moving ahead without losing the memories. He always maintained a positive outlook.

The scale at which our friendship grew was logarithmically advanced following a trip that Sadanand made to the U.S. Naval Submarine Base in Groton, Connecticut. He came to learn about the speech perception research going on at the navy base. By that point in time, he had amassed a series of studies on perception of speech based on classic linguistic categories such as frication, voicing, and so forth. The U.S. Navy was interested in speech analysis using acoustic information that was transmitted with various types of distortions such as submarine noise, divers wearing face masks, and transmission in helium-oxygen breathing mixtures. The early work of Sadanand and his colleagues was devoted to the identification of the phonetic and phonemic similarities of vowels and consonants (Danhauer & Singh, 1975; Mitchell & Singh, 1974; Singh & Woods, 1971; Singh, Woods, & Becker, 1972). The results of these and other studies by Sadanand and his colleagues in the early 1970s resulted in a book, *Distinctive Features: Theory and Validation* (Singh, 1976), which outlines the concept of distinctive features as they relate to speech sounds and their use in production and perception of speech and in the diagnosis of speech disorders.

Given that Sadanand had worked with both typical speakers and those with articulation or voice disorders, his input was valuable to the ongoing projects at the medical research laboratory in Groton, Connecticut.

We discussed acoustic analysis of speech and how speech distortions were difficult to classify when talkers were under water, in helium environments, or wearing face masks that distorted the speaker's anatomy as well as caused the speaker to speak loudly over the noise of the breathing apparatus and the undersea environment. It was those discussions that led to the lifelong development of our friendship as both voice scientists and entrepreneurs. During that period, Sadanand went from Howard University, to Ohio University, and, finally, to the University of Texas Health Science Center in Houston. During that same period, I went from the U.S. Navy to the Veteran's Administration Medical Center in San Diego. It would be several more years before Sadanand and his family moved to California. We began our research and the publishing business over that 1,600 mile distance.

MULTIDIMENSIONAL SCALING

Features of Speech

Multidimensional scaling (MDS) is a powerful tool that allows investigators to gain insight into the underlying structure of relationships between or among entities and provides a weighted geometrical relationship of those entities. MDS is a method of identifying relationships and thus belongs to the general category of multivariate analysis. For complex signals such as speech, MDS offers a method of describing the most important features of the signal and their weights according to how they are measured, either by acoustic measure or by perceptual measures. The value of MDS is that it can provide a visual picture of the similarities or dissimilarities of data and then develop relationships to that data.

Psychophysics is the study of relationship between physical properties and the perception of those properties. Speech analysis falls into the realm of psychophysics—what is relevant to the listener and what properties of the signal provide the information relevant to the listener. The parameters of the speech signal and their interrelationships have been examined for over a century, at first one parameter at a time, such as the relationship between pitch and intensity (Stevens, 1935). More recently, MDS scaling has been used to understand the interrelationships of the complex speech signal involving multiple parameters simultaneously. MDS offers a tool for understanding the relationship among the perceptual parameters of the speech signal and a way to interpret the relationships between the perceptual parameters and the acoustic attributes associated with those perceptual parameters. Results from early works by Hecker and Kruel (1971) and by Emanual and Smith (1974) point to the importance of a multidimensional approach for analysis of complex speech signals. Their early studies suggest that the perception of pitch may be guided by such parameters as the degree of roughness or hoarseness in the signal, not only the absolute fundamental frequency of the signal.

Using a multidimensional approach does not require a listener to make a judgment about a specific parameter. Judges, whether they are listeners or viewers, only need to make a rating of the similarity (or dissimilarity) between a pair of stimuli. In speech analysis, two samples are played to a listener and the listener judges either how similar or dissimilar the two are. By playing all pairs within an array, each sample is judged against every other sample (Carroll & Chang, 1976). The judging of similarity is usually done on a 7-point Likert scale, with 1 being highly similar and 7 being highly dissimilar. The number of pairs to be judged is a function of the number of items in the array. For example, if there are 20 voices in the sample, the number of judgments is $N(N-1)/2$ or $20(19)/2 = 190$.

Studies of Voice Qualities

The discussions that Dr. Singh and I had about multidimensional scaling led to our investigations of voice qualities. Voice, like articulation, is also a complex concept. The severity of a voice disorder may be related to the fundamental frequency, the degree of noise relative to that of the harmonics, the degree of breathiness, etc. We used a multidimensional scaling technique called individual difference scaling (INDSCAL) to determine the perceptual attributes of a group of non-normal voices. Although previous investigators studied the perception of pitch as it relates to roughness (Emanual & Smith, 1974; Hecker & Kruel, 1971), we were interested in which perceptual attributes of the voice were prominent in making judgments about the voice and how those perceptual attributes were related to the acoustic parameters.

Method

Our first study focused on abnormal voices (Murry, Singh, & Sargent, 1977). We randomly selected 20 voice samples from a library of 200 voices recorded in a quiet room with high quality recording equipment. The voice samples consisted of a 3-second sustained /a/. Sixteen graduate students made similarity judgments of all 20 × 20 pairs of voices using a 7-point equal-appearing interval scale. In addition, a subgroup of seven experienced speech-language pathologists judged the samples for hoarseness, breathiness, and nasality. Also, sound spectrograms were made of each voice producing the vowel /a/ and aerodynamic measures of mean air flow rate were obtained from the participants with disordered voices. From the spectrograms, the voices were classified as most, moderately, or least severe. Thus, we captured the acoustic and perceptual judgments of the speech-language pathologists and then submitted the voice samples to similarity judgments for input into the INDSCAL computations. From the spectrograms samples, the perceptual judgments, and the similarity judgments we obtained distinct features of the voices that had physical and perceptual relevance.

Results

The perceptual judgments of hoarseness, breathiness, and nasality were compared with the aerodynamic and acoustic measures. Significant correlations were found for the perceptual judgments and the physical measures as shown in Table 2–1. In this group of disor-

Table 2–1. Significant Results of the Multiple Regression Analysis Between Six Physical Measures (F0, F1, F2, F2/F1, F2–F1, mean airflow rate in cc/sec) and Three Perceptual Measures (hoarseness, breathiness, nasality)

Perceptual Judgment	Significant Relationships		
Hoarseness	F0		
Breathiness	F2/F1 F2–F1	mean airflow rate	
Nasality	F1, F2		

F0 (Fundamental frequency), F1 (Formant 1), F2 (Formant 2)

dered voices, hoarseness was not related to the fundamental frequency or the other physical measures, which suggests that hoarseness cannot be scaled unidimensionally.

When the results of the INDSCAL analysis were obtained, the perceptual judgments of hoarseness, breathiness, and nasality correlated highly with dimensions retrieved by the INDSCAL analysis. The results of the INDSCAL analysis revealed consistent perceptual categories by the judges. A 5-dimensional space provided the explanation for the variance in the data.

The total variance accounted for by the 5-dimensional space was 48% (Table 2–2). Of this total, 24% of the variance was accounted for by one dimension. The other dimensions accounted for smaller portions of the variance.

In the original publication (Murry, Singh, & Sargent, 1977), we could not interpret the fourth dimension that accounted for 5% of the variance. Since that time, a number of studies have shown that there are possible solutions for the interpretation of the data. Among the possible interpretations of D4 from that initial study, aspiration noise (Klatt

& Klatt, 1990), spectral slope (Buder, 2000), and loudness of noise (Shrivastav & Sapienza, 2003) may account for that dimension.

Further Studies

Dr. Singh was genuinely interested in voice from that point. The study and understanding of the voice and voice disorders continued to be a focal point of his for the rest of his life. He and his students went on to do additional studies of voice using the INDSCAL approach. Hasek, Singh, and Murry (1980) analyzed the attributes of preadolescent voices in 1980 to identify both sex-related differences and age-related trends as a function of fundamental frequency. Prior to that time, data from children, ages 5 to 10 years, indicated that children of that age could be identified by gender, but the basis for those judgments had not been explored. Hasek et al. (1980) found that a significant difference between the average fundamental frequency of male and female children occurs at the age of 7 to 8 years of age. At that point, the fundamental

Table 2–2. Percentage of the Variance Accounted by the Five Dimensional Solution Provided by the INDSCAL Similarity Judgments

Dimension	Percentage of Variance Accounted For	Interpretation
D1	24%	Noise in the signal
		Absence of periodicity
D2	8%	Elevation of F2
		Presence versus absence of vocal fold mass
D3	6%	Mean airflow rate
		Breathiness
D4	5%	No interpretation
D5	5%	F_0

frequency of the males begins to drop while the female mean fundamental frequency remains relatively stable.

Studies of the voice using INDSCAL and other forms of multivariate scaling have continued to describe the psychophysical properties of the voice since the early work of Dr. Singh, his students, and colleagues. Buder (2000), Shrivastav (2006), Shrivastav and Camacho (2010), Childers and Lee (1991), and Gelfer (1993) have presented data on the relationships between physical and perceptual attributes of significant vocal parameters. These studies and others have demonstrated the value of multivariate analysis techniques when studying complex stimuli such as articulation and voice. It is clear that the early experiments of Sadanand and colleagues using multivariate analyses for speech and voice parameters provided a stepping stone to these current studies. The principles of those early experiments continue to be used to understand the psychophysics of speech and voice production and perception.

THE COURSE OF A LIFETIME

When one begins to examine the activities of Dr. Singh following his successful transition from university professor to department chairman to publisher, the areas of voice and laryngology stand out. The early catalogs of College-Hill Press and Singular Publishing Group featured new books on voice. And when Dr. Singh decided to move beyond speech-language pathology and audiology, voice became the pillar for new books in otolaryngology. When Plural Publishing was activated, Dr. Singh and Dr. Robert Sataloff teamed up to produce the landmark volume, *Professional Voice: The Science and Art of Clinical Care, Third Edition.*

Dr. Singh and I enjoyed many exciting times from our early meetings in academic settings to the most recent times in San Diego during the Plural years. We walked the La Jolla beach many mornings and evenings talking about prospective authors, topics, and titles. He was energetic, enthusiastic, and committed to bringing the "niche" books that no other publisher wanted to the audiences that needed them. During our walks, we reviewed our previous experiences in publishing, what was new, and how the world of book publishing would survive in the electronic age. Those discussions and walks ended all too soon, despite our 46 years of collaboration. And in our last telephone call on the Saturday before he was taken to the hospital, we discussed the future of the company, the employees, new book topics, and future projections. He encouraged me to work on a new series of books called "Here's How Series." That series has blossomed, thanks to his input at its infant stage.

From the Saturday morning lectures in the voice science laboratory at Ohio State University to the study of multidimensional scaling to the grand scale of publishing books on that topic and many others, Dr. Singh and I maintained a close personal and professional relationship that carried through our lives and our interests with us these many years.

REFERENCES

Buder, E. H. (2000). Acoustic analysis of voice quality: A tabulation of algorithms 1902–1990. In R. D. Kent & M. J. Ball (Eds.), *Voice quality measurement* (pp. 119–244). San Diego, CA: Singular.

Carroll, D., & Chang, J. J. (1970). Analysis of individual differences in multidimensional scaling via an N-way generalization of Eckkart-Young decomposition. *Psychometrica, 35,* 283–319.

Childers, D. G., & Lee, C. K. (1991).Vocal quality factors; analysis, synthesis and perception. *Journal of the Acoustical Society of America, 90,* 2394–2410.

Danhauer, J., & Singh, S. (1975). A multidimensional scaling of phonemic responses from hard of hearing and deaf subjects of three languages. *Language and Speech, 18,* 42–64.

Emanual, F., & Smith W. (1974). Pitch effects on vowel roughness and spectral noise. *Journal of Phonetics, 2,* 247–253.

Gelfer, M. P. (1993). A multidimensional scaling study of voice quality in females. *Phonetica, 50,* 15–27.

Hasek, C. S., Singh, S., & Murry, T. (1980). Acoustic attributes of preadolescent voices. *Journal of the Acoustical Society of America, 68,* 1262–1265.

Hecker, M. H. L., & Kruel, E. J. (1971). Descriptions of the speech of patients with cancer of the vocal folds. Part 1: Measures of fundamental frequency. *Journal of the Acoustical Society of America, 49,* 1275–1282.

Klatt, D. H., & Klatt, L. C. (1990). Analysis, synthesis and perception of voice quality variations among female and male talkers. *Journal of the Acoustical Society of America, 87,* 820–857.

Mitchell, L., & Singh, S. (1974). Perceptual structure of sixteen prevocalic English consonants sententially embedded. *Journal of the Acoustical Society of America, 55,* 1355–1357.

Murry, T., Singh, S., & Sargent, M. (1977). Multidimensional classification of abnormal voice qualities. *Journal of the Acoustical Society of America, 61*(6), 1630–1635.

Shrivastav, R. (2006). Multidimentional scaling of breathy voice quality. *Journal of Voice, 20*(2), 211–222.

Shrivastav, R., & Camacho, A. (2010). A computational model to predict changes in breathiness from variations in aspiration noise level. *Journal of Voice, 24*(4), 395–405.

Shrivastav, R., & Sapienza, C. (2003). Objective measures of breathy voice quality obtained using an auditory model. *Journal of the Acoustical Society of America, 114,* 2217–2224.

Singh, S. (1976). *Distinctive features: Theory and validation.* Baltimore, MD: University Park Press.

Singh, S., & Woods, D. R. (1971). Perceptual structure of 12 American English vowels. *Journal of the Acoustical Society of America, 49,* 1861–1866.

Singh, S., Woods, D. R., & Becker, G. N. (1972). Perceptual structure of 22 prevocalic English consonants. *Journal of the Acoustical Society of America, 52,* 1698–1713.

Stevens, S. S. (1935). The relation of pitch to intensity. *Journal of the Acoustical Society of America, 6,* 150–154.

ESSAY 3

Milestones and Cases Along the Way

John W. Oller Jr.

Sometimes paths cross, re-cross, and cross again at perfect moments in time. I first met Dr. Sadanand Singh in Palm Springs, California, April 17, 1998. I remember that sunny day and Singh's warm greeting, handshake, smile, and the light in his eyes. We had no further contact until I got a personally addressed letter from Singh dated October 6, 2004 inviting me to publish with his new company. I have framed it to keep always. He had sold Singular and was launching Plural Publishing.

In January, 2005, I called to see if the offer was still open. We talked about the books that would later appear under the titles *Milestones* (2006) and *Cases* (2010). I will never forget that cold January day in 2005. I started to introduce myself and but he said, "Don't worry. I remember you and I researched your record." He got a smile about the transition from "Singh-ular" to "Plural." I mentioned the junior colleagues I planned to invite to work with me, including my son Steve, and my colleague Dr. Linda C. Badon, CCC-SLP. He remarked on the benefits of involving junior colleagues and said, "I will treat you the same as I would one of my best authors" and he named one of the top producers in the nation.

That day I understood something that would be confirmed in years to come: Singh was one of those rare teachers who inspires. He treated every interlocutor as if he or she were the most important person in the room. Sadanand Singh saw future possibilities as realities in the present tense. In doing so, he inspired others to do the same. I will never forget his closing statement on that gray day in January. He said, "John, let's keep the positive energy flowing between us."

His statement was like a light in the distance on a dark and stormy night. Along with the books we talked about that day, some of the benefits he predicted—tenure promotions for both of my junior colleagues and additional publications, presentations, and research products by themselves, our students, and other colleagues—have been realized. Dr. Stephen D. Oller (the younger of my two sons, the third of four children and father to four of my 10 grandchildren, two of whom are featured in the *Milestones* book) is now an Associate Professor at Texas A&M (Kingsville) and Dr. Linda C. Badon, CCC-SLP, is a tenured colleague and a distinguished member of the Graduate Faculty here at the University of Louisiana (Lafayette).

Initially we committed to present the most current and relevant research and the most advanced theory for both books at an introductory level. We argued that understanding normal speech and language development, the introduction in *Milestones*, is critical to sorting out, classifying, and introducing communication disorders in their social contexts, the purpose of *Cases*. We determined to look to causes, prevention, and making things better rather than merely accepting things as they are. We promised to look at dental mercury and Thimerosal (better known to many by its commercial name, Merthiolate) as potential causal factors in autism, but the toxicology would force us to consider Alzheimer's, parkinsonism, multiple sclerosis, and a host of other disorders and disease conditions as well. It was clear that certain toxins cannot do otherwise than make neurological disorders worse across the board. Also, though the toxicology research on these chemicals alone would fill a small library, no book in the field of communication disorders, to our knowledge, had even suggested their potential role in neurological disorders. Much less had any books in our field ever suggested that such factors might commonly be primary causal factors in some of the most puzzling of communication disorders.

The *Milestones* project, which appeared in 2006, was possibly the first book published in our field that addressed the role of organic-mercurials in the causation of neurological disorders including such demyelinating conditions as adrenoleukodystrophy (the genetic disorder featured in the 1992 film, *Lorenzo's Oil*). The research cited in our books shows that organo-mecurials are also genotoxins that damage the genetics of plants, insects, lab animals, and humans. In 2005, David Kirby had published *Evidence of Harm: Mercury in Vaccines and the Autism Epidemic—A Medical Controversy* under the imprint of St. Martin's Press, but *Milestones* and *Cases* seem to be the

first coursebooks in communication disorders dealing with toxins, disease agents, and their interactions as causal agents in neurological and genetic damage in humans.

Although public concern about ethyl mercury injections in vaccines, immunoglobulin preparations, medicines, cosmetics, and so on, had been sparked by a paper published in *Medical Hypotheses* 2001 (Bernard et al.) linking it, hypothetically at least, to autism spectrum disorders, medical practitioners were shocked to discover the amount of ethyl mercury in required vaccines. Dr. Neal Halsey, MD, then Head of the Institute for Vaccine Safety at Johns Hopkins, recounted his astonishment to Arthur Allen in 2002:

> From the beginning, I saw Thimerosal [Merthiolate] as something different. . . . It was the first strong evidence of a causal association with neurological impairment. I was very concerned. . . . My first reaction was simply disbelief, which was the reaction of almost everybody involved in vaccines. . . . In most vaccine containers, Thimerosal is listed as a mercury derivative, a hundredth of a percent . . . a trace, a biologically insignificant amount. . . . But the fact is, no one did the calculation. (Allen, 2002, p. 2)

The year we were writing *Milestones*, Parran et al. (2005) showed that ethyl mercury in parts per billion damages DNA by fragmenting it, interferes with mitochondrial communications essential to a healthy immune system, and kills developing nerve cells. But the research in toxicology, on the one hand, was little known to clinicians and researchers in communication disorders, whereas, on the other hand, the widely published defenses of vaccine manufacturers, mainstream medical and dental practitioners, and eager promoters of vaccines, dental amalgam, and the like, were everywhere. They were in full-page advertisements in magazines, in pharmaceutically sponsored medical journals such as *Pediatrics*, the *Journal of the American Medical Association*, the *Journal of the American Dental Association*, and so forth. Although millions of dollars were spent by the American Dental Association claiming that dental mercury does no harm to the brain of adults, that it's safe for young children, pregnant women, and unborn babies, billions were being spent to quell concerns about the toxins, disease agents (measles in particular), animal viruses (e.g., the cancer-linked Simian 40 and dozens of others), protein fragments, preservatives, adjuvants (e.g., aluminum), and other "adventitious" components, not to mention all of the inevitable interactions in the increasingly "multivalent" vaccines.

With the controversy raging in the background, we submitted our *Milestones* manuscript of 12 chapters, with the instructor's data DVD, 600 text-linked multiple choice questions, and many video and other illustrations to Plural. Within a couple of months, we learned that Dr. Singh had been lobbied not to publish on account of our questions about dental mercury, vaccines, and Thimerosal. He urged us to take another pass through parts where these issues were discussed. We did so, reading every word of text, checking references, and with renewed confidence submitted our updated version for yet another peer-review. In the end, Dr. Singh and his reviewers went with the research rather than the politics.

Later, in *Cases*, we concluded on the basis of thousands of research studies that "toxins included in the vaccines—mercury, aluminum, and so forth" along with the "increasing effort to combine . . . multiple disease agents . . . simultaneously into a single shot, for the sake of convenience" increase the risk of undesirable interactions. Why had it taken so long to discover them? "It is just that the injuries are at the atomic and molecular levels of our bodily systems and are sometimes not readily noticed or easily detected even with complex medical tests" (p. 640). Research showed (Oller & Oller, 2010; Ratajczak, 2011) that the rising incidence of autism is correlated with the uptake of vaccines; that it is *unreasonable not to suspect* interactions occurring between disease agents and toxins in vaccines. They are evidently prime causal factors in infant mortality—"crib death," "sudden infant death syndrome," "sudden unexpected infant death," and the like. The research suggests that the infant mortality rate (IMR) in the United States is strongly associated with the increasing use of vaccines. The evidence points to the almost unthinkable conclusion that Dr. Neal Halsey feared: rising rates of autism diagnosis, neurological disorders, and infant mortality appear to be linked to the increasing number of mandatory vaccine doses being administered to infants. On May 4, 2011, Miller and Goldman published research showing a strong correlation ($.70, p < 0.0001$) between the infant mortality rate (IMR) and number of doses of vaccines (NDV) administered in the 34 countries with the lowest IMRs. Of the countries included in their study, the United States has the highest IMR and the highest NDV. A grouping that reduced error variability by computing mean IMRs and NVDs produced a correlation at $.992$ ($p < 0.0009$). Increasing the vaccine doses seems to cause an increase in the number of infant deaths. In 2009, the IMR in the United States was 6.2 per 1,000, a rate roughly equivalent to the prevalence of autism 10 years ago.

By March 1, 2005 contracts for both the *Milestones* and the *Cases* books had been issued and by May 5, 2006, the first copies of the *Milestones* book had arrived in the Plural warehouse. Dr. Singh's twins, Sapna and Sanjay (then at age 10), appear on the cover of that book along with Dr. Badon's grandson, Cole (the baby crawling), Dr. D. Kimbrough Oller's youngest child, Lia Oller (the tiny infant), my daughter Ruthie and her friend Ashley (the two teenagers), my wife's dad, Tom Chavez (the septuagenarian), and an unknown baby in the womb (thanks to Dr. Stuart Campbell at Create Health Clinic in London). The green *Milestones* cover was jointly designed by Ruth Marie Toce and Mrs. Angie Singh. The cover itself shows that the *Milestones* project was more than a team effort; it was a family affair.

The *Cases* project, reclassifying and re-examining disorders across the board at an introductory level, though started earlier, would take longer to pretest and to complete. The proposal was sent to Dr. Singh on February 11, 2005, and the same day he wrote back referring to it as "a visionary approach to this very important course" (personal communication to J. Oller). The first draft of *Cases* was submitted electronically on January 15, 2008, and on February 25, 2008, I talked with Dr. Singh in a conference call that lasted the better part of an hour. At the end of that conversation, he suggested that we should let the book "age like a fine wine" and possibly return to it at a later date. At the time, I thought that we might have reached the end of the road for the *Cases* project. Then, on August 6, 2008, almost six months later, I received a call from Plural indicating that Dr. Singh himself had read the "most controversial chapters" of *Cases* and was eager to publish it. He was quoted as saying, "I have read the most controversial parts and it must be published." Not only was he himself a man of vision, but also of courage, integrity, and determination to make a difference for the better.

Research updates and new references were incorporated. Summary sidebars were added at Dr. Singh's insistence and when he kidded that the book was "much longer than promised" I replied that he "should therefore be willing to pay more for it!" Changes included a hardcover, two colors, and putting all 600 multiple choice items on the DVD. The latter was justified by research to be published (Yan, 2009) showing that advance access to test questions increased both the reliability and validity of tests based on those text-linked multiple choice items. A little under a year after the recommitment to proceed, the first copies of *Cases* arrived in the Plural warehouse on July 31, 2009. We had the entire book, DVD, and all relevant materials in time for the 2009 fall classes across the United States.

The last time I saw Dr. Singh was on November 2, 2009, at a Plural book signing. He was greeting people as warmly as he did on that sunny afternoon not so long ago in Palm Springs. Dr. Steve Oller called on March 9, 2010, to say he had seen the obituary for Dr. Singh as published in the *Washington Post*. On March 10, 2010, I wrote a tribute following the *Washington Post* that can still be seen on the website today. The descriptors I would apply now are still the same: Sadanand Singh was a visionary who inspired those he worked with to reach beyond themselves. He touched the world with love, enthusiasm, and grace. When I read the story of his life as told by the American Academy of Audiology (2010), I realized that our meetings were more than chance, and I longed to hear his voice once more and to see again the courage and determination in his eyes.

REFERENCES

Allen, A. (2002). The not-so-crackpot autism theory. *New York Times*, November 10, 2002. Retrieved May 11, 2009, from http://query .nytimes.com/gst/fullpage.html?res=9B03EFD 7153EF933A25752C1A9649C8B63&sec=&s pon=&pagewanted=1

American Academy of Audiology. (2010). In Memorium: Sadanand Singh, PhD (1934–2010). Retrieved May 10, 2011, from http:// www.audiology.org/news/Pages/20100302 .aspx

Bernard, S., Enayati, A., Redwood, L., Roger, H., & Binstock, T. (2001). Autism: A novel form of mercury poisoning. *Medical Hypotheses, 56,* 462–471.

Kirby, D. (2005). *Evidence of harm: Mercury in vaccines and the autism epidemic: A medical controversy.* New York, NY: St. Martin's Press.

Miller, N. Z., & Goldman, G. S. (May 4, 2011). Infant mortality rates regressed against number of vaccine doses routinely given: Is there a biochemical or synergistic interaction? *Human and Experimental Toxicology,* DOI: 10.1177/ 0960327111407644. Retrieved May 10, 2011, from http://het.sagepub.com/content/early/ 2011/05/04/0960327111407644

Oller, J. W., Jr., & Oller, S. D. (2010). *Autism: The diagnosis, treatment, and etiology of the undeniable epidemic.* Sudbury, MA: Jones and Bartlett.

Oller, J. W., Jr., Oller, S. D., & Badon, L. C. (2006). *Milestones: Normal speech and language development across the life span.* San Diego, CA: Plural.

Oller, J. W., Jr., Oller, S. D., & Badon, L. C. (2010). *Cases: Introducing communication disorders across the life span.* San Diego, CA: Plural.

Parran, D. K., Barker, A., & Ehrich, M. (2005). Effects of thimerosal on NGF signal transduction and cell death in neuroblastoma cells. *Toxicological Science, 1,* 132–140.

Ratajczak, H. V. (2011). Theoretical aspects of autism: Causes—a review. *Journal of Immunotoxicology, 8*(1), 68–79.

Yan, R. (2009). *Assessing English language proficiency in international aviation: Issues of reliability, validity, and aviation safety.* Saarbrücken, Germany: VDM Verlag.

My Personal Journey with a Good Friend and Scholar

My Tribute to Dr. Sadanand Singh

Jon K. Shallop

It was a cool fall day in 1963 in Columbus, Ohio, when I met Sadanand. We were both new doctoral students in the OSU Speech and Hearing Sciences Program with Prof. John W. Black as our advisor. Dr. Black said, "Shallop, you teach him English and he will teach you about Hindu philosophy." Indeed, that was just the beginning of many years of friendship that so many others have experienced. He already had a PhD in Hindu philosophy but I never did get to read his dissertation! I wondered why he wanted a second PhD and how he had selected Ohio State as his university of choice to study speech and hearing sciences.

Sadanand's English was quite limited for a few months but he developed his oral and written language skills very quickly. He would try to get all of us to learn words in Hindi and greet each other daily with "numestay." There were many other words he tried to get us to pronounce including his name. "It's easy, Jon, just slowly say 'suh don ond sing.' That's it Jon, now say it all together, fast!" Many people, including Dr. Black, could not pronounce Sadanand's name, so they just called him Singh. But many of us did master the

pronunciation of his first name. He thought it very humorous when someone would mispronounce his name, and he would laugh in his unique way that made all of us smile.

Our class was international. In addition to Sadanand, our fellow students included Yukio Takefuta from Japan and Oscar Tosi from Argentina. Early in September, the four of us went to the Graduate School Office to fill out some required papers. As we worked on page 1, Oscar suddenly said, "Jon, what is this, they want to know my age and color?" I looked at Oscar's arm and I said, "You look tan to me, just write tan." I continued, "Sadanand you are brown, Yukio you are light yellow, and I am light pink." A few days later the four of us were all called into Dr. Black's office, and he was chuckling about our responses, after the Dean's office had called him about our answers. There are so many other joyful stories about graduate school with Sadanand.

After Sadanand and I graduated, we both took our first teaching positions as assistant professors at Ohio University in Athens. Sadanand was quick to get his publication stream going in psycholinguistics and speech science. He made good friends in the Department of Linguistics (Dr. Zinny Bond) and Psychology (Dr. Danny Moates). He was also enjoyed working closely with Dr. JoAnn Folkes. They worked very well together, and many of their graduate students benefited.

I recall the day that he told me that he had decided to buy a publishing company, University Park Press. He told me that he was tired of other people making money on his publications. So with the help of his brother Vidia, Sadanand was in the publishing business. The rest is history, and I am sure others will write on this topic.

Sadanand and his family were from the Punjab area of northern India. They were farmers. Sadanand was very proud of his family, and made visits to India many times. Perhaps this is part of the reason that he decided to buy a small farm in rural Ohio. He and Kala had their first two children about this time. Their closest neighbor was Mr. Nixon. We all had a lot of fun in our discussions. He liked to tell the unsuspecting that he lived next to the President. One day Mr. Nixon asked Sadanand if he could continue to cut the hay on their farm and then share the bales of hay as he did with the previous owner. Sadanand said, "Sure, you keep 50% and I will get the other 50%." Mr. Nixon replied, "No percentages. I will count you 5 bales for you and 5 for me until they are all counted." Sadanand loved to tell this story and then he ended with his signature laughter.

I maintained contact with Sadanand and his family after we both left Ohio University. I recall a wonderful summer with Sadanand and his family in Washington, DC, when he was Chair of the Speech and Hearing Program at Howard University. He had invited me to teach for a summer session, which was a great experience for me. One of the students from Howard University enrolled and earned his PhD from Ohio University.

After the tragic death of his wife, Kala, and personal injuries to Sadanand and his children from that tragic 1986 Pan Am Flight 73 hijacking, Sadanand's life changed dramatically. But as usual, he rebounded and started a new family in California. I remember the day he called to tell me that he and Angie would soon have twins! He remarked, "And I am only in my 60s, isn't that great!" It was great, my dear friend. You have left this world for a better place of rest. So many people miss you, but none more than your wonderful family. Numestay, Sadanand.

PART II

The Nature of Translational Research

ESSAY 5

Models and Concepts of Translational Research

Ray D. Kent

Words do not suffice to describe Sadanand Singh, but words are all we have. I recently came across the following expression that meets at least part of the challenge: "The best measure of a person is not what he does but what he gives of himself." Sadanand certainly did a great deal, but, more importantly, he gave of himself. Many of us who were privileged to know him can testify to the truth of that statement. Sadanand gave of his resources, hospitality, advice, encouragement, friendship, and love. I remember him especially for the way he gave of himself to the fulfillment of others: to colleagues, students, and aspiring authors. Sadanand was scholarly, philosophical, gentle, generous, encouraging, and visionary. Above all, he was a friend. Sadanand and I had many conversations about research, especially about how it can transform clinical practice, and how clinical practice, in turn, can transform research. This chapter pertains to that issue and I humbly submit it in his memory.

OBJECTIVES OF THIS ESSAY

The topic at hand is translational research (TR), with the object of explaining what this kind of research is all about and why it is attracting so much interest. The essence of TR has been crystallized in the simple phrase "discovery to delivery." The sine qua non of TR is to move knowledge and discovery gained from the basic sciences (discovery) to applications in clinical and community settings (delivery). This concept also can be expressed as "bench-to-bedside" (T1) and "bedside-to-community" (T2) research, so that two types of translation, T1 and T2, are recognized in the fulfillment of TR. But this basic description has been criticized. Woolf (2008, p. 211) wrote, "Referring to T1 and T2 by the same name—translational research—has become a source of some confusion. The 2 spheres are alike in name only." Woolf's comment is a warning that simple definitions may create unintended problems and fail to capture the full dimensionality and scope of TR. In fact, TR can be conceived more broadly to include several phases of translation and to allow for bidirectional, if not multidirectional, influences (e.g., bench to bedside and back again). This paper summarizes models of translational research and discusses examples of this kind of research in communication sciences and disorders (CSD).

FORCES DRIVING TRANSLATIONAL RESEARCH

The motivation behind TR has been succinctly and strongly stated. Frances Collins, Director of the National Institutes of Health (NIH) expressed the challenge and goal of TR as follows: "Despite dramatic advances in the molecular pathogenesis of disease, translation of basic biomedical research into safe and effective clinical applications remains a slow, expensive, and failure-prone endeavor" (Collins, 2011, p. 1). To address this imbalance, the NIH has established a National Center for Advancing Translational Sciences (NCATS), the mission of which is "to catalyze the generation of innovative methods and technologies that will enhance the development, testing, and implementation of diagnostics and therapeutics across a wide range of diseases and conditions." This recognition of TR by the NIH has been duly noted by investigators in the various types of science supported by NIH. But enthusiasm for TR is rooted not only in NIH initiatives but also in ground-shifting advances, including remarkable progress in the basic sciences, especially molecular biology and genetics, and in the adoption of evidence-based medicine (and, more generally, evidence-based practice in a variety of specialties).

Another signal, among many, of the importance of translational research in medicine is that new journals are dedicated to the topic. One of these describes itself as follows (taken from the journal Web site): "To promote human health by providing a forum for communication and cross-fertilization among basic, translational, and clinical research practitioners and trainees from all relevant established and emerging disciplines" (Science Translational Medicine, n.d.).

TR is the center of much discussion and planning. To understand more about what TR is and what can be expected from its pursuit, we begin with a definition.

DEFINITION OF TRANSLATIONAL RESEARCH

The NINDS Cooperative Program in Translational Research defines TR as follows: "Translational research is the process of applying ideas, insights, and discoveries generated through basic scientific inquiry to the treatment or prevention of human disease" (NINDS Cooperative Program in Translational Research, n.d.). This definition introduces the essential nature of TR. But giving a precise definition of the term is difficult because different conceptions of it have been put forth. Gunnar and Cicchetti (2009, p. 5) observed that, "it is easier to describe the goals than the precise definition of *translational research* because the process of moving basic information along the path from discovery to the testing of novel treatments and interventions is a bit like the game of telephone." They explain that there are many points of information exchange, each involving translation. Therefore, the process is one of multiple translations needed to move discoveries in basic science to clinical application. Hörig and Pullman (2004, p. 2) were similarly reticent to propose a simple definition, noting that there are many ways of defining TR. They identified its core thesis to be "that information gathered in animal studies can be translated into clinical relevance and vice versa, thus providing a conceptual basis for developing better drugs." Their concept of TR applies to pharmaceuticals but not the wider range of interventions including behavioral methods. What is needed is a definition that encompasses all sciences related to human health, including biomedical and behavioral approaches, and not only for treatment, but also for prevention and assessment.

Rubio et al. (2010) crafted a rather lengthy definition of TR: "Translational research fosters the multidirectional integration of basic research, patient-oriented research, and population-based research, with the long-term aim of improving the health of the public. T1 research expedites the movement between basic research and patient-oriented research that leads to new or improved scientific understanding or standards of care. T2 research facilitates the movement between patient-oriented research and population-based research that leads to better patient outcomes, the implementation of best practices, and improved health status in communities. T3 research promotes interaction between laboratory-based research and population-based research to stimulate a robust scientific understanding of human health and disease" (p. 473). This definition identifies 3 types of translation but, as discussed in the following section, other conceptions of TR recognize up to 5 types. We examine next different models of TR.

MODELS OF TRANSLATIONAL RESEARCH

Block diagrams are one way to depict the processes and relationships in different conceptions of TR. The conceptual models of TR differ not only in the number of translations but also in the nature of knowledge that is translated. A few selected examples are shown in Figures 5–1, 5–2, and 5–3, which consist of block diagrams based on various descriptions of TR. The number of translations in these diagrams varies from 1 to 2 in Figure 5–1, and from 3 to 5 in Figures 5–2 and 5–3. That is, the complexity of the diagrams increases across the 3 figures. The variance in the number of translations does not necessarily mean

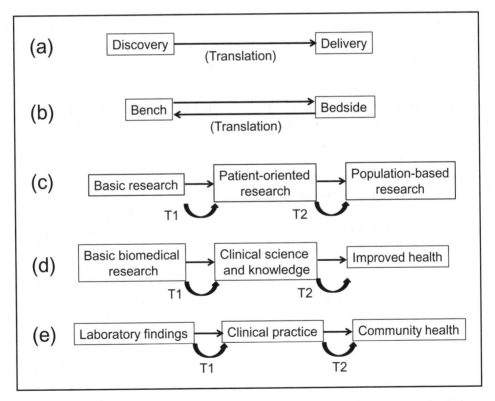

Figure 5–1. Models of TR that recognize 1 or 2 translations (T1 and T2 for the latter). The basic concepts in (a) and (b) are given fuller expression in (c), (d), and (e). Drawn from various sources including: Center for Clinical and Translational Sciences; Marincola (2003); Rubio et al. (2010); Sung et al. (2003); Translational Research Working Group of the National Cancer Institute; Woolf (2008).

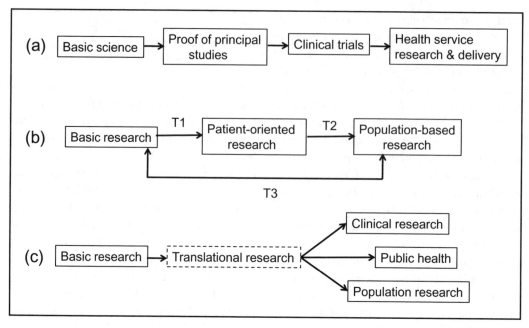

Figure 5–2. *Models of TR that recognize 2 or 3 translations (T1, T2, T3, as appropriate) with different interpretations of the nature of these translations. Drawn from various sources including: Dougherty and Conway (2003); Fleming, Perkins, Easa, and Conde (2008); Tabak (n.d.); University of Arkansas Medical School Translational Research Institute; University of Massachusetts Medical School and UMass Memorial Health Care, Academic Health Sciences Center.*

fundamental disagreement in concept, but rather differences in the degree of unfolding of the concept or differences in the kinds of interactions identified in the overall process. The variance also helps to explain why it is difficult to create a simple, all-inclusive definition. TR as an enterprise ultimately is more than a unidirectional translation of knowledge from basic science to clinical application. Science is rarely that simple in the nature and scope of its applications. Clinical application can take several forms, one being the services delivered to an individual patient or client ("bedside"), another being the delivery of services to populations of individuals ("community health"), and still another being the shaping of public health policy with the goal of optimizing methods of prevention, assessment, and treatment ("health policy"). The translations from bedside to community and from community to public health policy are

not necessarily accomplished in a sequential manner ("a pipeline model"), although they can be. There is good reason to emphasize integration rather than separation (Selker, 2010). Box and arrow diagrams like those in Figures 5–1, 5–2, and 5–3, may not capture the interaction and integration of the components; a diagram built from overlapping, staggered boxes may be appropriate.

The essential question is not which model of TR is correct, but rather which model is suited to a particular perspective or purpose. Some models are suited to pharmaceutical research involving early studies on animals and subsequent studies involving humans. Other models are suited to the study of communication processes, where the basic science is concerned with human behaviors and not necessarily with molecules or animal models as the starting point. Some models are better at capturing the spectrum of applica-

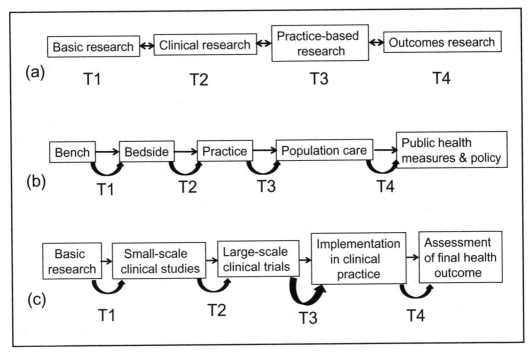

Figure 5–3. *Models of TR that recognize more than 3 translations T1, T2, T3, and T4). Drawn from various sources, including: Institute for Clinical and Translational Research, University of Iowa; Institute of Translational Health Sciences; Koury, Gwinn, Yoon, Moore, and Bradley (2007); Office of Translational and Applied Research, The Ohio State University Medical Center; Selker (2010), The University of Texas Southwestern Medical Center at Dallas, University of Massachusetts.*

tions to include not only care of the individual patient but also health care policies for large populations.

TRAINING FOR TRANSLATIONAL RESEARCH

To the extent to which TR demands skills and knowledge beyond those needed for earlier conceptions of basic and applied research, the training programs must gear up to meet the challenge of personnel preparation. Exactly what the training needs are, and how they might be accomplished, is yet to be fully determined, but some ideas have been proposed. As a beginning point, is important to note that the training is not entirely or sufficiently

accomplished by interdisciplinary research training. Interdisciplinary research certainly can be helpful, but it does not ensure confident and competent TR. Rubio et al. (2010) discuss aspects of training needed to ensure competence in TR.

EXAMPLES OF TRANSLATIONAL RESEARCH IN CSD

Even before the term TR was widely used, many researchers and clinicians in CSD were concerned with the timely and efficient transfer of knowledge from basic science to clinical populations and health policy. TR is not a newly discovered aspect of science, but rather one that is receiving a fresh emphasis that enhances its visibility and prospects for financial support. Considered in this section are contemporary examples of TR in the study of disorders of human communication. The articles included make explicit mention of TR and therefore reflect current thinking about how TR can be promoted in the field of CSD. Companion papers in this volume are also valuable indicators of progress in TR in CSD.

HEARING AND BALANCE

A good example of how discovery in basic science may lead to a clinical application is investigation of how the ears of a parasitoid fly (*Ormia ochracea*) inspired the development of microfabrication techniques to create a directional microphone for hearing aids (Miles & Hoy, 2005). The clinical application is underlain by two critical efforts in basic science: the study of the fly's ears and the development of silicon microfabrication technologies. In another example of TR, Witsell et al. (2011) reviewed the development of a practice-based research network (PBRN) called Creating Healthcare Excellence through Education and Research (CHEER) focused on patients with tinnitus and dizziness. Russ, Dougherty, and Jadadish (2010) discuss the means by which evidence-based research can be translated into service delivery for children with early hearing loss. Examples of TR focused on prevention are described in several articles in 2 special issues of the journal *Hearing Research* (Canlon, Henderson, & Salvi, 2007).

VOICE

A special issue of *Voice and Voice Disorders* in 2008 was given to translational science. The titles of the articles give a flavor of the top-

ics included (authors are given in parentheses): Voicing a vision of translational research (Stemple & Thomas), From bench to bedside: translational research on vocal fold hydration (Sivasankar & Leydon), Rheometers, bioreactors, and vocalization forces: using basic investigations to help the voices of teachers (Klemuk), Bench to bedside: research review in vocal fold extracellular matrix (Thibeault), and Recepter mediated uptake of pepsin: significance in otolaryngology (Johnston). The titles by themselves are sufficient to show the bench to bedside perspective in this special issue.

LANGUAGE

Although much of the discussion of TR has focused on the development and delivery of pharmaceuticals and biotechnologies, the need for TR in behavioral science has not been neglected. Beeghly (2006) considers the essential question: "How can results from longitudinal crosspopulation research on early language development in at-risk and atypical groups be "translated" into more effective evidence based clinical practice?" (Beeghly, 2006, p. 751). She points to 5 basic areas of research that provide substantial answers to this question.

NEUROSCIENCE

Several notable articles have been published on the translational opportunities in neuroscience. Among these are three papers growing out of a conference on neurorehabilitation, one focused on speech (Ludlow et al., 2008), another on language (Raymer et al., 2008), and a third on swallowing (Robbins et al., 2008). A common theme to these contributions was the clinical application of advances in the understanding of neuroplasticity.

Another series of articles appeared as a special feature in the *ASHA Leader*; see Rogers (2007) for an introduction and summary. Interactions among various stakeholders include basic and clinical scientists, clinicians, and patients. In an article on restorative neurosciences in stroke, Cheeran et al. (2009) emphasize the interactions needed for progress: "These interactions can be facilitated by funding research consortia that include basic and clinical scientists, clinicians and patient/carer representatives with funds targeted at those impairments that are major determinants of patient and carrer outcomes" (p. 97).

CONCLUSION

TR is not a novel and revolutionary development in science directed to improve human health. What is new is the emphasis given to it and the potential resources that could be available to support efforts in this direction.

REFERENCES

Beeghly, M. (2006). Translational research on early language development: Current challenges and future directions. *Development and Psychopathology, 18*, 737–757.

Canlon, B., Henderson, D., & Salvi, R. (Eds.) (2007). Special issues on: Pharmacological strategies for prevention and treatment of hearing loss and tinnitus. *Hearing Research, 226*(1–2), 1–254.

Center for Clinical and Translational Sciences. (n.d.). What is translational research? Retrieved September 21, 2011, from http://ccts.uth.tmc.edu/

Cheeran, B., Cohen, L., Dobkin, B., Ford, G., Greenwood, R., Howard, D., . . . Wolf, S. (Cumberlin Consensus Working Group). (2009). The future of restorative neurosciences in stroke: Driving the translational research pipeline from basic science to rehabilitation of people after stroke. *Neurorehabilitation and Neural Repair, 23*, 97–107.

Collins, F. S. (2011). Reengineering translational science: The time is right. *Science Translational Medicine, 3*, 1–6.

Dougherty, D., & Conway, P. H. (2008). The "3T's" road map to transform US health care. *Journal of the American Medical Association, 299*, 2319–2321.

Fleming, E. S., Perkins, J., Easa, D., Conde, J. G., Baker, R. S., Southerland, W. M., . . . Norris, K. C. (2008). The role of translational research in addressing health disparities: A conceptual framework. *Ethnicity and Disease, 18*(2 Suppl. 2), S2-155–160.

Gunnar, M. R., & Cichetti, D. (2009). Meeting the challenge of translational research in child development. In D. Cicchetti & M. R. Gunnar (Eds.), *Minnesota symposia on child psychology: Meeting the challenge of translational research in child psychology* (Vol. 35, pp. 1–27). New York, NY: Wiley.

Hörig, H., & Pullman, W. (2004). From bench to clinic and back: Perspective on the 1st IQPC translational research conference. *Journal of Translational Medicine, 2*, 44. doi: 10.1186/1479-5876-2-44

Institute for Clinical and Translational Research, University of Iowa. (n.d.). What is translational research? Retrieved September 12, 2011, from http://www.icts.uiowa.edu/content/what-translational-research/

Institute of Translational Health Sciences. (n.d.) Translational research. Retrieved September 21, 2011, from https://www.iths.org/about/translational

Johnston, N. (2008). Receptor mediated uptake of pepsin: Significance in otolaryngology. *Perspectives on Voice and Voice Disorders, 18*, 134–142.

Klemuk, S. (2008). Rheometers, bioreactors, and vocalization forces: Using basic investigations to help the voices of teachers. *Perspectives on Voice and Voice Disorders, 18*, 119–125.

Koury, M. J., Gwinn, M., Yoon, P. W., Moore, C. A., Bradley, L. (2007). The continuum of translational research in genomic medicine: How can we accelerate the appropriate integration of human genome discoveries into health care and disease prevention? *Genetics in Medicine, 9,* 665–674.

Ludlow, C. L., Hoit, J., Kent, R., Ramig, L. O., Shrivastav, R., Strand, E., . . . Sapienza, C. M. (2008). Translating principles of neural plasticity into research on speech motor control recovery and rehabilitation. *Journal of Speech, Language and Hearing Research, 51,* S240–S258.

Marincola, F. M. (2003). Translational medicine: A two-way road. *Journal of Translational Medicine, 1,* 1.

Miles, R. N., & Hoy, R. R. (2006). The development of a biologically-inspired directional microphone for hearing aids. *Audiology and Neurotology, 11,* 86–94. doi: 10.1159/000090681

NINDS Cooperative Program in Translational Research. (n.d.). Part I overview information. Retrieved September 11, 2011, from http://grants.nih.gov/grants/guide/pa-files/par-05-158.html

Office of Translational and Applied Research, The Ohio State University Medical Center. (n.d.). Translational research. Retrieved from http://medicalcenter.osu.edu/research/translational_research/Pages/index.aspx

Raymer, A. M. Beeson, P., Holland, A., Kendall, D., Maher, L. M., Martin, N., . . . Gonzalez Rothi, L. J. (2008). Translational research in aphasia: From neuroscience to neurorehabilitation. *Journal of Speech, Language and Hearing Research, 51,* S259–S275.

Robbins, J., Butler, S. G., Daniels, S. K., Diez Gross, R., Langmore, S., Lazarus, C. L., . . . Rosenbek, J. (2008). Swallowing and dysphagia rehabilitation: Translating principles of neural plasticity into clinically oriented evidence. *Journal of Speech, Language and Hearing Research, 51,* S276–S300.

Rogers, M. (2007, September 4). Translational neuroscience: An introduction. *ASHA Leader,* pp. 4–5.

Rubio, D. M., Schoenbaum, E. E., Lee, L. S., Schteingart, D E., Marantz, P. R., Anderson, K. E., . . . Esposito, K. (2010). Defining translational research: Implications for training. *Academic Medicine, 85,* 470–475.

Russ, S. A., Dougherty, D., & Jagadish, P. (2010). Accelerating evidence into practice for the benefit of children with early hearing loss. *Pediatrics, 126*(Suppl. 1), S7–S18.

Science Translational Medicine. (n.d.). *Science Translational Medicine* Mission Statement. Retrieved September 21, 2011, from http://stm.sciencemag.org/site/about/mission.xhtml

Selker, H. P. (2010). Beyond translational research from T1 to T4: Beyond "separate but equal." *Clinical and Translational Science, 3,* 270–271.

Sivasankar, M., & Leydon, C. (2008). From bench to bedside: Translational research on vocal fold hydration. *Perspectives on Voice and Voice Disorders, 18,* 112–118.

Stemple, J. C., & Thomas, L. B. (2008). Voicing a vision of translational research. *Perspectives on Voice and Voice Disorders, 18,* 105–111.

Sung, N. S., Crowley, W. F., Genel, M., Salber, P., Sandy, L., Sherwood, L. M., . . . Rimoin, D. (2003). Central challenges facing the national clinical research enterprise. *Journal of the American Medical Association, 289,* 1278–1287.

Tabak, L. A. (n.d.). The challenge of translation research at the NIDCR. Retrieved September 19, 2011, from http://www.nidcr.nih.gov/GrantsAndFunding/TechnologyTransfer/Pathway/Conference

Translational Research Working Group (TRWG), National Cancer Institute. (n.d.) Retrieved September 19, 2011, from http://www.cancer.gov/researchandfunding/trwg/TRWG-definition-and-TR-continuum

Thibeault, S. I. (2008). Bench to bedside: Research review in vocal fold extracellular matrix. *Perspectives on Voice and Voice Disorders, 18,* 126–133.

University of Arkansas Medical School Translational Research Institute. (n.d.) Translational research. Retrieved September 11, 2011, from http://www.uams.edu/TRI/cctrcore/cctrTranslatnalRsrch.asp

University of Massachusetts Medical School and UMass Memorial Health Care. Academic Health Sciences Center strategic plan (FY 2009–2014). (n.d.). Retrieved September 11, 2011, from http://www.ahscstrategicplan.org/index.aspx

University of Texas Southwestern Medical Center at Dallas. (n.d.). What is translational research? Retrieved September 19, 2011, from http://www.utsouthwestern.edu/utsw/cda/dept440996/files/489751.html

Witsell, D. L., Schulz, K. A., Moore, K., & Tucci, D. L. for the CHEER investigators. (2011). Implementation and testing of research infrastructure for practice-based research in hearing and communication disorders. *Otolaryngology-Head and Neck Surgery*. Published online ahead of print on May 18, 2011. doi: 10.1177/0194599811406369

Woolf, S. H. (2008). The meaning of translational research and why it matters. *Journal of the American Medical Association, 299*, 211–213.

ESSAY 6

❧ The Science of Dissemination ❧

John C. Rosenbek

Sadanand Singh spent hours staring across the gap between science and practice in all of healthcare. He worried that belief, tradition, and habit were often more powerful than data as motivators of clinical activity. Like Domino and colleagues (2009), he understood that "The slow diffusion of empirically supported treatments and the rapid diffusion of treatments lacking empirical support play a significant role in the quality gap in the care of people . . ." (p. 701) with a variety of disabilities. He recognized that this gap was both wide and potentially destructive because most people with disease and disability are willing to go anywhere and do anything to improve or recover their health and function. Fortunately for those of us in speech-language pathology, audiology, and the other health care professions served by Sadanand's three publishing houses: College-Hill Press, Singular Publishing, and Plural Publishing, he was motivated to provide publications, materials, money, and energy to help bridge the gap, and he had unwavering positive regard for those joining him in the effort.

Although we never talked about it specifically, I think he appreciated the difficulty of dissemination (building a bridge of data and action between laboratory and clinic), beyond even the obvious and considerable challenges of successful publishing. He would have agreed with Berwick's (2003) assessment that dissemination is as complex as the sciences producing

the data to be disseminated. Singh spent a bit of time in the clinic and much of his professional life talking with practitioners. He had to know and have heard about the shock many newly trained clinicians feel when they begin that first job. Armed with the latest innovations, they are sobered by the sometimes ancient attitudes and technologies they encounter. No clinician, however, has ever taken a job or persisted in one out of a desire to be inefficient or out of date. The problems are not with the practitioners, but with education; in other words with dissemination.

DISSEMINATION WAS SINGH'S PASSION

Because he had an unobstructed view of professional activity for nearly five decades he realized publishing; providing improved access to published data; supporting educators, clinicians, and researchers; and underwriting their professional meetings provided only a portion of the trusses necessary for a bridge across the know-do gap. Thus he was not surprised by data (Oxman, Thomson, Davis, & Hayes, 1995) confirming that clinical practice is insufficiently altered by publication and continuing education alone. He also understood instinctively that getting efficacious, effective care to those needing it required principles and procedures as robust as those governing the data collection and materials he published. A science of dissemination needed to be linked to the science of discovery. The rest of this essay describes the science of dissemination, and links that might bind the sciences of dissemination and discovery, and contains a few thoughts about how all this could benefit from Singh's particular genius.

Dissemination science, like other sciences, depends on definitions and models. A typical definition of dissemination is "a planned process that involves consideration of target audiences and the setting in which research findings are to be received, and where appropriate, communicating and interacting with wider policy and health service audiences in ways that will facilitate research uptake in decision-making processes and practices" (Wilson, Petticrew, Calnan, & Nazareth, 2010, p. 2). This definition highlights some of the important components: planning, identification of target audiences and settings, and convincing communication. Models convert components like those above into relationships that can guide action. Models of dissemination are conceptual rather than mathematical, physical, or animal. Conceptual models, according to Brandt and Pope (1997), assist understanding by allowing one to "examine and think about something that is not the real thing but may be similar to the real thing" (p. 62) and they help "people think about behaviors of components in complex systems" (p. 62). Adopting a model of the structure and potential interactions of this complex process's components is a first step. Multiple models are available. Three seem to predominate: persuasive communication, diffusion of innovations, and social marketing (Wilson et al., 2010). Anyone fresh from vowing never ever to write another book only to be convinced by Singh

that one more effort (at least) was critical to a profession's survival can identify the one most likely to have appealed to him — persuasive communication.

Persuasive communication features five related components critical to dissemination: source of communication, message to be communicated, channels of communication, characteristics of audience(s), and setting in which communication is received. General meanings of these components are self-evident. Source, for example, refers to the site from which the data arise, laboratory or clinic, and person delivering the message about those data. In general, procedures already moved from the laboratory to one or more clinics staffed by early adopters and delivered by a spokesperson with clinical credentials are more likely to appeal to other, more tradition bound clinicians. Regardless of who is delivering it, the message needs to be relatively simple and specific, and to include data on risk-benefit and cost. The message also needs to include vignettes and demonstrations, be delivered to clinicians where they work, and be supplemented by easily accessible Web-based and hard copy materials, including protocols. Clinicians, supervisors, fiscal officers, CEOs, and patient groups must be targeted, beginning with those expected to be early adopters of new approaches. Convention papers miss most of these targets.

In addition, the five components of persuasive communication interact. Because health care is delivered in a variety of facilities with different values and restraints, messages need to be tailored to these differences. The message to staff in a rehabilitation facility will be different from one for home health care providers. Indeed, some procedures may be inappropriate for some settings, and time spent bringing a message to those settings is wasted. An audience of administrators will respond to a message that a new treatment will cost the same or less than the present standard (Torrey et al., 2001). Clinicians will want to know that the new treatment is better for patient progress than the standard, that initiating the treatment is relatively straightforward, and that a mechanism for their acquiring any new skills has administrative support, is in place, and is effective. Further consideration of the model is outside this paper's purview, but the interested reader can consult Wilson et al. (2010).

Models alone, however, are inadequate to solving what Kilbourne and colleagues (2007) identify (and most scientists and clinicians recognize) as the failure of new developments to pass from academic to nonacademic affiliated settings. The fault lies not solely with clinicians. Gown and town are different, not in value but in values, and the differences matter. Kilbourne et al.'s (2007) solution is the Replicating Effective Programs (REP) project, a product of the Centers for Disease Control and Prevention (CDC). REP has four phases: preconditions, preimplementation, implementation, and maintenance and evolution. The preconditions phase dictates: (1) establishing the need for a new intervention; (2) guaranteeing that an intervention corresponds to local conditions, such as availability of resources to comply with the treatment protocol and presence of a population in need of the treatment; (3) an analysis of barriers or resistance to introducing the new procedure; and (4) preparing a manual.

If the science of dissemination is to wed the science of discovery, researchers must vow to use at least selected components of the four phases, and especially that of the preconditions, in the design of any clinically oriented research. The first component, establishing the need for a new procedure, is, of course, uppermost in the minds of all scientists whose motivation is to enhance practice. Not so the others. Most studies are designed with validity, not translation in mind. Study validity dictates rigid subject selection and administration of the protocol, with little regard for the similarity of study and clinical patients or whether clinicians have time, tools, and motivation to adhere to the protocol. An irony is that the greater the study's validity, the less likely the transfer into regular clinical practice. Thus the second and third of the preconditions, guaranteeing that the treatment corresponds to local conditions, and that barriers and resistance are analyzed, should influence the design of treatment research before any data are collected. Validity need not be threatened.

A researcher could begin by establishing a treatment's active ingredient(s), those parts of the treatment critical to its effects, and therefore to be preserved even in the erratic, rough and tumble world of the clinic. Clinicians' promises to provide those ingredients would guarantee fidelity to the treatment protocol, and would free them to otherwise adapt the treatment to local circumstances. For example, measurement of maximum expiratory pressures (MEPs) and training at 75% or some other of that maximum may not be critical to expiratory muscle strength training's (EMST) effect (Troche et al., 2011). Thus, adopters could be reassured that additional equipment to measure MEPS is unnecessary when initiating EMST. Reducing the instrumentation requirements would make the treatment quicker, easier, cheaper, and thus more attractive to busy clinicians.

As a publisher, Singh understood the tension between fidelity and translation, because it was critical to his success. He knew what clinicians wanted because he asked them, and he struggled daily to recruit the right authors, price the work appropriately, and reach target audiences with attractive, useful books and materials. Some researchers are equally insightful; many are not. That funding agencies are forcing the issue by requiring model-driven plans for dissemination may help if these plans are evaluated as rigorously as is the science of discovery. Helpful as well would be funding priority for those clinically oriented studies promising a programmatic search for active ingredients.

Scientists cannot do it all, however. Despite hundreds of journals and thousands of papers, presentations, press releases, and personal visits, the most frequent sources of information about how to treat an individual patient or client are the treating clinician's own experience and the opinion of colleagues. This same clinician, however, is likely to place a high value on data when asked about the importance of evidence-based practice. So why are researchers, books, articles, systematic reviews, practice guidelines, and meta-analyses not more frequent sources for what to do? The reasons are well known (Majid et al., 2011; Salbach, Jaglal, Korner-Bitensky, Rappolt, & Davis, 2007; Zipoli & Kennedy, 2005). These include a lack of resources, including time to retrieve and read the literature; lack of confidence about being able to interpret statistical analyses; and the perception of an abyss between laboratory and clinic. However, treatments designed for conditions resistant to traditional approaches, whose fidelity can be preserved with minimal alterations to the often hectic, resource-poor clinic environments where most clinicians practice, and whose effects have been established for the medically complex persons now dominating the caseload of most clinicians would fly across the abyss. Especially if researchers follow up their visits to find out what clinicians need with visits to teach these same clinicians how to do the treatments and monitor fidelity, followed by yet another set of visits to reinstruct and reward.

Like the science of discovery, the science of dissemination requires resources. Funds to support the data collection can sometimes be stretched to fund some portion, such as the creation of dissemination toolkits. An effective toolkit would contain a discussion of the treatment's active ingredients and those ingredients that can be modified to accommodate local conditions and elaborate, step-by-step, and user-friendly treatment protocols, ideally so specific that a reader could complete the protocol with little additional instruction. Among the other contents would be tools for determining fidelity of treatment delivery and directions about mechanisms for monitoring and rewarding fidelity to the protocol and for redressing protocol violations. Toolkits are as likely as books, however, to be neatly stored on a shelf, forgotten food for silverfish. Thus, successful dissemination requires usually more resources than can be squeezed from the typical grant.

The additional requirements are costly. They include Web-based guidance to all parts of protocol delivery; identification of likely, early adopters of new approaches; and face-to-face education and negotiation with administrators, and the training of clinicians. The costs do not end here, however. Follow-up visits to address fidelity, correct drift, reward compliance, and deal with the unexpected are critical as well. Finally, protocol developers need to be available for additional consultation until they and the users are convinced the protocol has become the new standard of practice. Researchers and funding agencies are unprepared by tradition and habit to go so far and do so much. In truth, data may be easier and cheaper to collect than to disseminate.

People worldwide get inadequate, inefficient, or inappropriate care. No practitioner would admit to providing such care on purpose, and most can be believed. The failure is not with the providers. The failure is in ignoring that evidence-based practice is as much about making evidence relevant and available as it is about collecting it. The answer is a union of the sciences of discovery and dissemination. Sadanand knew this, and he doubtless wonders why the dissemination empire he helped create is not more tightly united to the discovery he respected. Our apologies, Dr. Singh; we will get right on it.

REFERENCES

Berwick, D. M. (2003). Disseminating innovations in health care. *Journal of the American Medical Association, 289,* 1969–1975.

Brandt, Jr, E. N., & Pope, A. M. (1997). *Enabling America: Assessing the role of rehabilitation science and engineering.* Washington, DC: National Academy Press.

Domino, M., Donohue, J., Horvitz-Lennon, M., & Normand, S-L. T. (2009). Improving quality and diffusing best practices: The case of schizophrenia. *Health Affairs, 28,* 701–712.

Kilbourne, A. M., Neumann, M. S., Pincus, H. A., Bauer, M. S., & Stall, R. (2007). Implementing evidence-based interventions in health care: Application of the replicating effective programs framework. *Implementation Science, 2,* 42. doi:10.1186/1748-5908-2-42

Majid, S., Foo, S., Luyt, B., Zhang, X., Theng, Y-L., Chang, Y-K., & Mokhtar, I. A. (2011). Adopting evidence-based practice in clinical decision making: Nurses' perceptions, knowledge, and barriers. *Journal of the Medical Library Association, 99,* 229–236.

Oxman, A. D., Thomson, M. A., Davis, D. A., & Hayes, R. B. (1995). No magic bullets: A systematic review of 102 trials of interventions to improve professional practice. *Canadian Medical Association Journal, 154,* 1423–1431.

Salbach, N. M., Jaglal, S. B., Korner-Bitensky, N., Rappolt, S., & Davis, D. (2007). Practitioner and organizational barriers to evidence-based practice of physical therapists for people with stroke. *Physical Therapy, 87,* 1284–1303.

Torrey, W. C., Drake, R. E., Dixon, L., Burns, B. J., Flynn, L., Rush, A. J., . . . Klatzker, D. (2001). Implementing evidence-based practices for persons with severe mental illnesses. *Psychiatry Services, 52,* 45–50.

Troche, M. S., Okun, M. J., Rosenbek, J. C., Musson, N., Fernandez, H. H., Rodriguez, R., . . . , Sapienza, C. M. (2011). Aspiration and swallowing in Parkinson disease and rehabilitation with EMST: A randomized trial. *Neurology, 75,* 1912–1919.

Wilson, P. M., Petticrew, M., Calnan, M. W., & Nazareth, I. (2010). Disseminating research findings: What should researchers do? A systematic scoping review of conceptual frameworks. *Implementation Science, 5,* 91. doi: 10.1186/1748-5908-5-91

Zipoli, Jr., R. P., & Kennedy, M. (2005). Evidence-based practice among speech-language pathologists: Attitudes, utilization, and barriers. *American Journal of Speech-Language Pathology, 14,* 208–220.

ESSAY 7

Promoting Resilience in Young Children

A Role in Prevention of Communication Disorders

Lauren K. Nelson

I met Dr. Sadanand Singh in my first university position shortly after graduating from a Ph.D. program. At that time I knew him only through his earlier books, Distinctive Features: Theory and Validation, *and* Phonetics: Principles and Practices. *What struck me most was how approachable, gracious, and encouraging Dr. Singh was. This positive first impression was reinforced through our subsequent interactions in the preparation and publication of my book. Dr. Singh had a talent for offering guidance in the most constructive manner possible and I sincerely appreciate the opportunity he gave me to be part of the "Plural family."*

INTRODUCTION

Although assessment and treatment of individuals with communication disorders are the principal professional roles for most audiologists and speech-language pathologists, prevention is within the scope of practice for both professions (American Speech-Language-Hearing Association [ASHA], 2007). One approach to prevention has the aim of reduc-ing risk factors associated with communication disorders and other developmental disabilities, and in turn, reducing the prevalence of communication disorders (ASHA, 1991; Robinson, 2000). Examples include public health programs such as those to reduce the number of low birth weight infants by increasing access to prenatal care and reducing maternal smoking during pregnancy, programs to reduce childhood lead poisoning through lead abatement efforts in older housing, or programs to reduce the occurrence of traumatic brain injury by promoting children's use of helmets.

Another approach to prevention has the aim of promoting factors that contribute to positive developmental outcomes, even for children who face considerable adversity in their early childhood (Goldstein & Brooks, 2005; Masten & Powell, 2003; Rutter, 2006). This approach to prevention has ties to research on resilience and protective factors (Masten, 2001; Masten & Powell, 2003; Werner, 2000). Resilience emerges from two coexisting conditions: (1) experiencing substantial adversity such as economic disadvantage, perinatal complications, or parental mental illness or substance abuse; and (2) evidence of overcoming this adversity in one or more developmental domains such as academic success and social competence (Luthar, Cicchetti, & Becker, 2000; Luthar, Sawyer, & Brown, 2006). Rutter (2006) noted that the unique contribution of research on resilience was the initial focus on individual variation in response to adversity by identifying subgroups of individuals who overcame adversity, that is, individuals who showed resilience. Condly (2006) and Wright and Masten (2005) provide extensive reviews of the literature on resilience.

EVIDENCE FOR RESILIENCE AND PROTECTIVE FACTORS

Evidence for resilience and protective factors came initially from several longitudinal, cohort studies, and more recently from intervention studies designed to promote resilience in groups of children experiencing one or more risk factors. The Kauai Longitudinal Study was one of the first longitudinal, cohort studies to provide information on resilience (Werner, 1993, 2000, 2005). The study included nearly 700 children; approximately half were from economically disadvantaged homes. Families were recruited when their children were born, and data were gathered several times during the childhood years, as well as at ages 32 and 40 years. The researchers documented multiple adverse factors including "perinatal complications, parental psychopathology, family instability, and chronic poverty" (Werner, 2000, p. 117). A subgroup within this birth cohort showed better than expected outcomes, despite being exposed to multiple risk factors. Further examination of data from this subgroup revealed several internal and external factors that separated the resilient group from children with less optimal outcomes. Examples of within child or inter-

nal factors included having an easy-going temperament as an infant; being alert, responsive, and independent as young children; as well as having superior communication and self-help skills (Werner, 2000, 2005). Internal factors for school-age children included superior problem-solving and communication skills. Examples of external factors included having a close relationship with a parent or alternate caregiver such as grandparent or older sibling, a relationship with a mentor such as a favorite teacher, and friendships with peers (Werner, 2000, 2005).

A series of studies conducted by researchers at the University of Minnesota, referred to as Project Competence, focused on childhood competence in children experiencing one or more types of adversity and those who were not high-risk (Masten & Powell, 2003). The core study included over 200 children who were followed during their school years to young adulthood. The researchers identified competent children by looking for average or above average performance on developmental tasks such as academic achievement; relationships with peers; and behavior at home, in school, and in the community. An overall finding of the study was that children who experienced more cumulative risks, such as economic disadvantage, single-parent household, and maltreatment, also exhibited more difficulties with developmental tasks. However, Masten and Powell (2003) noted that some of the competent children in the study came "from a childhood characterized by great risk and adversity" (p. 9).

Identifying the unique characteristics of competent children who achieved positive developmental outcomes despite adversity could have implications for prevention programs. Masten and Powell (2003) described three categories of protective factors: (1) individual factors such as a child's intellectual skills, temperament, and personality; (2) relationship factors such as the quality of parenting, availability of other adults as mentors or substitute parents, and friendships with competent peers; and (3) community factors such as memberships in prosocial organizations, high quality schools, and access to social services and health care. A resilience approach to prevention would have an emphasis on promoting or increasing these protective factors, in addition to reducing risk factors and treating deficit areas of functioning.

Recent research on the topic of resilience and protective factors has focused on the effects of intervention programs (Greenberg, 2006; Klebanov & Brooks-Gunn, 2006; Merrell, 2010; Winslow, Sandler, & Wolchik, 2005). One of these studies included an intervention component for low birth weight (LBW) infants. The study focused on 228 infants from low-income households, who were randomly assigned to either a comprehensive intervention program or to a control condition with medical follow-up only. The intervention program participants received services such as home visits, child care, and parent group meetings through age three. The researchers determined the presence of several risk factors for each child, including economic disadvantage and unemployment, maternal age and education, mother's mental health, stressful life events, availability of social support, teenage mother, absent father, and family density (Klebanov & Brooks-Gunn, 2006). The dependent measure was the child's score on a cognitive test at ages 3, 5, and 8. Klebanov and Brooks-Gunn (2006) reported that cumulative risk had a significant association with child cognitive abilities. The researchers grouped the risk factors into "human capital" and "psychological" risks. The human capital risks included economic disadvantage, maternal education, and employment; the psychological risks included maternal mental health, stressful life events, and social support. For a subgroup of "heavier" LBW children (>2,000 to 2,500 g), human capital risks, but not psy-

chosocial risks, had a negative association with cognitive test scores.

Klebanov and Brooks-Gunn (2006) also examined the moderating effects of treatment on the negative association between human capital risks and cognitive abilities. The researchers divided the children into four levels of risk based on the number of cumulative risks they experienced. At age three, children in the intervention group had higher cognitive test scores than children in a control group across all levels of cumulative capital risk; however, for the two older age groups, intervention resulted in higher cognitive test scores only for the moderate levels of capital risk. In discussing their findings, Klebanov and Brooks-Gunn noted that higher human capital, such as higher parental education and employment, could relate to better parenting and a better home environment. Regarding the finding that early intervention resulted in sustained benefits primarily for children from families with moderate levels of cumulative risk, the authors speculated that families with the highest level of cumulative risk had difficulty sustaining the benefits of early intervention on their own, once the program ended.

Greenberg (2006) described prevention research aimed at reducing aggression and other behavior problems in children. The program, Promoting Alternative Thinking Strategies (PATHS), targeted the social-emotional domain by teaching children, ages 4 to 11, appropriate strategies for self-control and expressing feelings. A series of randomized control trials supported the effectiveness of the PATHS program for decreasing behavior problems in school. Differences between intervention and control groups were still observed at a one-year follow up. Greenberg suggested that the PATHS program led to improved executive function, "effective inhibitory control, emotion regulation, and planning skills" (Greenberg, 2006, p. 145). Greenberg also suggested that future research might go beyond the link between executive function and behavior, and include a neuroscience component to investigate changes in activation in the prefrontal cortex.

The Oregon Resiliency Project is a third example of a prevention program that emphasized protective factors and resilience. Merrell (2010) described research conducted through the Oregon Resiliency Project and the components of a curriculum that emerged form this research, Strong Kids/Social and Emotional Learning (SEL). Components of the SEL curriculum included self-awareness and self-management, social awareness, relationship skills, and responsible decision-making (Merrell, 2010). The Strong Kids curriculum includes five separate programs developed for children from pre-K and kindergarten through grades 9 to 12. Research demonstrated the program had benefits not only for the social-emotional domain, but also for academic success and school behavior (Merrell, 2010).

Although not designed as a study of resilience, the High Scope/Perry Preschool study is one of the most notable examples of research on early intervention and prevention in the literature (Barnett, 2000; Schweinhart, Barnes, & Weikart, 1993). This study is noteworthy for several reasons. The study included long-term follow-up of participants from preschool to adulthood, included information about the effects of the preschool program in many developmental domains, and provided sufficient information on program costs to allow a cost-benefit analysis (Barnett, 2000; Schweinhart et al., 1993). This study included 123 participants who were preschoolers at the beginning of the study. The participants were African-American children from low-income families. The children also had low IQ scores, ranging from 70 to 85, based on testing conducted at the beginning of the study. The researchers randomly assigned participants to a preschool program group or a no program control group. The preschool program was relatively intensive with a 2½-hour classroom experience five days per week, and a 1½-hour weekly home visit. The children participated in the preschool program at ages three and four. This longitudinal study included annual data collection from ages 4 through 11, and additional follow up data collection during adolescence through age 27 (Barnett, 2000; Schweinhart et al., 1993).

The researchers documented many benefits for children who participated in the program, compared to those in the control group. The program participants had higher mean IQ scores at age 5, spent significantly less time in special education programs during their school years, had higher high school graduation rates, and were more likely to have some postsecondary education. Program participants had significantly lower rates of juvenile delinquency, and had higher monthly earnings at age 27 (Barnett, 2000; Parks, 2000; Schweinhart et al., 1993). Barnett (2000) noted that the effects of the Perry Preschool program were both immediate and persistent, with positive effects observed from the preschool through adult years. A cost-benefit analysis of the program revealed that a dollar spent on the preschool program for facilities, staff, supplies, and so forth, provided more than eight dollars in benefits over the time of the study. From a public policy viewpoint, the most notable effects were the benefits to society. These included reductions in education costs associated with less need for special education services, increased earnings in adulthood and reduced need for welfare payments, and a substantial decrease in the costs of crime and delinquency (Barnett, 2000; Parks, 2000).

Researchers have generated a considerable body of evidence on resilience and protective factors, and their role in prevention of childhood disorders (Condly, 2006; Winslow et al., 2005; Wright & Masten, 2005). Audiologists and speech-language pathologists would profit from similar research, particularly research like the High Scope/Perry preschool program that demonstrated that our services are cost effective and provide an ultimate benefit to society.

IMPLICATIONS FOR COMMUNICATION SCIENCES AND DISORDERS

The research on resilience and protective factors provides a possible direction for future prevention research in the field of communication disorders. First, many of the populations examined in these studies are populations that speech-language pathologists and audiologists serve, including children with language and learning disabilities (Mather & Ofiesh, 2005), children from economically disadvantaged backgrounds, and children with perinatal complications (Werner, 2000). Additionally, the protective factors identified in resilience research are similar to skills targeted in speech and language intervention, such as children's problem-solving and communication skills, executive functions, and parent-child interactions.

Greenberg (2006, p. 140) noted that the problems children face in today's society are complex and require "interventions at the level of economic and social policy as well as the ability to strengthen the skills of educators, parents, and youth themselves." The fields with the strongest base of prevention research include public health, nursing, psychology, social work, medicine, and child and family development (Merrell, 2010). However, this type of research certainly is relevant for other fields such as education and communication disorders. In designing studies oriented toward prevention and resilience, researchers and clinicians in communication sciences and disorders should consider the following:

1. Studies to investigate causal relationships between resilience interventions and developmental outcomes are vital. Ideally these would be well-designed experimental studies with random assignment to treatment and control groups (Greenberg, 2006; Merrell, 2010). Alternatively, these studies could include random assignment to an enhanced treatment group and a usual treatment control group. The enhanced treatment would have greater emphasis on factors that contribute to resilience, such as parent-child interactions and children's communication and social skills with peers.

2. Well-designed prevention studies include measurement of effects outside the immediate domain of treatment. Speech-language pathologists should determine if their interventions have an impact beyond the areas of speech, language, and communication. These might include measures of school achievement, ability to establish relationships and friendships, success in regular education classrooms, and so forth. Early speech, language, and communication intervention possibly could have the kind of impact into adult life observed in the Perry Preschool Project. However, we lack well-designed intervention studies that document those kinds of broad effects.

3. The best prevention studies have employed longitudinal designs to determine how the effects of intervention change or persist over time. Long-term follow-up is important because individuals must accomplish different developmental tasks at various stages in life (e.g., early childhood, elementary school-age, adolescents, young adult), and the effects of intervention could vary over time.

4. Prevention research is most likely to succeed if researchers and clinicians collaborate in the design and conduct of the studies. Researchers can suggest the types of interventions most likely to have an impact based on current evidence; whereas clinicians have a strong presence in every day environments such as schools, community service agencies, and medical centers. Clinicians could provide insight into the most relevant developmental tasks and facilitate long-term follow up of participants.

5. Researchers should carefully document the costs of any intervention programs they deliver to allow for a cost-benefit analysis. The Perry Preschool Project provided an example of how to document the significant financial benefits of early childhood intervention and prevention programs (Barnett, 2000; Schweinhart et al., 1993). Cost-benefits analyses are important for informing legislative and public policy debates and securing adequate funding for clinical services.

CONCLUSIONS

Professionals in communication sciences and disorders might view the ideal type of prevention research as a highly ambitious undertaking. However, the research literature on resilience and protective factors includes some examples of projects conducted with relatively modest levels of funding (Merrell, 2010), and prevention research could have a substantial impact on the lives of persons who receive audiology and speech-language pathology services.

As they look to the future, resilience researchers note the importance of greater interdisciplinary focus in their research, particularly including perspectives from the fields of genetics and neuroscience (Cicchetti & Blender, 2006; Greenberg, 2006: Werner, 2005). This type of interdisciplinary work should be a future consideration for communication sciences and disorders as well.

REFERENCES

American Speech-Language-Hearing Association. (1991). *Prevention of communication disorders tutorial* [Relevant paper]. Retrieved September 26, 2011, from http://www.asha.org/docs/pdf/RP1991-00211.pdf. doi: 10.1044/policy.RP1991-00211

American Speech-Language-Hearing Association. (2007). *Scope of practice in speech-language pathology* [Scope of practice]. Retrieved September 26, 2011, from http://www.asha.org/policy/type.htm. doi:10.1044/policy.SP2007-00283

Barnett, W. S. (2000). Economics of early childhood intervention. In J. P. Shonkoff & S. J. Meisels (Eds.), *Handbook of early childhood intervention* (2nd ed., pp. 589–610). Cambridge, UK: Cambridge University Press.

Cicchetti, D., & Blender, J. A. (2006). A multiple-levels-of-analysis perspective on resilience: Implications for the developing brain, neural plasticity, and preventive interventions. *Annals of the New York Academy of Sciences, 1094,* 248–258. doi: 10.1196/annals.1376.029

Condly, S. J. (2006). Resilience in children: A review of literature with implications for education. *Urban Education, 41*(3), 211–236. doi: 10.1177/0042085906287902

Goldstein, S., & Brooks, R. B. (2005). Why study resilience. In S. Goldstein, & R. B. Brooks (Eds.), *Handbook of resilience in children* (pp. 3–16). New York, NY: Springer.

Greenberg, M. T. (2006). Promoting resilience in children and youth: Preventive interventions and their interface with neuroscience. *Annals of the New York Academy of Sciences, 1094,* 139–150. doi: 10.1196/annals.1376.013

Klebanov, P., & Brooks-Gunn, J. (2006). Cumulative, human capital, and psychological risk in the context of early intervention: Links with IQ at ages 3, 5, and 8. *Annals of the New York Acad-*

emy of Sciences, 1094, 63–82. doi: 10.1196/annals.1376.007

Luthar, S. S., Cicchetti, D., & Becker, B. (2000). The construct of resilience: A critical evaluation and guidelines for future work. *Child Development, 71*, 543–562. doi: 10.1111/1467-8624.00164

Luthar, S. S., Sawyer, J. A., & Brown, P. J. (2006). Conceptual issues in studies of resilience: Past, present, and future research. *Annals of the New York Academy of Sciences, 1094*, 105–151. doi: 10.1196/annals.1376.009

Masten, A. S. (2001). Ordinary magic: Resilience processes in development. *American Psychologist, 56*(3), 227–238. doi: 10.1037//0003-066X.56.3.227

Masten, A. S., & Powell, J. L. (2003). A resilience framework for research, policy, and practice. In S. S. Luthar (Ed.), *Resilience and vulnerability: Adaptation in the context of childhood adversities* (pp. 1–25). Cambridge, UK: Cambridge University Press.

Mather, N., & Ofiesh, N. (2005). Resilience and the child with learning disabilities. In S. Goldstein & R. B. Brooks (Eds.), *Handbook of resilience in children* (pp. 239–256). New York, NY: Springer.

Merrell, K. W. (2010). Linking prevention science and social and emotional learning: The Oregon resiliency project. *Psychology in the Schools, 47*(1), 55–70. doi: 10.1002/pits.20451

Parks, G. (2000, October). The High/Scope Perry preschool project. *Juvenile Justice Bulletin.* Retrieved September 28, 2011, from https://www.ncjrs.gov/pdffiles1/ojjdp/181725.pdf

Robinson, J. L. (2000). Are there implications for prevention research from studies of resilience? *Child Development, 71*, 570–572.

Rutter, M. (2006). Implications of resilience concepts for scientific understanding. *Annals of the New York Academy of Sciences, 1094*, 1–11. doi: 10.1196/annals.1376.002

Schweinhart, L. J., Barnes, H. V., & Weikart, D. P. (1993). *Significant benefits: The High/Scope Perry preschool study through age 27.* Ypsilanti, MI: High/Scope Press.

Werner, E. E. (1993). Risk, resilience, and recovery: Perspectives from the Kauai Longitudinal Study. *Development and Psychopathology, 5*, 503–515. doi:10.1017/S095457940000612X

Werner, E. E. (2000). Protective factors and individual resilience. In J. P. Shonkoff & S. J. Meisels (Eds.), *Handbook of early childhood intervention* (pp. 115–132). Cambridge, UK: Cambridge University Press.

Werner, E. E. (2005). What can we learn about resilience from large-scale longitudinal studies? In S. Goldstein & R. B. Brooks (Eds.), *Handbook of resilience in children* (pp. 91–106). New York, NY: Springer.

Winslow, E. B., Sandler, I. N., & Wolchik, S. A. (2005). Building resilience in all children. In S. Goldstein & R. B. Brooks (Eds.), *Handbook of resilience in children* (pp. 237–256). New York, NY: Springer.

Wright, M. O., & Masten, A. S. (2005). Resilience processes in development. In S. Goldstein & R. B. Brooks (Eds.), *Handbook of resilience in children* (pp. 17–38). New York, NY: Springer.

ESSAY 8

The Artistry of Practice-Based Evidence (PBE)

One Practitioner's Path—Part I

Wendy Papir-Bernstein

In 1980 when College-Hill Press was established, I was a staff developer for the organization that hired and provided training and supervision to speech therapy professionals in the NYC public schools. College-Hill Press published just about every book I used to develop my training packages. When Dr. Singh founded Singular Publishing in 1990, I was supervising many of the professionals who provided the speech therapy services to students with severe and profound disabilities.

One day I received an advance copy of one of Singular's books, and instantly bonded with this book in a way that I had with none other. I developed a series of workshops for speech supervisors and speech providers that wound up having wide implementation. I now use this text for one of my courses as well, and following Dr. Singh's death decided to contact the author and tell him about the impact that his research and writing had on my professional life.

HOW IT ALL BEGAN

We all have preferences, ways of thinking and patterns of behavior that generate self-comfort, and which dominate our professional lives as well as our personal ones. One of my beliefs is that everything is connected. Information is all around me, and my job is simply to look for, receive, and translate it toward some practical purpose in my life. This "information" comes to us at the most unexpected times, from the most unexpected sources, and crosses over from one field to another. In 1970 my first professional supervisor came back from a theatre arts staff development workshop, and her description of that workshop became my first memorable translational experience. It was at this training session that I learned theater games such as *mirroring* and *vocal symphony*. My job was to figure out how to integrate these techniques with articulatory placements, repetitive production, and bombardment. No one talked about the research; we were imaginative, we were creative, and our enthusiasm sold success.

I continued to use these and other "unusual" activities in my speech therapy program. One day a student looked up at me with a brace-filled smile and in all of his lateral emission glory spurted out, "I don't know what this is, but it's *not* speech therapy." This student grew up to become a world-famous comedic film actor, lisp-less of course. And I was hooked on the glories of implementing research and discovering techniques with demonstrated success from other disciplines.

IN THE EARLY DAYS

Through most of the 1970s, I was the speech-language therapist in a New York City Department of Education school program called School for Language and Hearing-Impaired Children (SLHIC). Many of these students were the original "rubella babies," born of mothers who had contracted German measles in their first trimester of pregnancy. Although rubella and congenital rubella syndrome (CRS) are currently of very low incidence in this country, such was not the case in the early to mid 1970's. In 1964 over 12 million cases of rubella were diagnosed in the U.S., and epidemics were occurring in 6- to 9-year cycles. (Orenstein, 1988) The MMR vaccine (measles, mumps and rubella) was not licensed in the United States until 1971, and it was not until 1989 that a second dose was introduced to school-age children who had not developed immunity after the first dose.

Needless to say, this population was largely underrepresented in research. The same was true for the second population of students I worked with beginning in the early 1980s, now as a speech therapy supervisor — children with Autism Spectrum Disorder (ASD) and/or Pervasive Developmental Disability (PDD). Although in both of these instances, I had access to fascinating populations of low-incidence students, research in these and other areas of our field was sorely lacking and what we now call evidence-based practice (EBP) had not yet been born.

EBP began in the field of medicine during the 1990s, and met with such success in improving services that the procedures became integrated (or translated) into an increasing number of disciplines. The definition most of us are familiar with includes the integration of best research evidence with clinical expertise and patient values. Although these principles are often depicted as the three points on a triangle, the weight or clinical significance of each point changes depending on perspective. For example, universities and clinical training institutions will certainly be emphasizing best research evidence, whereas practitioners working in schools will be citing the importance of clinical expertise and student/caregiver values when making decisions about assessment and intervention approaches.

TRANSLATIONAL RESEARCH

Although research ultimately guides intervention by transforming science into practice, most practitioners perform certain professional activities before they are in vogue or even have a name. At best, professional practices should make sense prior to having become legally mandated or professionally sanctioned as best practices. In much the same way, assessment and intervention practices would hopefully make sense before the research and evidence has been generated.

Translational research (sometimes called outcomes research or clinical research) has evolved over the years as a result of time and practice, and the translational continuum has expanded. The types or phases of translation are usually represented as *T-phases*, and research institutions have described these phases as interacting on a linear as well as circular plane. Woolf (2008) describes why the term itself conjures up different meanings to different professionals. Initially, the term "translational research" was thought of as movement in one direction (from bench to bedside). The newer model expands the number of T-phases from

2 to 4 or sometimes 5, and emphasizes the importance of bi-directionality and overall interaction throughout the phases.

The Clinical Research Roundtable at the Institute of Medicine convened for the first time in June 2000. As a result of those deliberations, two major categories of obstacles or *translational blocks* (Sung et al., 2003) relating to the clinical research environment were identified. The first block impeded the translation of a scientific discovery into a clinical study (T1), and the second impeded the translation of a clinical study into clinical practice and decision making about patient care (T2). At that time, additional challenges were identified, and included enhancing public participation in clinical research, as well as increasing staff development efforts and workforce training (Sung et al., 2003).

In the field of translational research, there is much discussion about the National Institutes of Health (NIH, 2009) Roadmap for Medical Research. This NIH Roadmap initially included these same two transitional steps and two research laboratories, bench (basic science research) and bedside (human clinical research). However, they proposed the addition of one more research laboratory, practice-based research, as an essential link between discoveries at the bench, bedside efficacy, and everyday effectiveness in the clinical arena (Westfall, Mold, & Fagnan, 2007). The additional research laboratory would set the stage for one more translational step, T3 or clinical practice (practice-based research), which is hallmarked by dissemination and implementation of research.

In recent articles about genomic medicine (e.g., Khoury et al., 2007, 2010), a framework for a 4-phase continuum of multidisciplinary translation research was presented. T1 moves a scientific discovery into a health application. T2 moves the health application into evidence-based guidelines. T3 moves the guidelines into health practice

through dissemination and diffusion research. The last phase of translation, T4, would move the health practice into the public sector and continues to remain one of our greatest challenges. In our own field as well, T1 and T2 research studies are more common than T3 and T4 studies. Justice identifies the need for additional studies addressing the issues of diffusion and dissemination, studies that are "truly translational" (Justice, 2010, p. 96).

THE PRACTICE-BASED CONTEXT

The Centers for Disease Control and Prevention (CDC) have defined translational research in public health as it relates to accepted and evidence-based public health interventions. The principal that research is important and needs to be translated is not in dispute, but the remaining questions relate to everyday applications in clinical practice. Cases have been made for the synthesis of evidence from practitioners working in other sectors (such as architects and teachers), input from a wider range of disciplines, and expansion of practice-based applications. (Ogilvie et al., 2009; Westfall, Mold, & Fagnan, 2007)

Although practice-based research networks (PBRNs) have been part of the NIH roadmap vision, they have served largely as a recruitment vehicle for clinical trials, because they provide access to large groups of patients. However, the practice-based context provides another laboratory for data collection via observational studies, surveys, and qualitative analyses. Intervention studies can contribute crucial knowledge that takes us beyond evidence of efficacy.

One of the best explanations about the importance of practice-based arenas is stated by Westfall, Mold, and Fagnan (2007), who refer to the *blue highway*, and the need to increase the use of practice-based research and evidence to better serve the people living on those highways. The blue highway often denotes the back roads on a map, the places where the majority of people live.

In the field of medicine, the blue highway is where most of the health care is delivered, and a far cry from the medical centers and universities where research is funded and takes place. In the field of education, blue highway or practice-based evidence takes place in the schools. The dissemination, implementation, and diffusion of research occur through staff development programs and enhanced clinical practices of the professionals who are both supervising the programs and directly working with the students.

According to the CDC, *dissemination* refers to the spread of knowledge and distribution of the information, resulting in behavioral change. *Implementation* refers to the integration of activities and strategies for adoption within specific settings (such as a community center or school), and *diffusion* refers to the study of factors necessary for successful adoption and use of new practices (NIH, 2009). Dissemination, implementation, and diffusion will be greatly impacted by individual and organizational variables, such as readiness for change, packaging of information, organizational leadership attitudes, and staff resources (Flay, 2005). In addition, before dissemination, implementation, and diffusion of translational research can begin, two factors need to be considered: knowledge management and information design.

KNOWLEDGE MANAGEMENT

Knowledge, in any of its manifestations, is one of the most valuable commodities that we have. The knowledge systems of local communities are sometimes referred to as Indig-

enous Knowledge Systems or IK. IK systems are dynamic, and encompass the skills, experiences, and insights of individual community members, as influenced by internal creativity and experimentation on the part of those individuals. IK contrasts with the knowledge systems generated by universities and research institutions, and yet is often the basis for local level decision-making in agriculture, health care, food preparation, and education. In fact, our Western thought process about the scientific method sometimes results in IK being undervalued, because it lacks scientific validation (Sahai, 1998).

The scientific discipline called Knowledge Management (KM) has existed since the early 1990s and is utilized in fields of public health, information sciences, and business administration. KM efforts lead to successful knowledge creation, dissemination and application, improvement of performance, an increase in innovative thinking, and greater integration of newly learned information (Addicott, McGivern, & Ferlie, 2006). In 1999, the term *personal knowledge management* was introduced, (as distinguished from *organizational knowledge management*), which refers to the management of knowledge at the individual level.

INFORMATION DESIGN

The process of structuring data, presenting information, leading to integrative knowledge and eventual evaluative wisdom is called information design (Shedroff, 2000). The greatest challenge of information design is for the manager or director to build a meaningful experience for the user, and that can only happen if the information is organized, translated /transformed, and presented in a way that gives it meaning. It must make sense.

Information design specialists focus on four areas: data, information, knowledge and wisdom. *Data* are discovered, researched, and gathered. They involve sensory input without much reflection. The problem is that data easily overwhelm us, and most users of information are not terribly interested in seeing the raw data. That is the job of the design specialist: to provide context through meaning.

Although data can be the building blocks of meaning, there is no context aside from a relationship to other bits of data. In isolation, data can float disconnected and meaningless to the user. In order to make sense, data must be connected and contextualized, assume a form, and become converted to information. Their purpose is to change and/or impact someone's perception, behavior, or judgment. *Information* is there to be learned, and learning is a change in behavior due to our experience with information (Ormrod, 1999). The change can be internal or external, but must be observable in some fashion.

Because the amount of information available to us is enormous, information needs to be organized and presented in ways that make sense and can be connected to what is already known. The LATCH principle is one group of strategies that may be used for organizing information (Wurman & Bredford, 1996). The acronym stands for location, alphabet, time, category, and hierarchy.

In addition to using organizational strategies, another role that the information design specialist assumes is to structure the information to facilitate its share-ability. *Share-ability*, a term used in experimental psychology, refers to the extent to which information can be communicated to others (Freyd, 1993). Share-ability is highest when there is little loss of fidelity as information moves from person to person. According to Freyd's research, external or written information has the highest level of share-ability.

EXPLICIT VERSUS TACIT KNOWLEDGE

Some types of knowledge are more easily communicated than others. One type of knowledge framework distinguishes between tacit or personal knowledge and explicit or formal knowledge. Whereas tacit knowledge represents internalized and often unconscious knowledge, explicit knowledge represents information that is consciously held in mental focus, and can be easily communicated to others (Alavi & Leidner 2001). Tacit knowledge, which is difficult to quantify, is thought of as *knowhow*, as opposed to *know-what* (the facts), *know-why* (the science), or *know-who* (the networking).

Explicit knowledge is codified and conveyed through dialogue or some type of written media. Tacit knowledge is deeply personal and consists more of experience, perceptions, insights, and knowhow that can more easily be implied than directly expressed.

Nonaka and Hirotaka (1995) describe the relationship of these two types of knowledge systems: tacit knowledge is communicated best through shared experience, and tacit knowledge is converted to explicit knowledge through the creation of formal models or instructional frameworks. Whereas both explicit and tacit knowledge are valuable to any organization, one of the most vital responsibilities is to protect and enhance the sources of tacit knowledge by creating a culture of knowledge sharing, knowledge exchanges, and knowledge conversion (Nonaka & Hirotaka, 1995).

Wisdom, the final step in the design process, can be thought of as the ultimate level of understanding. It is achieved when we see enough patterns in our knowledge base so that we can synthesize and use the information in novel ways. It is through patterns of information that we are able to make inferences and predictions, and move our thinking from the present to the future. We see what is missing, and wisdom enables us to create something new (Shedroff, 2000). Our ability to self-reflect, evaluate and interpret knowledge leads to personal growth and the acquisition of wisdom. Wisdom, in this sense, implies a larger vision, and the ability to connect holistically that vision with the well-being of the larger community (Allee, 1997).

Allee points out that organizational systems expert Gene Bellinger summarized it beautifully when he drew an analogy to data-information-knowledge-wisdom from the Tao quotation "Find the path, enter the path, travel the path, become the path." We must first find and build on the data, develop the information from the data, isolate the knowledge as we travel through it, and sift through it all as we ultimately model those enduring truths and become the wisdom (Allee, 1997).

The remaining questions to be discussed in Part II (Essay 12) are:

1. How do we identify, generate and share the personal (tacit) and formal (explicit) knowledge systems within our organization? and
2. How do we translate useful information into professional knowledge and finally into clinical wisdom?

REFERENCES

Addicott, R., McGivern, G., & Ferlie, E. (2006). Networks, organizational learning and knowledge management. *Public Money and Management*, 26(2), 87–94.

Alavi, M., Leidner, D. (2001). Review: Knowledge management and knowledge management systems: Conceptual foundations and research issues. *MIS Quarterly*, 25(1), 107–136.

Allee, V. (1997). *The knowledge evolution: Expanding organizational intelligence.* Oxford, UK: Butterworth-Heinemann Press.

Flay, B. R., Biglan, A., Boruch, R. F., Castro, F. G., Gottfredson, D., Kellam, S., . . . Ji, P. (2005). Standards of evidence: criteria for efficacy, effectiveness and dissemination. *Prevention Science*, 6(3), 151–175.

Freyd, J. (1993). Five hunches about perceptual processes and dynamic representations. In D. Meyer & S. Kornblum (Eds.), *Attention and performance XIV: Synergies in experimental psychology, artificial intelligence and cognitive neuroscience.* Cambridge, MA: MIT Press.

Justice, L. (2010). Truly translational research. *American Journal of Speech-Language Pathology*, 19, 95–96.

Khoury, M. J., Gwinn, M., & Ioannidis, J. (2010). The emergence of translational epidemiology: From scientific discovery to population health impact. *American Journal of Epidemiology*, 172, 517–524.

Khoury, M. J., Gwinn, M., Yoon, P. W., et al. (2007). The continuum of translation research in genomic medicine: How can we accelerate the appropriate integration of human genome discoveries into health care and disease prevention? *Genetics in Medicine*, 9, 665–674.

National Institutes of Health. (2009). Translational research. Retrieved July 11, 201 from http://nihroadmap.nih.gov/clinicalresearch/overview-translational.asp

Nonako, I., & Hirotaka, T. (1995). *The knowledge creating company: How Japanese companies create the dynamics of innovation.* Oxford, UK: Oxford University Press.

Ogilvie, D., Craig, P., Griffin, S., Macintyre, S., & Wareham, N. J. (April 28, 2009). A translational framework for public health research. *BMC Public Health*, 9, 116, 1–10.

Orenstein, W., Bart, K., & Hinman, A.(1988). The opportunity and obligation to eliminate rubella from the United States. *Journal of the American Medical Association*, 251(15), 1988–1994.

Ormrod, J. E. (1999). *Human learning* (3rd ed.). Englewood Cliffs, NJ: Prentice-Hall.

Sahai, S. (August, 1998). *Indigenous knowledge is technology: It confers rights on community.* Paper presented at the conference on Gender and Technology in Asia, Bangkok.

Shedroff, N. (2000). Information interaction design: A unified field theory of design. In R. Jacobson (Ed.), *Information design.* Cambridge, MA: MIT Press.

Sung, N., Crowley, W., Genel, M., Salber, P., Sandy, L., Sherwood, L. M., . . . Rimoin, D. (2003). Central challenges facing the national clinical research enterprise. *Journal of the American Medical Association, 289*(10), 1278–1287.

Westfall, J., Mold, J., & Fagnan, L. (2007). Practice-based research: Blue highways on the NIH road map. *Journal of the American Medical Association, 297*(4), 403–406.

Woolf, S. (2008). The meaning of translational research and why it matters. *Journal of the American Medical Association, 299*(2), 211–213.

Wurman, R. S. (1996). *Information architects.* Zurich, Switzerland: Graphic Press Corp.

ESSAY 9

SoCal BRIDGE Collaborative

Across Treatment Disciplines

Karyn Lewis Searcy, Aubyn Stahmer, and Lauren Brookman-Frazee

Although I only had an opportunity to interact with Dr. Singh very briefly, those who knew him well and with whom I have worked since that time have created a colorful and inspirational profile that has touched my life. He died before I completed my contribution to Plural's Here's How series, which recognizes the significance of clinical experience as well as research. Spirits such as his inspires writers to reach beyond the familiar and value instinct, intuition, and perception. Dr. Singh's commitment to nurture new authors and his recognition that clinically driven research is worthy of respect leaves me wishing I had gotten to know him. I am, however, grateful for this opportunity to contribute to a testimony to his endeavors, and share his passion for clinical application of research. My collaboration with research psychologists, Aubyn Stahmer, PhD, and Lauren Brookman-Frazee, PhD, has broadened the scope of my work as an SLP, which reflects Dr. Singh's vision.

—KLS

One of the major challenges facing our field today is the translation of evidence-based practices into clinical care in a manner that is both effective and fits the needs of the children and families with whom we work. Collaboration among stakeholders, including researchers, clinicians, families, and funders is essential to translational efforts, but can be very challenging. In this essay, we discuss theoretical rationales supporting such collaboration, and provide an example of an effective and productive model of working together that has led to improved care for children and families in our community.

TRANSLATIONAL SPEECH-LANGUAGE THERAPY AND COMMUNITY-BASED PARTICIPATORY RESEARCH IN EARLY INTERVENTION

To maximize therapeutic efficacy, scientific research outcomes must be translated into practical and functional application (National Institute of Health, 2011). The time it takes to do this can often be frustrating to therapists who are seldom aware of the time and resources involved in the research process needed before an intervention becomes publicly available. It often takes 10 to 20 years for research findings to be translated reliably into clinical practice (U.S. Department of Health and Human Services Public Health Service, 2001), which is clearly too slow a pace for families involved in early intervention (EI).

Scientists are beginning to recognize the value of translational research, which is a bi-directional exchange of information between researchers and clinicians (National Institute of Health, 2011). This process can expedite the access to functional and evidenced-based interventions for children with developmental delays who need immediate treatment and can improve the research process as well. There has been a call for an exchange of knowledge involving active partnership at all stages of the research-to-practice transfer process between researchers and community stakeholders, including clinicians, parents, and funders (Addis, 2002; Beutler, Williams, Wakefield, & Entwistle, 1995; Wells & Miranda, 2006). This collaborative approach to establishing a research and functional foundation for evidence-based practices (EBP) that values the perspectives, experience, and skills of all participants is particularly relevant to EI speech-language therapists who work closely with parents (Figure 9–1).

With the progressive increase in prevalence of developmental delays (Boyle et al., 2011), including autism spectrum disorders (ASD), techniques that require expensive training have multiplied. Many agencies race to ensure that their therapists are certified in the latest program, some of which have popular marketing and name recognition, but not necessarily a sound empirical basis. It is often difficult to determine when research trumps clinical instinct or, conversely, when commercial hype distorts the value of a truly innovative approach (Searcy, 2012). Therapists struggle

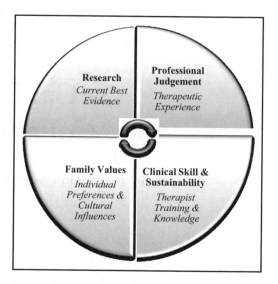

Figure 9–1. Evidence-based practice (EBP).

to find an effective way to integrate empirical data with family, therapeutic values, and experience (Dollaghan, 2004; Guyatt, Meade, Jaeschke, Cook, & Haynes, 2000), as well as interpret the frequently abstract language of the research itself. Ideally, intervention for young children with communication disorders should match empirically based techniques to individual parent-child dynamics and cultural differences, as well as to therapist style, intuition, and experience.

One method of promoting EBPs and maximizing collaboration between researchers-therapists, therapists-therapists, and therapists-parents is through community-based participatory research (CBPR) (Israel, Eng, Schulz, & Parker, 2005), which has the potential to integrate research and practice at all levels of intervention development, and the testing of methodology (Brookman-Frazee, Stahmer, Searcy, Feder, & Reed, in press). CBPR specifically supports efforts to implement evidence-based practices in community-based settings (Jones & Wells, 2007), and values the clinical knowledge of the therapist and the input of families.

THE BRIDGE COLLABORATIVE: AN EARLY INTERVENTION CBPR

The diagnosis of ASD has increased at an astounding rate, due in part to increased access to early intervention, improved screening tools, and heightened community awareness. Therapists working with this unique population have become increasingly aware of the need to identify children at risk as quickly as possible, although eligibility criteria and treatment techniques have not traditionally been clearly defined for infants and very young toddlers.

As the general public becomes more aware of ASD, many speech-language therapists are becoming overwhelmed by the numbers of families with young children entering their practices and considered at-risk for ASD. Very young children, however, are not always found eligible for treatment, with funding agencies struggling to find ways to catalogue their needs. Growing requests for services at local funding agencies, in community service settings, and even in research settings led us to form a group to examine possible models for a community-wide collaboration that would build capacity for preventative interventions appropriate for infants/toddlers at risk for autism and their families in our community.

Composed of more than 15 community members, including parents, providers, researchers, and funding agency representatives, this collaborative began meeting formally in 2007 and continues to meet monthly. In order to enhance visibility and impact in the community we named ourselves the SoCal BRIDGE Collaborative to signify the bridge we were building between research and practice, and to represent our identified early intervention values: **B**ond-**R**egulate-**I**nteract-**D**evelop-**G**uide-**E**ngage). Our mission statement became *"to build a community dedicated to improving the earliest intervention for children with challenges in relating and communicating,"* with a primary objective to bridge the gap between research and practice. The challenges we faced included moving what we knew about ASD from research into the community at a fast enough pace to keep up with the growing numbers of at-risk children, to identifying interventions that effectively addressed the individual needs of families, and to maximizing the use of EBP in the community.

The BRIDGE Collaborative rapidly became a research-community partnership based on the CBPR framework that brought together a transdisciplinary team. In 2009 we received funding from National Institute for Mental Health (NIMH) to select an evidence-based intervention to adapt for implementation in the community for 12- to 24-month-old children at risk for disorders of relating and communicating, such as ASD.

Selecting a Model Program

Our first step was to determine what we were looking for in an intervention (Stahmer et al., 2011 for a complete description of the process) and we achieved consensus on the following elements: parent-implemented; brief/short-term treatment; appealing to many therapists and parents (behavioral/developmental combination); evidence-based for early intervention; practical in terms of community resources and need; and met community values. These elements included a parent-implemented focus, introducing a brief/short-term treatment time lines, appeal to many therapists and parents (behavioral/ developmental combination), a strong evidence-base for early intervention, being practical in terms of community resources and need, and finally that it meet community values.

After reviewing more than 20 programs, the collaborative narrowed the field to three highly respected treatment models. To obtain community input, we hosted three, half-day conferences at which the developer of each approach presented their program to our selected focus groups, as well as to collaborative members and the public.

Focus Groups

The collaborative identified two groups of community members to participate in the final selection: parents who had been through the early intervention system; and providers who worked with early intervention families. Ten participants were selected for each of the two focus groups. They were first asked to develop a list of priorities for an early intervention treatment program, including the strengths and weaknesses of those currently available in our community (Table 9–1).

Table 9–1. Questions to Stakeholders

Valued Components of Early Intervention Programs
1. What factors do you consider when choosing services to provide to children with risk for ASD between ages 12 to 18 months?
2. What are your thoughts on the efficacy of early intervention services specifically for children with risk for ASD between ages 12 to 18 months?
3. How are parents involved/included in services you currently provide to children with risk for ASD ages 12 to 18 months?
4. What do you like about existing early intervention services for children with risk for ASD ages 12 to 18 months?
5. How might existing services be improved?
6. Do you see gaps or limits in current services?
7. What would the "ideal" intervention for children with risk for ASD ages 12 to 18 months and their families look like?

Immediately following each conference, facilitators met separately with both focus groups to obtain feedback on each intervention and collaborative members met the presenters to clarify specific points, including: process and cost for training; flexibility for adaptation; ongoing training options; and available training materials for therapists and for parents.

Final Selection

Analysis of the focus group feedback indicated substantial overlap between parent and provider perspectives (Table 9–2). Both groups believed in the importance of an early start to intervention that should be both individualized and comprehensive. Both stated that interventions must be evidence-based; however, they were more influenced by the intervention presenters' method of presenting evidence than the scientific strength of the evidence given. Parents and providers did have some areas where their focus differed. Parents wanted flexibility in choosing their provider, opportunities to include siblings in the intervention, and more support in understanding and navigating services. Providers wanted comprehensive training, including on-going supervision, and coaching. Analysis of the focus group responses (see Table 9–2) revealed significant overlap between what researchers, parents and providers were looking for in a treatment design (Searcy, 2012; Stahmer et al., 2011).

The collaborative reviewed the community input and the elements previously identified as important in an early intervention program. A specialist in consensus-building helped objectify what was quickly becoming an emotional process: some of us felt strong connections to one program, whereas others were torn between two or all three. Although elements of all three intervention programs were highly respected, our group selected one model as the best fit for our identified

Table 9–2. Values Identified by SoCal BRIDGE Focus Groups

Parents	Providers
Early identification	Earlier the better
Accessible	Accessible
Intervention fits family needs	Family-focused collaborative process
Proactive, engaging provider with background in autism	Experiential training & ongoing support for provider
Efficient	Efficient
Evidence-based	Evidence-based
Parent involvement	Parent/family involvement
Collaborative	Comprehensive
Comprehensive	Support for parents
Parent support	Engaging/Fun
Effective	Play-based
	Individual & group
	Culturally relevant

needs. The process was a little like *American Idol*, with some of us grumbling under our breaths but everyone agreeing in the end that the selection was fair (Searcy, 2012).

Project ImPACT (Improving Parents as Communication Teachers-PI; Ingersoll & Dvortcsak, 2010) was selected, in part because it was recognized as a blended program that teaches families naturalistic developmental and behavioral intervention techniques to increase their child's social and communication skills. Another feature of *PI* was that it included both a therapist manual and a parent manual with specific guidelines for implementation.

Pilot Program

After selecting *PI*, 10 therapists from multiple disciplines at agencies participating in BRIDGE

(at least 4 being speech-language pathologists), were selected for training. BRIDGE members served as supervisors. The pilot study would follow these therapists as they learned the intervention and implemented *PI* with families in the community.

As *PI* was originally designed for older children, training included treatment enhancements developed by BRIDGE members to address those areas identified as unique to our younger population (parent/child relationship; sensory issues; reflective supervision). The process of developing the enhancements required a great deal of cross-discipline collaboration to determine the most important aspects to cover, as well as coordination with the program developer and research team to ensure the integrity of the intervention. In the end, we achieved the art of blending our philosophical approaches, because we actually listened to each other, had a history of working together toward a common goal, and began to recognize the value of our open collaboration (Searcy, 2012).

OUTCOMES TO DATE

Collaborative Outcomes

To ensure that our collaborative is sustainable, we have been careful to monitor our interactions. We assess group process through monthly check-in at meetings and quarterly surveys of members. Thus far, a majority report on partnership process surveys indicated that the amount of trust between BRIDGE members had grown (90%) and our capacity to work together had increased (70%). Ratings of trust, collaborative decision-making, and the value of the research team to community programming are consistently rated positively by over 80% of the members. All members who began with the group have remained active participants, and 100% of agencies have committed to ongoing participation, indicating good sustainability of the collaborative.

Therapist, Child, and Family Outcomes

Eight out of ten therapists met fidelity (indicating that they had implemented the treatment as intended). One did not complete the program because of maternity leave, and the Health Maintenance Organization's therapist data were not available. Ninety percent of the therapists have reported confidence in their use of strategies, liked the materials and format, and would recommend the program.

A total of 13 families have completed intervention. The average age of children at entry is 16 months. Data indicate increases in communication scores on standardized assessments and improvements in parent/child

interaction for 90% of children. Eighty percent of parents met fidelity of implementation criteria by the end of intervention. Families rated the intervention, materials, and therapists very positively. The BRIDGE Collaborative achieved and maintained interdisciplinary, interagency, and research-clinician collaboration. It also provided direct examination of treatment techniques for very young children at risk for communication and social-relating disorders such as autism at a very early age. This parent-implemented intervention is still being used in our community.

NEXT STEPS

The current focus of our research includes examining the longer term sustainability of the BRIDGE collaborative model to implement an evidenced-based program (EBP) for infants and toddlers at-risk for ASD. It is hypothesized that the BRIDGE model can be successfully adopted and replicated in a new community with high acceptability, penetration of collaboration, shared leadership, and shared decision making (Brookman-Frazee et al., in press).

The BRIDGE Collaborative is currently focused on the next step in their program development, including working with new funding agencies, developing improved training methods (including designing a training manual for parents and therapists specific to infants at risk for autism), and expanding to outside new communities.

LESSONS LEARNED

Collaboration among disciplines allows therapists and researchers to speak a universal language, minimize use of jargon, provide a more cohesive and comprehensive program for children, and meet extensive and diverse family needs (Brown, Amwake, Speth, & Scott-Little, 2002; Bruner, 1991). Collaboration with parents maximizes generalization of skills across environments. Collaboration between researchers, funding agencies, parents, and therapists promotes development of more functional programs that can be implemented with greater speed than isolated research allows.

Long-term benefits of collaboration are found in the development of relationships, rather than in the achievement of the goals themselves (Huxham, 2003), and treatment agencies have documented improved clinical skills in their staff after they have participated in research projects. Similarly, clinicians report that these collaborative experiences have provided significant professional enrichment, often more powerfully than attending isolated workshops or continuing education courses. Just as parents are more apt to alter their manner of communication and interaction with their young children when they are directly involved in the treatment process, therapists may more eagerly integrate new techniques when they are integrally involved in the development of those techniques.

REFERENCES

Addis, M. E. (2002). Methods for disseminating research products and increasing evidence-based practice: Promises, obstacles, and future directions. *Clinical Psychology: Science and Practice, 9,* 381–392.

Beutler, L. E., Williams, R. E., Wakefield, P. J., & Entwistle, S. R. (1995). Bridging scientist and practitioner perspectives in clinical psychology. *American Psychology, 50*(12), 984–994.

Boyle, C. A., Boulet, S., Schieve, L. A., Cohen, R. A., Blumberg, S. J., Yeargin-Allsopp, M.,

. . . Kogan, M. D. (2011). Trends in the prevalence of developmental disabilities in U.S. children, 1997–2008. *Pediatrics.* Published online May 23, 2011. doi: 10.1542/peds.2010-2989.

Brookman-Frazee, L., Stahmer, A., Searcy, K., Feder, J., & Reed, S. (in press). Building a research-community collaborative to improve community care for infants and toddlers at-risk for autism spectrum disorders. *Journal of Community Psychology.*

Brown, E. G., Amwake, C., Speth, T., & Scott-Little, C. (2002). The continuity framework: A tool for building home, school, and community partnerships [Electronic version]. *Early Childhood Research and Practice, 4.* Retrieved March 15, 2007, from http://ecrp.uiuc.edu/v4n2/brown.html

Bruner, C. (1991). *Thinking collaboratively: Ten questions and answers to help policy makers improve children's services.* Washington, DC: Education and Human Services Consortium. (ERIC Document Reproduction Service No. ED 338 984).

Dollaghan, C. A. (2004). Taxometric analyses of specific language impairment in 3- and 4-year-old children. *Journal of Speech, Language, and Hearing Research, 47,* 464–475.

Guyatt, G. H., Meade, M. O., Jaeschke, R. J., Cook, D. J., & Haynes, R. B., (2000). Practitioners of evidence based care: Not all clinicians need to appraise evidence from scratch but all need some skills. *British Medical Journal, 320,* 954. doi: 10.1136/bmj.320.7240.954

Huxham, C. (2003). Theorizing collaboration practice. *Public Management Review, 5*(3), 401–423.

Ingersoll, B., & Dvortcsak, A. (2010). *Teaching social communication to children with autism: A practitioner's guide to parent training.* New York, NY: Guilford Press.

Israel, B. A., Eng, E., Schulz, A. J., & Parker, E. A. (Eds.). (2005). *Methods in community-based participatory research for health.* San Francisco, CA: Jossey-Bass.

Jones, L., & Wells, K. (2007). Strategies for academic and clinician engagement in community-participatory partnered research. *Journal of the American Medical Association, 197*(4), 407–410.

National Institute of Health (NIH), Division of Program Coordination, Planning, and Strategic Initiatives. (2011). Translational research. Retrieved from http://commonfund.nih.gov/clinicalresearch/overview-translational.aspx

Searcy, K. L. (2012). *Here's how to do early intervention for speech and language: Empowering parents.* San Diego, CA: Plural.

Stahmer, A. C., Brookman-Frazee, L., Lee, E., Searcy, K. L., & Reed, S. (2011). Parent and multidisciplinary provider perspectives on earliest intervention for children at risk for autism spectrum disorders. *Infants and Young Children, 24*(4), 344–363. doi: 10.1097/IYC.0b013e31822cf700

Wells, K., & Miranda, J. (2006). Promise of interventions and services research: Can it transform practice? *Clinical Psychology: Science and Practice, 13*(1), 99–104.

PART III

Public Health, Education, and Clinical Policy

ESSAY 10

Community and Office-Based ❧ Oral, Head, and Neck Cancer ❧ Screening and Education

Our Role and Responsibilities

Edie Hapner

For many years, I would see Dr. Singh at conferences and meetings as I made my stop at the Singular Publishing, now Plural Publishing booths for a hug and the always heard words, "When are you going to write something for us?" My response was always the same, "When the kids are older; when I finish my PhD; when the voice center is not taking so much of my time." Then during one of my stops by the Plural booth in 2009, my response changed to, "Dr. Singh, it's time." Of course, he wasted no time in having one of his team contact me, sign a contract, and sent me off to develop my first published project. We lost Dr. Singh before I finished the FEES project. That will forever sadden me. But my essay in honor of Dr. Singh and his work to educate the speech-language pathology community, addresses another initiative for speech-language pathologists regarding our roles and responsibilities in increasing awareness of head and neck cancer, and incorporating prevention initiatives into our patient care environments.

The people who make a difference are not the ones with the credentials, but the ones with the concern.

Lucida, 2010

COMMUNITY AND OFFICE-BASED ORAL, HEAD, AND NECK CANCER SCREENING AND EDUCATION: OUR ROLE AND RESPONSIBILITIES

Head and neck cancers are among the fifteen most common cancers according to the National Cancer Institute Cancer Trends Progress Report Update 2009/2010 (National Cancer Institute, 2011), and accounting for 2.8% of all new cancers each year. Head and neck cancers are responsible for $3.2 billion dollars in health care expenditures and approximately 4.4% of all cancer treatment expenditures. Head and neck cancers are more common in men than women (2:1) and usually present after age 60 years. However, younger, nonsmokers under the age of 50 years are the fastest growing population of persons with oral cancer (Schantz & Yu, 2002). Factors identified as posing a risk for the development of oral, head, and neck cancers include tobacco use, HPV, and racial disparities due to cultural practices and lower socioeconomic status. Seventy-five percent of head and neck cancers are related to tobacco use including smokeless tobacco. Cultural practices of reverse smoking (smoking with the burning end of the cigarette in the mouth) in the Hispanic population, and the practice of placing betel nut in the buccal mucosa in the Indian population are related to the increased incidence of head and neck cancers in these groups.

Morbidity and mortality from head and neck cancer has changed little in the past 30 years, despite significant advances in diagnosis (NCI, 2011). Studies confirm that survival rates of head and neck cancer are closely related to the extent of cancer progression and the stage of cancer at diagnosis. Early detection of oral and head and neck cancers does save lives, as described by the multistep carcinogenesis model (Petruzzelli, 2011). The model describes a molecular progression of head and neck cancer from early stages of hyperkeratosis to dysplasia to cancer in situ, and finally progressing to invasive carcinoma as time progresses. This means that early detection of hyperkeratotic lesions may prevent progression of the cells to invasive carcinoma. Yet, the National Guidelines Clearinghouse (NCG), a Web-based guidelines resource for physicians to remain up to date on the use of screening, evaluating, and treating many health conditions, provides no U.S. initiative for screening of oral, head, and neck cancer (Scottish Intercollegiate Guidelines Network, 2006).

FACTORS RELATED TO ADVANCED DIAGNOSES

Lower socioeconomic status, lack of insurance, lack of knowledge in health care providers regarding head and neck cancer, and lack of knowledge in the public including personal risk perceptions and knowledge base regarding head and neck cancer have all been linked to advanced stage diagnoses and higher morbidity and mortality figures in the United States (Hapner, Bauer, & Wise, 2010). Chen, Schrag, Halpern, Stewart, and Ward (2007) examined whether patients without insurance were more likely to present with advanced-stage laryngeal cancer. Results of their study indicated that patients with advanced-stage laryngeal cancer at diagnosis were more likely to be uninsured or covered by Medicaid, as compared with those with private insurance coverage. They found that patients who were African American or from lower socioeconomic areas were more likely to be diagnosed with larger tumors. The conclusion from the study was that individuals lacking insurance or having Medicaid are at greatest risk for presenting with advanced laryngeal cancer. In another study, Chen and Halpern (2007) examined factors that may be predictive of improved survival among a large group of patients with advanced laryngeal cancer. Survival rate was lower among men, African Americans, and those who were uninsured.

In several large surveys of adults in two distinct regions of the United States, over 15% of the respondents had never heard of head and neck/oral cancer and 40% knew very little about it. The most disturbing finding was that only 19% of the respondents reported having an oral exam within the last 12 months (Cruz, Geros, Ostroff, Hay, Kenigsberg, & Franklin, 2002; Tomar & Logan, 2005). A total of 448 nurse practitioners (NP) in the state of Florida, an area with one of the highest oral cancer rates in the country, were surveyed regarding their knowledge of oral cancers and their use of oral cancer screenings for their patients. Only 30% of the respondents thought their knowledge about oral cancer was current and less than 30% of respondents used oral cancer examinations in their clinical practice (Meng, Duncan, Porter, Li, & Tomar, 2007).

White, Chin-Quee, Berg, Wise, and Hapner (2011) surveyed 507 people regarding head and neck cancer risk perception while comparing smokers to nonsmokers. Both smokers and nonsmokers had little worry about their risk of head and neck cancer, little perceived danger of the disease, and limited knowledge of their personal risk of developing head and neck cancer, despite a high prevalence of at-risk behaviors.

SCREENING FOR HEAD AND NECK CANCER

The U.S. Preventive Services Task Force (USPSTF) (2004), a federally funded health care initiative, makes recommendations for preventative medical initiatives and the usefulness of screenings for a variety of health problems. A systematic review of the oral and head and neck cancer literature was conducted to update the USPSTF's 1996 recommendations on oral cancer screenings. Results of the review determined that there were no studies that provided information regarding treatment efficacy of early detection for oral cancer, and there were no studies that indicated that screening for head and neck cancer leads to reduced morbidity and mortality. The USPSTF concluded that there was limited evidence in the literature for determining the efficacy of early detection of head and neck cancer and did not recommend routine screening for these cancers. The problem is not the usefulness of early detection, but that the literature lacks studies to support its use.

Although there are several reports of large scale community-based oral cancer screenings in Japan and other European countries, there are limited reports of community-based

screenings for oral or laryngeal cancer in the United States (Nagao, Warnakulasuriya, Ikeda, Fukano, Fujiwara, & Miyazaki, 2000; Zain, Ikeda, Razak, Axell, Majid, Gupta, & Yaacob, 1997). In one large office-based screening for oral and laryngeal cancer in the United States, 4,911 people underwent screening for head and neck cancer. Although diagnosis of cancer was rare in the screening (less than 3%), over 70% of the participants were sent for further workup due to abnormal findings (Prout, 1987). Hapner and Wise (2011) studied the incidence of abnormal findings in a large-scale community-based screening for head and neck cancer in an at-risk population of NASCAR fans. NASCAR (National Association of Stock Car Auto Racing) is the largest sanctioning body of motorsports in the United States. It has become a popular sport, ranking second only to football. The demographics of NASCAR fans indicate that they are at high risk for head and neck cancers with a significantly higher incidence of smoking and the use of smokeless tobacco. Market research indicates that NASCAR fans smoke at a rate 28% higher than in the general public (Simmons Market Research, 2005). In the Hapner et al. (2011) study, 568 male and female participants, ages 18 to 73 years, were screened for oral and laryngeal cancers during three NASCAR race weekend events. A total of 43% of the screening participants were daily alcohol users; 54% had a history of tobacco smoking, whereas 28% were current smokers; and 13% were current users of smokeless tobacco. The mean years as a smoker was 19.9 years and the mean number of packs of cigarettes smoked per day was 2 ppd. Results of the screenings indicated that 43% of participants with a history of smoking had abnormal findings and were instructed to contact their physician for follow-up. Those individuals who exhibited abnormal findings were significantly older and smoked significantly more packs of cigarettes per day. The only significant predictor of the presence of abnormal findings was tobacco use. Specifically, for every pack of cigarettes smoked per day, an individual was 1.95 times more likely to evidence abnormal findings, even after controlling for alcohol use, family history of cancer, personal history of head and neck cancer, gender, age, and occupation.

PREVENTION, EDUCATION AND THE SPEECH-LANGUAGE PATHOLOGIST

Although the responsibility of prevention, awareness, and education has fallen on the shoulders of otolaryngologists in the past, few people see the otolaryngologist without referral from other healthcare professionals. The lapse in time from initial patient complaint to otolaryngology assessment poses a threat to the early detection and improved survival from head and neck cancer. The reality is that many front line medical professionals have the opportunity to impact the problem of early detection and limited education and awareness of head and neck cancer. By educating themselves on the risks, signs, and symptoms of this cancer, and by implementing simple visual oral examinations and adding case history taking questions that might identify the presence of concerning findings and the need for immediate otolaryngology follow-up, speech-language pathologists have the opportunity to impact the survival rates from this cancer.

Although speech-language pathologists do not diagnose head and neck cancers, they are the providers of treatment for the communication and swallowing disorders that accompany head and neck cancer. The simple fact is that head and neck cancers, whether surgically treated or medically treated with radia-

tion, result in disorders of communication and swallowing (Riegers, Zalmanowitz, & Wolfaardt, 2006). Consistent with the American Speech-Language-Hearing Association's (ASHA) core principles of the prevention of communication disorders, it is incumbent on speech-language pathologists to participate in programs to prevent communication disorders. ASHA writes:

> The American Speech-Language-Hearing Association (ASHA) has long accepted the prevention of communication disorders as one of the profession's primary responsibilities. Article II of the ASHA Bylaws states that one of the " . . . purposes of this organization shall be to . . . promote investigation and prevention of disorders of human communication." (ASHA, 1988)

ASHA directs speech-language pathologists to: (1) play a significant role in the development and application of prevention strategies, and (2) educate colleagues and the general public relative to personal wellness strategies as they relate to the prevention of communication disorders. Lubinski and Golper (2007), in their book on professional issues in speech-language pathology, direct the speech-language pathologist that it is their professional obligation to educate the public, promote healthy lifestyles, and develop community outreach for dissemination of this information to prevent communication disorders.

Speech-language pathologists routinely examine the oral cavity and the laryngeal cavity for the assessment of speech/voice/resonance and swallowing disorders. It is incumbent on the speech-language pathologist to be familiar with the normal and abnormal structure and function of the areas examined. It is also incumbent on the speech-language pathologist to know when structure and function is abnormal and requires medical attention in place or in addition to therapeutic management. Oral, pharyngeal, nasopharyngeal, and laryngeal lesions or functional impairments should be examined by a qualified physician in a timely fashion and the speech-language pathologist is in the perfect position to educate the patient/client on the immediate need for medical follow-up and to assist with the seamless transition to the physician. Educating oneself on the use of a visual oral examination for the presence of oral pathologies, developing the insight into swallowing complaints that may signal the presence of a tumor, and knowing the risks and signs of laryngeal cancers allows the speech-language pathologist to be a front-line health care provider actively engaged in the battle against head and neck cancer and the resulting speech and swallowing disorders.

The following resources will be helpful for the speech-language pathologist to utilize in implementing a head and neck cancer prevention and awareness program:

1. An oral cancer screening tool with pictorial directives that can also be copied and given to the patient for monthly self-examinations can be found at: http://www.mouthandthroatcancer.org, from the nonprofit organization Voices of Hope.
2. Beyond assessing for swallowing function only during FEES examinations: Training and Interpretation of FEES in Adults: Plural Publishing Group: http://www.pluralpublishing.com/publication_tif.htm
3. Interpretation of videostroboscopy:
   a. Videostroboscopy Manual: Rating Laryngeal Videostroboscopy and CAPEV Normal and Pathologic Samples: https://pluralpublishing.com/publication_rlvc.htm
   b. ASHA CEU product: Interpretation of Videostroboscopy: http://www.emoryvoicecenter.org

REFERENCES

American Speech-Language-Hearing Association. (1988). *Prevention of communication disorders* [Position statement]. p.1. Available from http://www.asha.org/policy. doi: 10.1044/policy.PS 1988-00228.

Chen, A. Y., & Halpern, M. (2007). Factors predictive of survival in advanced laryngeal cancer. *Archives of Otolaryngology-Head and Neck Surgery, 133*(12), 1270–1276.

Chen, A. Y., Schrag, N. M., Halpern, M., Stewart, A., & Ward, E. M. (2007). Health insurance and stage at diagnosis of laryngeal cancer: Does insurance type predict stage at diagnosis? *Archives of Otolaryngology-Head and Neck Surgery, 133*(8), 784–790.

Cruz, G. D., Geros, L., Ostroff, J. S., Hay, H. L, Kenigsberg, H., & Franklin, D. H. (2002). Oral cancer knowledge, risk factors, and characteristics of subjects in a large oral cancer screening program. *Journal of the American Dental Association, 133*(8), 1064–1071.

Hapner, E. R., Bauer, K. B., & Wise J. C. (2011). The impact of a community-based oral, head and neck cancer screening for reducing tobacco consumption. *Otolaryngology-Head and Neck Surgery.* Published online before print July 21, 2011. doi: 10.1177/0194599811415804

Hapner, E. R., & Wise, J. C. (2011). Results of large scale head and neck cancer screenings of NASCAR fans. *Journal of Voice, 25*(4), 480–483.

Lubinski, R., & Golper, L. A. (2007). Professional issues: From roots to reality. In R. Lubinski, L. A. Golper, & C. Frattali (Eds.), *Professional issues in speech-language pathology and audiology* (pp. 29–31). New York, NY: Thompson Delmar Learning.

Lucida, M. (2010). It's time for some heartwork. In D. Zadora (Ed.), *The heart of a volunteer* (p. 5). Seattle, WA: Compendium.

Meng, X., Duncan, R. P., Porter, C. K., Li, Q., & Tomar, S. (2007). Florida nurse practitioners' attitudes and practices regarding oral cancer prevention and early detection. *Journal of the American Academy of Nurse Practitioners, 19*(12), 668–675.

Nagao, T., Warnakulasuriya, S., Ikeda, N., Fukano, H., Fujiwara, K., & Miyazaki, H. (2000). Oral cancer screening as an integral part of general health screening in Tokoname City. *Journal of Medical Screening, 7*(4), 203–238.

National Cancer Institute. *Cancer trends progress report, 2009/2010 update*. Retrieved October 3, 2011, from http://progressreport.cancer.gov/

National Cancer Institute. *Surveillance epidemiology and end results: Cancer of the oral cavity and pharynx*. Updated 2008. Retrieved May 23, 2011, from http://seer.cancer.gov/statfacts/html/oralcav.html

Petruzzelli, G. *Epidemiology, etiology, pathogenesis, and staging adult head and neck tumors*. Retrieved October 5, 2011, from http://www.plasticsurgery.hyperguides.com/logreg/login.asp

Prout, M. (1987). Early detection of head and neck cancer. *Hospital Practice, 30*(22), 111–112, 114, 118.

Riegers, J. M., Zalmanowitz, J. G., & Wolfaardt, J. F.(2006) Functional outcomes after organ preservation treatment in head and neck cancer: A critical review of the literature. *International Journal of Oral Maxillo Facial Surgery, 3*(7), 581–587.

Schantz, S. P., &Yu, G. P. (2002). Head and neck incidence trends in young Americans, 1973–1997, with a special analysis for tongue cancer. *Otolaryngology-Head and Neck Surgery, 128*, 268–274.

Scottish Intercollegiate Guidelines Network (SIGN). (2006). *Diagnosis and management of head and neck cancer. A national clinical guideline.* Edinburgh (Scotland). Retrieved October 5, 2011, from http://www.guideline.gov/content.aspx?id=10043

Simmons Market Research. (2005). *What are the demographics for NASCAR fans?* Retrieved January 10, 2011, from http://answers.google.com/answers/threadview?id=476206

Tomar, S. L., & Logan, H. L. (2005). Florida adults' cancer knowledge and examination experience. *Journal of Public Health Dentistry, 65*(4), 221–230.

U.S. Preventive Services Task Force (USPSTF). (2004, February 4). *Screening for oral cancer: Recommendation statement.* Rockville (MD): Agency for Healthcare Research and Quality (AHRQ).

White, L. J., Chin-Quee, A., Berg, C., Wise, J. C., & Hapner, E. R. (2011). Differences in head and neck cancer risk perception between smoking and non-smoking NASCAR attendees. *Otolaryngology-Head and Neck Surgery, 145*(2 Suppl.), 63–64. doi: 10.1177/0194599811416318a74

Zain, R. B., Ikeda, N., Razak, I., Axell, T., Majid, Z. A., Gupta, P. C., & Yaacob, M. (1997). A national epidemiological survey of oral mucosal lesions in Malaysia. *Community Dental Oral Epidemiology, 25*(5), 377–383.

ESSAY 11

Fostering Patient Compliance by ❧ Nurturing Clinical Expertise in ❧ Graduate School

Alison Behrman

I had the honor of writing a textbook and co-editing a volume of therapeutic techniques under Dr. Singh's guidance. Each project presented unique challenges and opportunities for professional growth. Dr. Singh was sensitive to and perceptive of the scholarly needs of the academic and clinical communities. And he was equally attuned to the needs of his authors. I will always remember with gratitude his encouragement, support, and guidance.

CLIENT ADHERENCE TO SPEECH-LANGUAGE THERAPY

Client adherence, an individual's willingness and ability to comply with clinical advice (Murphy & Coster, 1997), is an important, yet underaddressed topic in our field. Nonadherence is a multidimensional and ubiquitous problem that can make good therapy ineffective. Clinical experience and some limited research suggest that, for any communication disorder, many therapy techniques have the potential to yield positive outcome, and that it is the client's ability to adhere to the therapy that most strongly predicts success (Behrman, Rutledge, Hembree, & Sheridan, 2008; Zinn, 2008). Therefore, teaching students in speech-language pathology how to facilitate client adherence is as important as teaching them any single therapeutic approach. Yet, we largely ignore the issue of adherence in our graduate school curricula.

As academicians, clinical supervisors, and mentors, our first step is to help our students to accept the majority of the responsibility for adherence. Instead of labeling the client as nonadherent, we must teach our students to ask, "What can I do differently to help this client to adhere with therapy and achieve therapeutic success?" Learning how to answer that question, and to act on the answer, is part of the gradual process of acquiring clinical expertise. In this essay, I explore the definition of clinical expertise and its relationship to adherence, and offer a few suggestions for nurturing the clinical expertise learning process in graduate students of speech-language pathology.

CLINICAL COMPETENCE AND EXPERTISE

Our ASHA certification is one of clinical *competence*, not expertise. Graduate school practicum hours, followed by the clinical first year, provide students and novice therapists with the knowledge and experience to be competent in their therapies. Common wisdom tells us that clinical expertise, encompassing both advanced knowledge and skills, comes only with practice and experience, counted in years and, often, in specialization.

The traditional attitude in our field is that one must first learn the basic craft of speech-language therapy; that expertise can only begin to develop after competency has been achieved. Buried within this notion of clinical expertise are a number of assumptions. One assumption is that expertise cannot be taught: that somehow, it is a spontaneous process resistant to being rushed. Second, the acquisition of expertise is an inherent characteristic of the therapist. An individual is either naturally talented, or not so much. And, finally, the assumption is made that basic competency and expertise are separate learning processes acquired sequentially.

These assumptions are overstatements, each having aspects of both truth and falsehood. The premise of this essay is that, although acquiring basic knowledge toward clinical competency, students and novice therapists can and should be learning skills that would allow them to optimize their exposure to the *clinical expertise learning process*.

THE RELATIONSHIP BETWEEN CLINICAL EXPERTISE AND PATIENT COMPLIANCE

Expertise is multifaceted. It is part of the foundation of evidence-based practice (EBP). The classic definition of EBP is, in part, a process of "*integrating individual clinical expertise* (my emphasis) with the best available external clinical evidence from systematic research" (Sackett, Rosenberg, Muir Gray, Haynes, & Richardson, 1996). Dollaghan (2007) makes the point well: EBP does not deny the validity of clinical experience, for without expertise in the application of external data, the evidence is of limited value.

Expertise gives us the ability to interpret and apply research data and experiential knowledge in a meaningful way that produces the desired therapeutic outcome for a specific client. It is manifested in the client-clinician interaction, which defines the nature of the therapy and, therefore, the patient's ability to adhere to the therapy (Kelham, Shaw, & Myners, 2006).

Expertise is also willingness to set aside the myth of our certainty of what is correct. In fact, a client's poor adherence may be a sign that the therapist is making the wrong decisions. Expertise is listening to what our clients have to tell us through their words and actions, including inactions (nonadherence), and to adapt our behaviors accordingly. Willingness to question one's own certainty, that we may serve our clients best by changing what we do, opens doors wide to clinical growth. Expertise must also include flexibility: the ability to revise a hypothesis, revisit the decision-making process, consider novel evidence from heretofore unexplored sources, and abandon or amend what is not working. Flexibility demands imagination in the ability to see different possible solutions (divergent thinking) and use of the information from diverse sources to solve clinical problems (convergent thinking). Clinical expertise is closely related to creativity and innovation, the ability to produce ideas, approaches, or actions applied to a specific context (Sternberg, 2005), in our case, applied to the clinical decision-making process to facilitate client adherence.

SEARCHING FOR THE NEUROBIOLOGY OF EXPERTISE

Expertise can appear to be magical, but it is not magic. It is the product of neurological activity. By studying the neurobiology of the skills that comprise expertise, we might better understand how and what to teach students to optimize their learning process. For this essay I have chosen to look briefly at the neurologic control of creativity, in part, because creativity, in all likelihood, plays a significant role in clinical expertise. In many respects, speech-language therapy is a creative enterprise between client and clinician.

In addition, common experimental tasks used in neurological research on creativity, divergent thinking, artistic and musical, and insight (Dietrich & Kanso, 2010), have some relevance to the clinical process. Divergent thinking has a long history of being considered a process that requires creative thinking (Guilford, 1950). We use divergent thinking in the therapy process when we consider many possible behavioral goals and techniques to achieve a long-term goal. Artistic and musical tasks have been explored in mental health counseling (Autry & Walker, 2011; Gladding, 2008), where the creative process can facilitate a deeper sense of self, and where that self-reflection is important in client-clinician rapport. The third common task used in experimentation of creativity is insight. Clinical expertise appears to offer us insights into our client's problems that influence our decision-making process.

Across all of these tasks, research data challenge the popular notion of right-hemisphere dominance for creativity. Many studies using electroencephalography demonstrate no cerebral dominance for divergent thinking tasks (Danko, Shemyakina, Nagornova, & Starchenko, 2009), insight tasks (Aziz-Zadeh, Kaplan, & Iacoboni, 2009), or artistic "thought" tasks such as mentally visualizing paintings or composing music or actually looking at a painting (Bhattacharya & Petsche, 2005; Petsche, Kaplan, von Stein, & Filz, 1997). Brain imaging studies (such as fMRI and PET) also demonstrate no laterality for divergent thinking (Fink et al. 2009; Gibson, Folley, & Park, 2009; Moore et al. 2009), artistic activities, such as playing improvisational jazz (Limb & Braun, 2008), and insight (Aziz-Zadeh et al., 2009).

The frontal lobe plays a prominent role in many of these experimental tasks, demonstrating activation particularly in the prefrontal cortex in brain imaging studies during activities that require significant mental concentration in novel tasks, including certain artistic activities, (Berkowitz & Ansari, 2008; Dietrich, 2004) and insightful problem solving (Aziz-Zadeh et al., 2009). In contrast, another study of a more intuitive, spontaneous task, jazz improvization (Limb & Braun, 2008), reveals increased activation of temporoparietal areas.

An all-encompassing neurobiological-theoretical framework for creativity does not exist. However, the evidence does suggest that creativity is not a single, uniform construct, but rather a number of different types of cognitive processes, such that creativity as an attribute cannot be localized to one specific area or set of related areas of the brain (Fink et al., 2009; Petsche, Kaplan, von Stein, & Filz, 1997). Creativity is a multidimensional phenomenon of cognition and emotion that is a product of diverse mental processes (Berkowitz & Ansari, 2008) and multiple phases (Fink et al., 2009). The interconnectivity between various brain areas during different phases of problem-solving may be one of the major processes of creative thinking (Sternberg, 2005).

NURTURING CLINICAL EXPERTISE IN ACADEMIA

If "no single brain area is necessary or sufficient for creativity or any of its component stages" (Dietrich & Kanso, 2010, p. 838), then let's take a mental leap, admittedly based on a slim body of data, and make two suppositions. First, no individual novice therapist can claim to be insufficiently creative to achieve the expertise necessary to facilitate client adherence. Every student should benefit, to some extent, from practicing skills that will enhance their ability to learn from their clinical experiences to facilitate adherence. Second, training students to draw upon a variety of creative abilities may help them to establish problem-solving skills that can be accessed to increase therapy success.

Following are suggestions for promoting the development of skills that may facilitate the clinical expertise learning process. Some suggestions are fully developed activities, each of which is framed to address a client's struggle with adherence. Other suggestions are listed briefly and the reader is encouraged to be creative in developing tasks. In all instances, students should engage in discussion about their experiences after completing an activity, and then relate what they learned to the adherence problem provided to them.

EXPLORE THE MULTIPLE STAGES OF THE CREATIVE PROCESS

Students work on a project that requires them to increase their explicit awareness (meta-awareness) of how they experience creativity. Adherence Problem: A client attends therapy inconsistently and complains that the sessions are boring. Task: The students are assigned a behavioral goal and must develop three different types of activities. (Alternatively, more advanced students can be given a case study and told to develop three activities appropriate for a behavioral goal that they also develop.) Each week, the students work on only one stage of the process and keep a daily journal of their progress through each respective stage. In the first week, they can only contemplate the three activities. In the second week, they may only conduct "field research" in diverse venues or contexts for inspiration, such as going to a toy store, a museum, or interviewing people. In the third week, the students construct their activities. The instructor must emphasize to the students that the journal entries that reflect their experiences are far more important than the final products.

TAKE AN INTROSPECTIVE JOURNEY TO EXPLORE ONE'S OWN PERSPECTIVES

Self-reflection, particularly in creative tasks, has been used in medical and health-related fields (Autry & Walker, 2011; Gladding, 2008; Rakel & Hedgecock, 2008) as a tool for strengthening an individual's ability to build strong clinical relationships. Adherence Problem: A client is not practicing exercises at home, and, as a result, is not making progress in therapy. Task: Students identify two different examples in which they, themselves, were nonadherent. They must identify as many factors as possible that caused their lack of adherence. Next, in pairs, each student reads the other's list of factors, and challenges the partner to go deeper. For example, students rank the major factors in their own list by importance, and play "devil's advocate" to help each other build a persuasive argument about the validity of each factor.

WALK IN THE CLIENT'S SHOES

Teach students to work hard to understand the current reality of their clients. This skill is necessary for client-centered therapy, a nonjudgmental, nondirective approach. Adherence Problem: A client is not practicing exercises at home, and, as a result, is not making progress in therapy. Task: Students are instructed to identify a situation (previous or current) in their own lives in which they tried to persuade someone to do something. (Example: A student wants to convince her parents to pay for a trip to Europe for a summer vacation.) Each student must create a detailed list of factors that would impede her from being successful in her argument: in other words, all of the reasons why the listener would say "No." A second list must then be created of all the factors that would help her reach her goal: all of the reasons why the listener would say "Yes." Next, in pairs, each student listens to the other's persuasive goal and list of positive and negative factors, and helps her partner develop additional items for each list. Finally, each student frames a persuasive argument based on the revised list of the listener's current reality. In this way, students are encouraged to think deeply about their listeners' assumptions, opinions, and fears that might factor into decision-making, and to modify their argument to account for the listener's point of view.

EXPLORE NEW IDEAS

Bernstein Ratner (2011) makes the point that openness to new ideas is connected strongly to exposure to new ideas. Projects that require students to move outside of their usual areas of interest may help encourage them to be more willing to do so in the future. Adherence Problem: A pediatric client does not partici-

pate well in therapy sessions, and the parents don't appear to understand the need to reinforce appropriate behavior and to participate in homework exercises. Task: Students explore literature in another field (psychotherapy or pediatric medicine, for example) to find possible solutions.

And Briefly

Foster self-efficacy to help students believe that they have the ability to be creative. Students find a photograph, drawing or piece of music that reflects how they feel at a given moment. They must explain the connection between the artwork and their feelings. Alternatively, students select an object (or are assigned one) and must create a novel use for it. It may be helpful, first, to assign students a video on creativity to view for inspiration. Many options can be found, at the time of this writing, at TED videos (http://www.ted.com/).

Help students learn to tolerate uncertainty and ambiguity, so that they may develop solutions when the problem is not clearly defined. Group students into teams, and give each team a problem situation in which they must develop one or more solutions. Provide incomplete information about the situation, so that the teams must guess or make assumptions about the missing information.

Help students recognize their own hidden assumptions. Provide students with a list of brief problem situations and ask them to provide quick solutions, together with the assumptions that they make in the problem-solving process. The focus is not on providing the correct answer, but on explaining the thought process that went into the answer. Follow up with discussion about the differences in assumptions among the students.

Foster generation of ideas without judgment. Help students learn that if an idea is thrown out too quickly, its potential to evolve into a great solution may be lost. Divide students into teams and present each team with a complex problem. Students must generate as many solutions as possible, no matter how outrageous and impractical, with no judgments made. Then, each team must choose five solutions and find ways to make them workable.

Assign a brief creative task each week. Students must do an activity that is new for them, and then report on the experience.

Assign a video of a therapy session for students to watch (either a successful session or one in which the client was resistant to participating or struggled with the tasks). Then, in pairs, they take on the client-clinician roles, first imitating what they saw, then recreating the session with a novel story.

LOOKING FORWARD

The skills with which the therapist manages the problem of client adherence are the very skills that comprise clinical expertise. The learning process of clinical competency and expertise is not sequential at all, but asynchronously simultaneous. As we develop expertise in some areas, we learn new skills and implement them as novices in other areas. Future neurobehavioral research will help us to understand better the organization and control of clinical expertise. With that information, we may be better equipped to know what types of activities to incorporate into our training programs. In the meantime, we must forge ahead somewhat blindly to find ways to nurture the clinical expertise learning process as it relates to client adherence in speech-language pathology.

REFERENCES

Autry, L. L., & Walker, M. E. (2011). *Journal of Creativity in Mental Health, 6*, 42–55. doi: 10.1080/15401383.2011.560076

Aziz-Zadeh, L., Kaplan, J., & Iacoboni, M. (2009). "Aha!": The neural correlates of verbal insight solutions. *Human Brain Mapping, 30*, 908–916. doi: 10.1016/j.cortex.2009.06.006

Behrman, A., Rutledge, J., Hembree, A., & Sheridan, S. (2008). Vocal hygiene education, voice production therapy, and the role of patient adherence: A treatment effectiveness study in women with phonotrauma. *Journal of Speech, Language, Hearing Research, 51*, 350–366. doi: 10.1044/1092-4388(2008/026)

Berkowitz, A., & Ansari, D. (2008). Generation of novel motor sequences: The neural correlates of musical improvisation. *NeuroImage, 41*, 535–543. doi: 10.1016/j.neuroimage.2008.02.028

Bernstein Ratner, N. (2011). Some pragmatic tips for dealing with clinical uncertainty. *Language, Speech, and Hearing Services in Schools, 42*, 77–80. doi: 10.1044/0161-1461(2009/09-0033)

Bhattacharya, J., & Petsche, H. (2005). Drawing on mind's canvas: Differences in cortical integration patterns between artists and non-artists. *Human Brain Mapping, 26*, 1–14. doi: 10.1002/hbm.20104

Danko, S., Shemyakina, N. V., Nagornova, Z. V., & Starchenko, M. (2009). Comparison of the effects of the subjective complexity and verbal creativity on the EEG spectral power parameters. *Human Physiology, 35*, 381–383. doi: 10.1134/S0362119709030153

Dietrich, A. (2004). The cognitive neuroscience of creativity. *Psychonomic Bulletin and Review, 11*, 1011–1026. Retrieved from http://pbr.psychonomic-journals.org.

Dietrich, A., & Kanso, R. (2010). A review of EEG, ERP, and neuroimaging studies of creativity and insight. *Psychological Bulletin, 136*, 822–848. doi: 10.1037/a0019749

Dollaghan, C. (2007). *The handbook for evidence-based practice in communication disorders.* Baltimore, MD: Brookes.

Fink, A., Grabner, R., Benedek, M., Reishofer, G., Hauswirth, V., Fally, M., . . . Neubauer, A. C. (2009). The creative brain: Investigation of brain activity during creative problem solving by means of EEG and FMRI. *Human Brain Mapping, 30*, 734–748. doi: 10.1002/hbm.20538

Gibson, C., Folley, B. S., & Park, S. (2009). Enhanced divergent thinking and creativity in musicians: A behavioral and near-infrared spectroscopy study. *Brain and Cognition, 69,* 162–169. doi: 10.1016/j.bandc.2008.07.009

Gladding, S. T. (2008). The impact of creativity in counseling. *Journal of Creativity in Mental Health, 3,* 97–104. doi:10.1080/1540138080 2226679

Guilford, J. P. (1950). Creativity. *American Psychologist, 5,* 444–454. doi: 10.1037/h0063487

Kelham, C., Shaw, J., & Myners, G. (2006). No quick fix: Shared decision-making and tailored patient support as the route to more effective medicine-taking. In M. Davies & F. Kermani (Eds.), *Patient compliance: Sweeting the pill* (pp. 179–196). Hamphsire, UK: Gower.

Limb, C., & Braun, A. (2008). Neural substrates of spontaneous musical performance: An fMRI study of jazz improvisation. *PLoS ONE, 3,* e1679. doi: 10.1371/journal.pone.0001679

Moore, D. W., Bhadelia, R. A., Billings, R. L., Fulwiler, C., Heilman, K. M., Rood, K. M. J., & Gansler, D.A. (2009). Hemispheric connectivity and the visual-spatial divergent-thinking component of creativity. *Brain and Cognition, 70,* 267–272. doi: 10.1016/j.bandc.2009.02.011

Murphy, J., & Coster, G. (1997). Issues in patient compliance. *Drugs, 54,* 797–800. doi: 10.2165/00003495-199754060-00002

Petsche, H., Kaplan, S., von Stein, A., & Filz, O. (1997). The possible meaning of the upper and lower alpha and frequency ranges for cognitive and creative tasks. *International Journal of Psychophysiology, 26,* 77–97. doi: 10.1016/S0167-8760(97)00757-5

Rakel, D. P., & Hedgecock, J. (2008). Healing the healer: A tool to encourage student reflection towards health. *Medical Teacher, 30,* 633–635. doi: 10.1080/01421590802220675 4

Sackett, D., Rosenberg, W., Muir Gray, J., Haynes, R., & Richardson, W. (1996). Evidence based medicine: What it is and what it isn't. *British Medical Journal, 312,* 71–72. Retrieved from http://cebm.jr2.ox.ac.uk/ebmisisnt.html

Sternberg, R. J. (2005). *Handbook of creativity.* New York, NY: Cambridge University Press.

Zinn, S. (2008). Patient adherence in rehabilitation. In H. Bosworth & E. Oddone (Eds.), *Patient treatment adherence: Concepts, interventions, and measurement* (pp. 195–238). Mahwah, NJ: Lawrence Erlbaum.

ESSAY 12

The Artistry of Practice-Based Evidence (PBE)

One Practitioner's Path—Part II

Wendy Papir-Bernstein

Translational research is well underway in our field; however, questions and challenges continue to pervade our efforts with T3 and T4 phases of the translational continuum (dissemination, implementation and diffusion of research). These translational research phases ultimately effect changes in professional beliefs, behaviors and practices.

In Part I (Essay 8), *knowledge management* and *information design* were introduced as two factors that influence knowledge dissemination within the "blue highway" of practice-based educational programs, where most of our children learn (Westfall, Mold & Fagnan, 2007). On these blue highways, the learning context becomes the laboratory and staff development and supervision become the tools that facilitate research dissemination, implementation, and diffusion.

THE SCHOLARSHIP OF TEACHING AND LEARNING (SoTL)

In light of recent evidence about the scholarship of teaching and learning (SoTL), the value and credibility of what is sometimes called "pedagogical scholarship" is now very much on our professional radar screens. It is defined as scholarly work about teaching and learning, published within fields *other than* education (Weimer, 2011). SoTL is based on both scholarly research and reports of practice-based experience, generated by and relevant to cross-discipline communities of professionals, which by definition occupies a seat in the translational arena.

SoTL research seeks to lessen the divide between research and practice by describing functional applications, and to enhance learning practices through process analysis and self-reflection (McKinney, 2007). For example, much of the current SoTL investigations relate to the spheres of higher education, college classrooms, and enhancement of student learning (Bowen, 2010; Boyer, 1990). However, the science of teaching and learning extends far beyond the academic setting. Many of the same tools identified and utilized in clinical and educational training programs may be applied to lifelong learning.

Weimer identifies one category of pedagogical scholarship as *wisdom of practice* or experience-based scholarship, which refers to published work based on professional experience. Such experience may include: personal accounts of change resulting from the implementation of new instructional practices or policies; recommended practices reports; and personal narratives, reflecting opinions and concerns (Weimer, 2011).

THE PRACTICE-BASED EDUCATIONAL ARENA

A translational school-based speech/language therapy program is a practice-based educational arena. As such, it becomes the ideal platform for the identification, dissemination, and integration of new knowledge to take place. In order for that to happen, application vehicles need to exist for the purpose of transferring knowledge to practice, increasing accessibility through information dissemination, helping professionals develop into active recipients of new knowledge, and developing strategies that will ultimately benefit students. Staff development is one application vehicle, the success of which is influenced by individual and organizational variables such as attitudes about leadership, learning, and commitment (Westfall, Mold, & Fagnan, 2007).

This essay describes one practitioner's path, using differentiated systems of supervision and professional development as the tools for change. As a result, a training approach was developed that modeled reflective practices, self-directive supervision, and ongoing self-assessment.

THE LEARNING ORGANIZATION

The creation of a learning organization begins by fostering a climate that allows personal mastery to be valued as well as practiced, and then reframing our definition of *accountability* (Senge, 1990). Senge popularized the concept of learning organizations as structures within which both individual and collective learning can take place. A learning organization encourages people to develop personal mastery through commitment to the development of a personal vision. Most often, what passes for commitment is simply organizational compliance. Commitment, however, refers to the state of feeling fully responsible for making a vision happen, and the creation of structures to support it (Papir-Bernstein, 2001; Senge, 1990).

In most bureaucratic settings, when people express feelings about accountability within the larger organization, they often view their individual responsibilities in isolation (Connors, Smith, & Hickman, 1994). Responsibilities tend to fall through the cracks if they fall outside the boundaries drawn around independent aspects of their job and the job of others. However, when we view our accountability as something larger, we are more apt to take responsibility for what lies beyond the literal interpretation of job descriptions.

These more expansive views prompt us to consider the effectiveness of speech therapy programs from the perspective of the larger school organization. Schools have been described as *complex host environments* that can potentially impact our work with the students in a variety of ways (Schmitt & Justice, 2011). Peer influence and teacher self-efficacy (feelings about effectiveness) are two variables that impact our intervention. Schmitt and Justice (2011) suggest using strategies that maximize the quality of the school environments, such as becoming an integral part of school committees and increasing awareness of our own self-efficacy related to student outcomes.

The importance of adopting this expanded view of commitment and accountability is supported by cognitive science research in the areas of single-loop learning (SLL) and double-loop learning (DLL) (Argyris & Schon, 1974).

SLL involves action without reflection. We act compliantly and efficiently, but with no understanding of assumptions or values that underlie the original intent for action. Only with DLL is there potential for real change, because we evaluate assumptions through reflection, which better align ideas with actions and actions with outcomes (Osterman & Kottkamp, 1993). In essence, we become more skilled at gathering information, and develop greater awareness of the impact of our actions.

REFRAMING SUPERVISION

Within a learning organization, differentiated supervisory approaches support the design of self-directed professional development plans. Supervision has been broadly defined as the process of facilitating another individual's professional growth. Anyone involved with professional development—whether supervisor, staff development specialist, or speech-language therapist—has the potential for bringing about real change in three areas: beliefs and attitudes, instructional and clinical practices, and student outcomes (Papir-Bernstein & Legrand, 1993).

The ultimate goal of supervision is the creation of professional autonomy and the ability to self-monitor, self-analyze, and self-evaluate. Anderson's model of supervision is frequently cited in our field as describing a continuum of changing relationships for both the supervisor and supervisee (Anderson, 1988). The basic premise of Anderson's continuum is that as the supervisee becomes more autonomous, the type of supervision changes from supervisor-directed to self-directed.

One of the strongest arguments for use of differentiated supervision is that professionals have different growth needs and learning styles. However, even more basic are two principles from adult learning theory. First, most adults have a strong and basic desire to be self-directing. Second, individual differences increase with age as they relate to style, time, place, and pace of learning (Ormrod, 1999). A self-directed program is more likely to elicit a positive response, because it acknowledges individual differences. In addition, professionals who believe they have the capability and opportunity to affect what happens to them are more likely to be high achievers and self-directed individuals, who initiate and take responsibility for their goals (Senge, 1990).

In typical school districts, research, development, and diffusion models look fairly similar. Experts are hired, and practice implementation often assumes a subordinate relationship to theoretical knowledge acquisition. Knowledge comes from the outside in, whereas in reflective practice, knowledge is gained from the *inside* first (Geller & Foley, 2009; Osterman & Kottkamp, 1993). In the traditional model, the practitioner becomes a passive consumer of knowledge. In the reflective practice model, the practitioner becomes a researcher and engages in a continuing process of self-education and lifelong learning.

FACILITATING SELF-DIRECTION AND REFLECTIVE PRACTICE

A self-directed supervisory program was created that allowed individuals to assume primary responsibility for their own professional growth (Anderson, 1988). The self-directed process has four steps: professional growth objectives are identified; a professional growth plan including analysis of strengths, weaknesses and targeted areas for growth is completed; an action plan is developed that identifies objectives, methods, resources, and time lines; and some type of summative conference or self-evaluation is performed (Papir-Bernstein, 2001).

Self-assessment and self-directed professional development planning are two approaches that facilitate reflective practice, since both encourage thinking about our own learning objectives (Osterman & Kottkamp, 1993). Through reflective practice, we develop an increased level of self-awareness about the impact of our work, and create openings for previously unseen opportunities for professional growth.

As part of a professional development program, any type of reflective practice strategy is effective in achieving behavioral change (Tremmel, 1993). Whereas the primary purpose of traditional staff development (SD) is knowledge acquisition, in reflective SD the ultimate purpose is behavioral change leading to improved performance. The knowledge transmitted is useful, and allows practitioners to make better sense of their experiences.

When we learn what is useful and functional, we are acquiring knowledge of the artistry of our craft, and what Schon calls *knowing-in-action* (Schon, 1983). Schon compares two knowledge systems: *technical rationality,* or the formal science of knowledge; and *reflection-in- action*, or the knowledge based on the art and intuition surrounding and framing our practice. It has been suggested that practitioners across disciplines limit the artistry of their practice when they adhere to a strict policy of technical rationality (Dilollo, 2010; Schon, 1983).

Clinical decision making must include craft as well as theory, and needs to be intuition-driven as well as science-driven (Justice & Fey, 2004). Schon refers to the *art* of problem framing and improvisation in everyday practice as necessary neighbors to the *rigor* of the science and research. Whereas technical rationality is based on the results of research, usually conducted off site, reflection generates knowledge directly from experience. The artistry of practice is influenced by the knowing that comes from doing, and eventually by the development of *intuitive knowing* (Schon, 1983). The practitioner acts as a researcher on site, and the practice site becomes the laboratory.

STAFF DEVELOPMENT CONTENT

The decision of what type of information to include in staff development programs is important, not only for the recipients of the information but for the organization it serves. The content of professional *education training* programs, and their emphasis on technical training, can and should influence the structure of professional *work training* programs. However, as important as technical knowledge is, intuitive or reflective knowledge is at least equally important (DiLollo, 2010; Shepard & Jensen, 1990).

One way of analyzing staff development content is to consider a model proposed for evaluating curricula (Eisner, 1985). Eisner differentiates between the types of information contained within an explicit curriculum and implicit curriculum. The explicit curriculum contains the courses and most of the technical information. The implicit curriculum, however, includes values, beliefs, attitudes, and expectations. Implicit variables influence professional actions, behaviors, and ways of thinking that ultimately enhance or inhibit professional growth.

Self-reflection has been described as a process that facilitates self-evaluation and self-directed behavioral change, and ultimately leads to increased clinical competence. Reflective functioning demands a level of awareness that streams across cognitive as well as affective or emotional domains. Feelings play a large influential factor in one's ability to interpret and respond to situations, and so professional development needs to address this emotional dimension (Geller & Foley, 2009; Schon, 1993; Tremmel, 1993).

EMOTIONAL COMPETENCY IMPACTS PROGRAM EFFECTIVENESS

As part of the self-directed supervisory process, the professionals under my supervision identified their own professional growth objectives. Two interesting patterns emerged. First, most felt comfortable with their knowledge of professional or technical content. However, they felt hampered by competencies related largely to those programmatic accountability issues that interfered with the perception of a smoothly running therapy program, or program effectiveness. The other area that appeared on numerous action plans fell under the heading of what Goleman (1988) calls *emotional intelligence*: emotional and social competencies that relate to managing feelings and handling relationships (Papir-Bernstein, 2001).

Goleman (1988) studied the relationship that personal and social competencies have on job performance across fields. His framework is broken down into five elements: Personal competence determines how we manage ourselves, and includes self-awareness, self-regulation, and motivation. Social competence relates to our ability to handle relationships, and includes empathy and social skills.

As part of the reflective process, and because self-assessment is facilitated through the use of attitude questionnaires and professional competency checklists, two questionnaires were constructed using a Likert scale from 1 to 5 (Cascella & Vogel, 2008; McCarthy, 2010; Meilijson & Katzenberger, 2009). They were offered to the speech providers as pre- and post-self-assessments in their first year of differentiated (reflective and self-directed) supervision, and became an active component of our ASHA-endorsed continuing education (CE) program that year and in years to follow. The Emotional Competency (EQ) questionnaire was constructed from Goleman's (1988) emotional intelligence framework, and the Program Effectiveness Questionnaire was constructed from variables gathered through meetings and discussions with speech providers and their supervisors (Papir-Bernstein, 2001).

At the end of the year the following trends were revealed. As *personal competence* improved (how we manage ourselves), a variety of program effectiveness variables improved as well: *self-awareness* impacted self-advocacy, awareness of student progress, and self-image; *self-regulation* impacted balance of service delivery, space organization, use of materials, student independence, and paperwork management; and *motivation* impacted student outcomes, professional growth, and staff development implementation.

As *social competence* improved (our ability to handle relationships), so did the following program effectiveness variables: *empathy* impacted communication with administrators, the school-home connection, diversity consciousness and involvement with school community; and *social skills* impacted classroom involvement, peer communication, relationship with evaluation and instructional support teams, integration of curriculum and standards, and student carryover (Papir-Bernstein, 2001).

LESSONS LEARNED ON THE PATH

The lessons learned on the path of practice-based evidence are clear. Continuous learning involves the ability to reflect on action. In practice-based professional learning settings, individuals are better able to learn from their own professional experiences. Reflection encourages professionals to recognize gaps in their own knowledge and attend to their own learning needs, fostering lifelong professional exploration and growth.

Reflection supports change, and awareness is the first step in any change process. Identification of problems is never easy. Problems are often seen as indicators of failure or incompetence. Through self-directed supervision and the use of self-evaluations, the professionals in my organization were able to target their own social and emotional areas for improvement, and experience the resulting impact on their program effectiveness. As we practiced reflection, problem finding became more natural. Supervisors were able to identify and address mismatched supervisor-supervisee styles, and speech providers were able to identify and improve social and emotional variables that were impacting the clinical effectiveness of their therapy program.

REFERENCES

Anderson, J. L. (1988). *The supervisory process in speech-language pathology and audiology.* Boston, MA: College-Hill Press.

Argyis, C., & Schon, D. (1974). *Theory in practice: Increasing professional effectiveness.* Oxford, UK: Jossey-Bass.

Bowen, G. (2010). Service learning in the scholarship of teaching and learning: Effective practices. *International Journal for the Scholarship of Teaching and Learning, 4*(2), 1–15.

Boyer, E. L. (1990). *Scholarship reconsidered: Priorities of the professoriate.* Princeton, NJ: Carnegie Foundation for the Advancement of Teaching.

Cascella, P., & Vogel, D. (2008). Student self-directed professional development as a formative assessment skill. *ASHA Perspectives on Issues in Higher Education, 11*(1), 4–8.

Conners, R., Smith, T., & Hickman, C. (1994). *The Oz principle: Getting results through individual and organizational accountability.* Paramus, NJ: Prentice-Hall.

DiLollo, A. (2010). The crisis of confidence in professional knowledge: Implications for clinical education in speech-language pathology. *ASHA*

Perspectives on Administration and Supervision, 20(3), 85–91.

Eisner, E. (1985). *The educational imagination: On design and evaluation of school programs.* New York, NY: Macmillan.

Geller, E., & Foley, G. M. (2009). Broadening the "ports of entry" for speech-language pathologists: A relational and reflective model for clinical supervision. *American Journal of Speech-Language Pathology, 18*(1), 22–41.

Goleman, D. (1988). *Working with emotional intelligence.* New York, NY: Bantam Books.

Justice, L. M., & Fey, M. E. (2004). Evidence-based practice in schools: Integrating craft and theory with science and data. *ASHA Leader* (Electronic version). Retrieved June 10, 2011, from http://www.asha.org/Publications/leader/2004/040921/f040921a.htm.

McCarthy, M. P. (2010). Promoting reflective practice using performance indicator questionnaires. *ASHA Perspectives on Administration and Supervision, 20*(2), 64–70.

McKinney, K. (2007). *Enhancing learning through the scholarship of teaching and learning: The challenges and joys of juggling.* San Francisco, CA: Jossey-Bass.

Meilijson, S., & Katzenberger, I. (2009). Reflections on reflections: Learning processes in speech and language pathology students' clinical education. *ASHA Perspectives on Administration and Supervision, 19*(2), 62–71.

Ormrod, J. E. (1999). *Human learning* (3rd ed.). Englewood Cliffs, NJ: Prentice-Hall.

Osterman, K. F., & Kottkamp, R. B. (1993). *Reflective practice for educators.* Thousand Oaks, CA: Corwin Press.

Papir-Bernstein, W. (2001, November). *Creating the perfect fit: Merging personal competence with program effectiveness.* ASHA Mini-Seminar, New Orleans, LA.

Papir-Bernstein, W., & Legrand, R. (1993, November). *Differentiated systems for staff development: Self-direction and reflection.* ASHA Mini-Seminar, Anaheim, CA.

Schmitt, M. B., & Justice, L. (2011). Schools as complex host environments: Understanding aspects of schools that may influence clinical practice and research. *ASHA Leader, 16*(7), 8–11.

Schon, D. A. (1983). *The reflective practitioner: How professionals think in action.* New York, NY: Basic Books.

Senge, P. M. (1990). *The fifth discipline: The art and practice of the learning organization.* London, UK: Random House.

Shepard, K. F., & Jensen, G. (1990). Physical therapist curricula for the 1990's: Educating the reflective practitioner. *Physical Therapy, 70*(9), 44–51.

Tremmel, R. (1993). Zen and the art of reflective practice in teacher education. *Harvard Educational Review, 63*(4), 434–458.

Weimer, M. A. (2011). A primer on pedagogical scholarship. *ASHA Perspectives on Issues in Higher Education, 14*(1), 5–10.

Westfall, J., Mold, J., & Fagnan, L. (2007). Practice-based research: Blue highways on the NIH road map. *Journal of the American Medical Association, 297*(4), 403–406.

ESSAY 13

The Interplay ❧ Between Legal Policy and ❧ Clinical Practice

Andrea F. Blau, Esquire

Sadanand Singh was one of the pioneers in supporting the advancement of best practices in the field of speech and hearing sciences. As a publisher, his passion and commitment to providing a forum of expression for authors in applied research has impacted both academia as well as the quality of care for thousands of people with communication challenges. As a theoretician, his advancement of translational research practices has made a significant influence on generations to come. This essay gives homage to this legacy.

WHAT DO WE MEAN BY TRANSLATIONAL RESEARCH?

Translational research, as embraced by the medical field, is a blending of theory and practice; making the results of research practicable for use for/by the population under study; insuring more meaningful outcomes; blending of ivory tower and lay public impact; and promoting "bench to bedside" (Goldblatt & Lee, 2010), from laboratory-based research to point of care patient applicability.

Different from the more straightforward commitment for communication between pure empirical and applied research or the promotion of mutual respect for the interplay between top-down and bottom-up approaches to analyses, a more interdisciplinary (cross discipline, multidisciplinary) perspective is a core part of the translational research perspective.

So in a sense it's both the integration of theory and practice as a research paradigm, while simultaneously integrating perspectives from related fields as essential for practical findings and future research.

HAS A BROADER DEFINITION OF TRANSLATIONAL RESEARCH PERHAPS EVOLVED?

Perhaps not part of the original definition, but certainly worth including in viewing translational research today, is respecting the dynamic nature and context within which the features under study are being viewed, both from a cross-sectional perspective (even from a short slice of time) as well as longitudinally (almost a life span perspective), giving homage to what has come before, what exists now, but perhaps most importantly when dealing with application, what lies ahead.

The elements of this fuller perspective have been acknowledged for decades by those of us in the field of speech and hearing sciences who have been working with the complex constellation of developmental and acquired communication challenges faced by the multiply disabled individual (Blau, 1986). There has never been any other way, effectively, to treat or understand individuals with such complex disorders than additionally to examine the world through their eyes, eyes which pragmatically see the world from a multidisciplinary vantage point. Whether doing basic research or analyzing best practices, ignoring the fuzzy boundaries and significant overlap, or attempting too ardently to disentangle the coexistence of different core disciplines (e.g., occupational therapy, physical therapy, speech and hearing sciences, movement science, neurology, linguistics, psychology, sociology, nutrition, and health sciences) creates only a false sense of the reality within which these heavily challenged people must function.

Perhaps equally limited is the perspective that focusing on a static unit of analysis or isolated learned skill, albeit from a multidisciplinary perspective, might have substantive merit without seeing where the unit of analysis or skill might fit within a broader spectrum or dynamic continuum of function (Rifkin, 2012.)

Over time, the relatively interchangeable terms *multidisciplinary, cross-disciplinary, transdisciplinary,* and *interdisciplinary,* evolved as an accepted standard or approach for viewing clinical work; not just for the severely challenged population but as a way for bridging the gap between theory and practice for most forms of human analyses.

Embedded within this perspective is an acknowledgment of how any unit of analysis is invariably influenced by the context within which it is viewed, especially when it comes to clinical practice. Neither the notion of pure nor applied research can be viewed as completely distinct from the context within which it exists. Yet, the statement is equally true that our units of analyses, and how we instinctively view them, influence the context within which they are embedded.

Similarly, our research or practice is embedded within our political climate. The focus of this essay is to explore a few examples of how public policy, as expressed through our legal system, impacts our clinical practice and how speech and hearing sciences, in turn, influence the practice of law.

HOW MIGHT THE PRACTICE OF LAW IMPACT UPON CLINICAL PRACTICE?

Where better to begin than with the Code of Ethics that guides legal practice? The first two sections in the Preamble of the New York Rules of Professional Conduct (effective April 1, 2009 and amended January 28, 2011) list the following:

1. A lawyer, as a member of the legal profession, is a representative of clients and an officer of the legal system with special responsibility for the quality of justice. As a representative of clients, a lawyer assumes many roles, including advisor, advocate, negotiator, and evaluator. As an officer of the legal system, each lawyer has a duty to uphold the legal process; to demonstrate respect for the legal system; to seek improvement of the law; and to promote access to the legal system and the administration of justice. In addition, a lawyer should further the public's understanding of and confidence in the rule of law and the justice system because,

in a constitutional democracy, legal institutions depend on popular participation and support to maintain their authority.

2. The touchstone of the client-lawyer relationship is the lawyer's obligation to assert the client's position under the rules of the adversary system, to maintain the client's confidential information except in limited circumstances, and to act with loyalty during the period of the representation.

As an attorney, as well as a speech-language pathologist, I am personally morally and ethically bound by the above. But most of us, whether seasoned practitioners or new clinicians entering the field of communication sciences and (re)habilitation might instinctively see the parallels between the sections above and the ethical obligations we hold as our clinical responsibilities.

Perhaps we might "translate" the sections above as follows:

1. An SLP, as a member of the speech and hearing science profession, is a representative of clients and of the speech and hearing profession with special responsibility for the quality of intervention provided. As a representative of clients, an SLP assumes many roles, including advisor, advocate, negotiator, therapist, and evaluator. As a representative of the speech and hearing profession, each clinician has a duty to uphold the therapeutic process; to demonstrate respect for the professional community; to seek improvement of the treatment of communication disorders; and to promote access to these interventions and its equitable administration. In addition, a clinician should further the public's understanding of and confidence in the role of intervention and available access to the services of the profession because, in a democratic society, the advancement of clinical services depend on popular

participation and governmental support to maintain their equitable accessibility.

2. The touchstone of the client-clinician relationship is the clinician's obligation to provide appropriate therapeutic services and assert the client's position under the rules of both a collaborative and an adversarial system, to maintain the client's confidential information except in limited circumstances, and to act with loyalty and respect during the period of the direct service and beyond.

This second point above might seem somewhat perplexing to the clinician just entering the work force. What do we mean by providing services under the rules of both a collaborative and adversarial system? What obligations do we, as clinicians, have within an adversarial system?

Subsections of two additional ethical "Rules" that have been adopted by the Appellate Division of the New York Supreme Court (22 NYCRR Part 1200) in respect to attorneys are of particular relevance in guiding some of our clinical decisions. Their subsequent "translation" might assist in answering the question above:

Rule 1.1: COMPETENCE

   c. A lawyer shall not intentionally:

      1. fail to seek the objectives of the client through reasonably available means permitted by law and these Rules;

Rule 1.3: DILIGENCE

   a. A lawyer shall act with reasonable diligence and promptness in representing a client.

   Comment

   1. A lawyer should pursue a matter on behalf of a client despite opposition, obstruction, or

personal inconvenience to the lawyer, and to take whatever lawful and ethical measures are required to vindicate a client's cause or endeavor. A lawyer must also act with commitment and dedication to the interests of the client and in advocacy upon the client's behalf.

And the translation to clinical practice:

Rule 1.1: COMPETENCE

   c. A clinician shall not intentionally:

      1. fail to seek the objectives of the client through reasonably available means permitted by law and these Rules;

Rule 1.3: DILIGENCE

   a. A clinician shall act with reasonable diligence and promptness in representing a client.

   Comment

      1. A clinician should pursue a matter on behalf of a client despite opposition, obstruction or personal inconvenience to the clinician, and to take whatever lawful and ethical measures are required to vindicate a client's cause or endeavor. A clinician must also act with commitment and dedication to the interests of the client and in advocacy upon the client's behalf.

As a speech-language pathologist (SLP) who has been providing interventions for children and adults with severe communication challenges since the early 1970s (35 years before I became an attorney), I've found myself almost consistently operating on two planes simultaneously. The first, and always at the heart of my commitment, is the provision of quality clinical intervention to my clients regardless of the severity and complexity of their challenges; and the second, which at times seems even more difficult than the first, is to ensure and secure my clients' rights to receive the aforementioned interventions.

This second commitment may seem to fall exclusively within my role as an attorney, but that is neither the case nor where many of these battles are fought and won. It is our commitment as clinicians, with our expertise in identifying our client's needs, our exclusive ability to provide the necessary justification for the prescribed treatment, and our willingness to stand our ground in advocating for the level of service required that has become nearly equal in importance to the provision of the services themselves.

Our ethical and moral responsibility, whether our services are funded through private or public sources, as translated above, requires diligently supporting our clients so that they may achieve the communicative competency we are committed to help them attain.

HOW MIGHT CLINICAL PRACTICE TRANSLATE INTO IMPROVED LEGAL OUTCOMES?

As clinicians responsible for creating dynamic solutions for people with extreme communication challenges, we are provided with a rich education on the impact these challenges have across all aspects of an individual's life. This increased sensitivity might translate into improved legal outcomes. As we become more committed advocates for our clients and are called upon as clinical experts (Blau, 2011) in litigation or mediation efforts (Blau, 2007a), or to serve on interdisciplinary committees responsible for promulgating regulations (Blau, 2007b), we have an opportunity to influence the legal/judicial system and ultimately change public policy.

Below are a few brief examples from my own clinical/legal experience that reflect how clinical sensitivity is beginning to translate into upgraded legal practices.

There exists, within the Supreme Court in New York County, a "dual Part" that exclusively deals with the protections needed for individuals with mental disabilities who are facing eviction (Hagler, 2012). Many of these people have minimal resources and are not able to represent themselves or communicate their needs adequately. To protect them, APS (Adult Protective Services) initiates a guardianship petition. One judge presides over both actions; the pending eviction and the guardianship petition (hence the "dual Part.") By staying the eviction the Court determines whether the AIP (alleged incapacitated person) has the capacity to take care of personal and property needs or requires supervision prior to having to relocate. To assist the Court in making this determination, a CE (Court Evaluator) is appointed. The CE is considered the eyes and ears of the Court, and is given full authority to access all records, to look into all available resources, and suggest solutions that might spare the AIP from being evicted, or if relocation is necessary, provide the individual with the necessary support to effectuate a suitable relocation plan (Mental Hygiene Law §81.09). I have had the opportunity to serve in this special capacity as Court Evaluator. My appointment was primarily based on my clinical experience and the Court's realization that the expertise that we provide, as clinicians, translates into effective legal outcomes for these respondents.

There has been an evolving focus within innovative legal clinics, offered by law schools providing free legal services to clients with disabilities, to incorporate better observation, memory assistance, and listening skills in their interview techniques. Students are being taught to see client interviewing as problem solving (Krieger & Neumann, 2003), a notion borrowed from the social sciences. Translating methodologies used by social workers and communication specialists in diagnosing clients' problems while identifying their goals, becomes key to developing trust between client and attorney, based on interview preparation, active listening and selective information reformulation. In my personal experience as a legal intern in these clinics, my extensive clinical experience as an SLP translated into almost an instinctual trust and comfort level that clients with complex disabilities seemed to experience. Clients with mental disabilities, such as Colliers (hoarders) and PTSD (post-traumatic stress disorder), who had refused to cooperate with other attorneys became much more compliant. This turnaround was based on their ability to respond more positively within a clinical model which incorporated painstaking patience and small steady facilitations, respecting the clients' perspective as the pivotal point from which to effect change.

AREA OF POTENTIAL INCOMPATIBILITY ACROSS CLINICAL AND LEGAL PRACTICES

Despite the noted congruity across clinical and legal domains, there is, at minimum, one inherent roadblock that merits our attention. Perhaps via open discussion we might collectively find a solution that translates into improved client outcome.

When litigating for a client as an attorney, the strongest legal arguments are not based on what is known to be true or even fair; rather they are based on the fact pattern of the case, the letter of the law, the decisions that have already been handed down by judges within the same jurisdiction or higher courts, and the evidence that is entered into record as admissible. It is not uncommon for a client who on appearance is undeniably disabled and deserving of disability benefits, equipment, or support services to be denied those benefits because of a technical error when a petition was filed, a statute of limitation violated, a medical report written by a less than savvy physician, or even an unfavorable decision that preceded the case with a similar fact pattern within the same jurisdiction.

As an SLP with years of experience in working with clients with a broad range of disabilities across the life span, my hands are often tied, as an attorney, in presenting evidence or even arguing a motion, based on information I have empirical data to support, but which falls outside the scope of legally permissible guidelines.

When appearing at a Hearing as an expert witness, rather than as an attorney, I may share my perspective to the limited extent that the Court allows. But as an attorney, my theory of the case and the arguments that I present may only reflect legal evidence, not clinical experience. Research outcomes when allowed on record may be persuasive but not determinative.

Perhaps an interesting area where a translational research model might effect change?

REFERENCES

Blau, A. F. (1986). *Communication in the backchannel: Social structural analyses of nonspeech/ speech conversations.* Unpublished PhD dissertation, CUNY. New York, NY.

Blau, A. F. (2007a). Available dispute resolution processes within the reauthorized individual with disabilities education improvement act (IDEIA) of 2004: Where do mediation principles fit in? *Pepperdine Dispute Resolution Law Journal, 7,* 65–86.

Blau, A. F. (2007b). The IDEIA and the right to an "Appropriate" education. *Educational Law Journal, Brigham Young University, 2007,* 1–22.

Blau, A. F. (2011). Advocating for "appropriate" special education services: Focusing on the IEP. *NYSBA, Elder and Special Needs Law Journal, 21*(3), 20–24.

Goldblatt, E. M., & Lee, W. H. (2010). From bench to bedside: The growing use of translational research in cancer medicine. *American Journal of Translational Research, 2,* 1–18.

Hagler, S. (2011, June 22). Innovative Part integrates guardianship and housing matters. *New York Law Journal, 4,* 9.

Krieger, S. H, & Neumann, Jr., R. K. (2003). *Essential lawyering skills: Interviewing, counseling, negotiation, and persuasive fact analysis.* New York, NY: Aspen.

Mental Hygiene Law §81.09. Appointment of Court Evaluator.

Part 1200 of the Joint Rules of the Appellate Division. (2011). *22 NYCRR Part 1200. New York rules of professional conduct, New York State unified court system.* Effective April 1, 2009, amended January 28, 2011.

Rifkin, A. J. (2012). The proper purpose of assessments in the IEP process: It's a lot more than reporting a score. *NYSBA, Elder and Special Needs Law Journal, 22,* 1.

Overdependence on ❧ Technology in the Management ❧ of Hearing Loss

Joseph J. Montano

This essay is dedicated, with thanks, to Sadan-and Singh. I feel fortunate to have been able to work with him and experience first-hand the dedication and beauty of a man committed to the fields of speech-language pathology and audiology. When Jaci Spitzer and I first approached Sadanand about our concept of a doctoral text on adult audiologic rehabilitation that would focus on the psychosocial impact of hearing loss, I was concerned he would reject our proposal. It would have been perfectly understandable. There already existed several outstanding AR textbooks, some published by his own company. Instead, Sadanand explored our thinking, evaluated our rationale, and supported our decision to embark on a different approach to presenting an AR textbook. I soon learned that Sadanand's commitment was not only to our book, but to us. I am proud to be one of hundreds, perhaps thousands who have been touched by the spirit of this great man, filled with dedication and love.

It may develop slowly over time, years, perhaps decades before an individual with hearing loss acknowledges changes in communication. The onset, behavioral manifestations, inter-personal, vocational, and social implications of hearing loss are extremely personal and the journey toward understanding its impact, indi-vidualized, and in some cases unpredictable. Developing an awareness of communication change is a process that weaves throughout a person's lifestyle with input from multiple sources: family, friends, coworkers, and even casual acquaintances. From direct comments from a spouse to nonverbal actions perhaps from the barista at Starbucks, people are pre-sented with clues alluding to their communi-cation failures and the possibility of hearing loss. Once acknowledged, the solution is often simplified by medical professionals, family, and friends as, "You need a hearing aid." Thus begins the process of introduction to the tech-nocentric world of the audiologist. Armed with the latest in technological developments, we may be prepared to improve hearing per-ception but fall far short of addressing com-munication loss.

Hearing loss is frequently oversimplified. The expectation is that technology will provide the solution. Our training as audiologists rein-forces this concept. The curriculum in most doctor of audiology programs emphasizes the diagnostic nature of our profession, and while aural rehabilitation (AR) is certainly present in doctoral training, it seems to take a back seat to assessment and amplification. Technology seems to be at the core in our training. Courses focusing on differential diagnosis, instrumentation, electrophysiology, acoustics, and hearing aids flood the curriculum while classes focusing on interpersonal communication and psychosocial issues related to hearing loss are few. Even counseling, which has been referred to as the essence of AR treatment (Erdman, 2009), may only be embedded in diagnostic academic offerings. Many academic programs do not offer specific coursework in this area, and when it is offered, is frequently limited to one or two credits. Ross (1997) provides a convincing argument that AR, despite its role in the foundation of our profession, is minimally present in the curriculum and even further in the background of our professional practice. Yet, most audiologists, academicians and clinicians alike, will tout the importance of AR in service provision. In fact, training and provision of AR is frequently cited by many as one of the primary factors that distinguishes the audiologist from the hearing aid specialist in the delivery of amplification.

There are many arguments audiologists make to support the lack of availability of AR service. Perhaps the most prevalent is the fact that it is not a reimbursable service by most third-party payers. Instead, we opt to sell hearing aids, another largely nonreimbursable service, without providing the necessary support to make them successful. But the question remains, can hearing loss be remediated simply by fitting hearing aids? While technological advances with hearing aids has been extraordinary over the past decade, device returns and patient satisfaction has essentially been stable for decades (Kochkin, 2009), not improving along with the available instrumentation. How can we account for this? What is the missing link? Most audiologists would agree that the provision of amplification to persons with hearing loss is a complex multilayered process involving much more that the fitting of hearing instruments, yet our service delivery system does not support this belief.

SERVICE DELIVERY MODELS

Many authors have advocated a review of the service delivery model for audiology and have recommended alternative possibilities for professional practice. Erdman, Wark, and Montano (1994) advocated the use of the rehabilitation model over the traditional medical model. They reported that the medical model presented a top-down authoritative process where the audiologist serves to provide a diagnosis and treatment. Patients' roles are largely passive and it is intended that they follow a recommended treatment plan, most often including the provision of amplification, to remediate their hearing loss. The rehabilitation model, on the other hand, was reported to be more of a horizontal delivery of service that was interactive and facilitative. The audiologist works with the patient to determine the appropriate goals for resolving the issues related to hearing loss. It is not meant to be prescriptive, but rather collaborative.

Duchan (2004) acknowledged the impact of the medical model of service delivery on the profession of audiology and advocated the inclusion of both social and narrative models as alternate considerations for the management of patients with hearing loss. In advocating a social influence on service provision, the author identifies the role society plays in a person's ability to cope with hearing loss within the context of the social settings. Hearing loss can impact a person's performance in a variety of events on many social levels, from listening to a lecture in a classroom to functioning in a noisy environment such as a restaurant. The underlying principle for her social model is the reduction of the obstacles that result in participation restrictions. This concept clearly identifies with the ASHA (2001) definition of AR as a process that aims to reduce activity limitations and participation restrictions. Furthermore, Duchan (2004) goes on to describe a narrative model that can be incorporated into audiology practice. The use of narrative allows for patient self-expression. It encourages a dialogue that can provide the audiologist with additional information on the impact of hearing loss on the patient's daily functioning. The use of the patient narrative can be a useful tool in determining treatment options and measuring outcomes.

The patient narrative is a key component of the biopsychosocial approach to service delivery described by Erdman (2009). In her discussion of the biopsychosocial approach to audiologic rehabilitation, she identifies the shortcomings of the biomedical model, emphasizing that this approach is a "band-aid solution." The provision of a hearing aid to resolve the issues related to hearing loss may not adequately address the underlying concepts that influence a person's behavior. Amplification alone is inadequate when patients present with significant psychosocial manifestations as a result of hearing loss. The role of the audiologist is more than just identifying the presence of hearing loss and "curing" it with hearing aids.

According to Erdman (2009), the heart of the biopsychosocial model of service delivery is the patient story. This narrative provides the audiologist with a better understanding of the patient's experiences with hearing loss. As a result, the audiologist and patient develop an interactive relationship that can lead to productive sharing. Together, treatment goals and recommendations can be formulated with an increased likelihood of adherence and increased satisfaction.

The medical model seems to be, by far, the most prevalent delivery system for audiologists. It is part of our identity and practice. Even within our training programs this concept of diagnosis and cure is fostered. Many

programs acknowledge the accomplishments of their doctoral students by holding "white coat" ceremonies. Here they are presented with their white coats to symbolize their entry into the professional realm of audiology. But what does the white coat represent? It is most associated with medical practice and has been the symbol for physicians for over 100 years (Hochberg, 2007). It immediately makes a statement to the patient and serves to set up the medical model of service delivery. The "white coat" audiologist is expected to diagnose hearing loss and treat it with, what else, the hearing aid. Once again, the aid is viewed by most as the cure to hearing loss.

I believe audiologists would agree with the concepts presented in all three recommended models: rehabilitation, social/narrative, and biopsychosocial. My experience tells me that most believe we must provide more rehabilitative services to our patients with hearing loss. It seems, however, we tend to focus on why we can't as opposed to how we can. One theory may be that we, as audiologists, with our educational background and experience with instrumentation, are more comfortable dealing with the more concrete concept of hearing loss rather than the abstract implication of feelings, emotions, and adjustment issues. But then, who better than the audiologist can address these issues?

The provision of AR services falls within the scope of two professionals, speech-language pathologists and audiologists. ASHA (2001) specifically addresses this issue by distinctly identifying the specific knowledge and skills for the provision of AR services for both professions. The professions have different roles in the identification and management of adults and children with hearing loss. The argument has been that, by training, the audiologist is better equipped to address the needs of people with hearing loss as a result of their educational background. Unfortunately, though, they have little to no experience with long-term patient interaction, therapeutic goal setting, and behavioral objectives. Speech-language pathologists have a great deal of experience in these areas of service, with their experience largely involved in the provision of therapeutic intervention but, unfortunately, they have little education and training in hearing loss. What is the result? Patients in need of AR have a difficult task ahead of them if they look to find a professional to provide these services. Although two professions claim to be qualified by virtue of their degrees and training, the truth is that AR services virtually go unprovided in the professional arena.

Audiologists have for years identified themselves with AR. In fact, the entire professional field is the result of early rehabilitative management of hearing loss as a result of military noise exposure. The Steering Committee of Special Interest Division 7 (1992) defined audiologic rehabilitation as audiology. It is the basis for our profession. Numerous definitions of AR exist and are all closely aligned with audiology. Even though our professional literature supports the belief that AR is indeed audiology and audiologists themselves identify AR as within their purview, practice seems to imply otherwise (Montano, 2009). Many consumers of our services report that we do not adequately address the needs and resolve the issues associated with hearing loss solely through the dispensing of hearing aids (Ida Institute, 2011). The relationship developed seems to emphasis the hearing aid rather than the person with hearing loss (Montano, 2011).

TECHNOCENTRIC VERSUS PATIENT CENTERED

Montano (2011) reported that the services provided by audiologists appear to be primarily technology focused, that is, instrumentation is the basis for decision making and recom-mendations. The technocentric model (Figure 14–1) represents this methodology. The figure illustrates the typical process a patient may experience when receiving treatment for hearing loss. Technology is the core of service provision. The initial contact with the audiologist usually involves obtaining a brief history consisting of closed-set questions, such as: "Do you have any ringing in your ears?" "Have you ever had ear surgery?" It is followed by an assessment of hearing loss, which is typically performed in a sound-treated environment with the patient and audiologist in different rooms. The audiogram then becomes the pivotal focus in counseling and resultant recommendations.

As a result of the identification of hearing loss, barring necessary medical intervention, hearing aids are the likely recommendation. This can either be accepted or rejected by the patient. Treatment includes a discussion of hearing aid technology, various styles and features, manufacturers, and costs. The model continues with hearing aid fitting and training. Frequently audiologists use hearing aid orientation to educate their patients in the care and maintenance of their hearing aids. In order to determine the appropriateness of the recommended amplification, verification is necessary. Real-ear measurement is used to verify the acoustic characteristics of the recommended hearing aids and is a formulaic process using prescriptive features and target measurements. Frequently, afterward the fitting may be accentuated by the provision of additional technology accessories, such as connectivity devices and remote controls.

This model emphasizes the assessment and importance of instrumentation in the management of hearing loss. It is technology driven and the patient appears to be in the periphery, while the hearing aid and assessment instrumentation is at the core. It allows little opportunity for the audiologist to explore the possible impact of hearing loss on daily living.

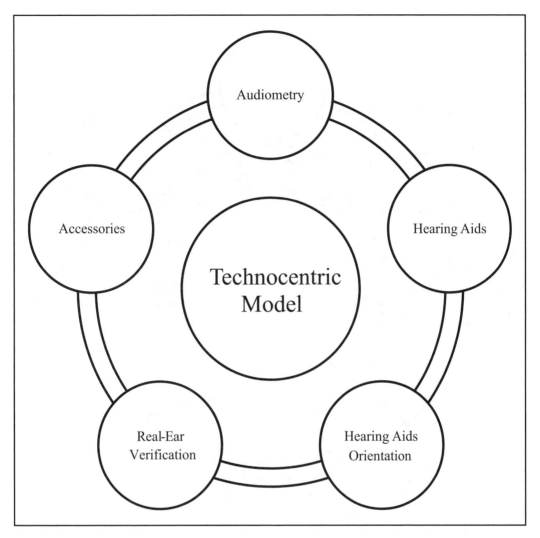

Figure 14–1. *Model representing a technology-focused service delivery. Used with permission from Montano (2011).*

By focusing on the hearing test or audiogram rather than the resultant manifestations of the loss itself, both the audiologist and patient are unable to properly identify crucial elements necessary for audiologic rehabilitation.

The person-centered model (Figure 14–2), on the other hand, emphasizes a cooperative exploration of the issues and needs associated with hearing loss. At the core of this model is the person, and although technology is certainly a component, it no longer serves as the central or focal point of the rehabilitation. Counseling is the key element of service delivery. The counseling relationship is established immediately at the onset of the interaction. Instead of the use of a history intact form, the audiologist explores the patient's story through open-ended dialogue. "What brings you here today?" "Tell me about your hearing loss." In fact, Gagne and Jennings (2011) reported that the patient narrative is critical and at the foundation of the person-centered

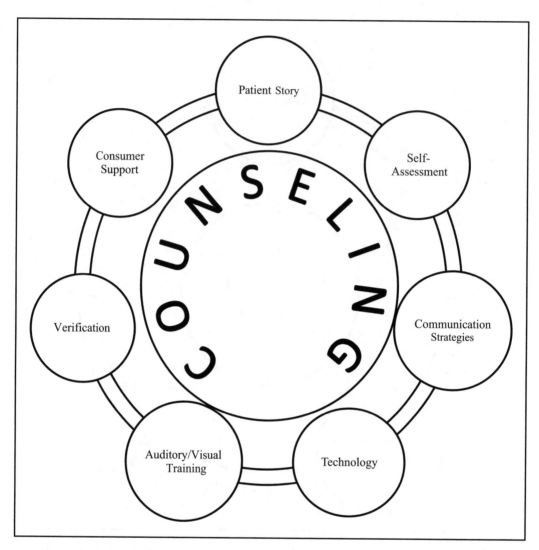

Figure 14–2. *Model representing a person-centered service delivery. Used with permission from Montano* (2011).

approach to treatment. In addition to the standard audiological evaluation, self-assessment becomes a valuable tool in the process. Self-assessment scales have been available for decades and many only require a few minutes to administer. The use of self-assessment will help the audiologist determine the impact the hearing loss is having on everyday functioning. For example, items on the *Hearing Handicap Inventory for the Elderly* (Ventry & Weinstein, 1982) can not only provide an assessment of self-perceived hearing handicap, but can invite further dialogue on the impact of hearing loss.

Understanding how an individual functions with hearing loss, in daily activities and communication environments, can prepare the audiologist to make better choices when determining amplification options. The person-centered model does not diminish the need for use of technology but rather, focuses on the patient/clinician relationship, problem resolution, and cooperative efforts. It is a process that engages the patient in his or her own rehabilitation. Yes, the hearing aid is important, as is real-ear verification and accessories, but these are merely tools designed to direct the patient toward improved communication. The hearing aid, undoubtedly, will not resolve all communication issues, and therefore equal importance must be placed on self-adjustment to hearing loss. According to Erdman (2009), patients must be engaged in their own rehabilitation if they are to adjust to hearing loss. Technology cannot substitute for a therapeutic relationship.

EMBRACING COUNSELING IN PRACTICE

Counseling has long been acknowledged as an important component to the AR process. We are all aware of the need to counsel parents when their child has been identified as hearing impaired or to help a patient adjust to a sudden sensorineural hearing loss. There are many books and articles by such esteemed authors in the realm of audiologic counseling as Luterman, English, Erdman, and Greer Clark, to name a few. Resources are available to help build a foundation from which to approach counseling and patient-centered service delivery. There appears, however, to be a growing number of audiologists throughout the world who have begun to acknowledge the limitations of technology, and are now embracing the underlying concepts of counseling. At the core of this movement is the Ida Institute.

The Ida Institute was established with a mission to foster a better understanding of the human dynamics of hearing loss. As part of its mission, the Ida Institute began to reach out to audiologists around the world, and, with the help of talented faculty and staff, began to offer interactive workshops designed to

address what many believed were the unmet needs of both audiologists and patients. As a result of these workshops and the collaborative efforts of all involved, tools were developed that would guide the audiologist in practice toward building relationships with patients with hearing loss. A series of tools such as the Patient Journey were designed to help the audiologist and patient reflect on the pathway that brought them together. Motivation tools such as the Line, the Box, and the Circle help the audiologist assess readiness for aural rehabilitation, technology, and improved communication. Communication rings and the GPS are designed to engage communication partners in the AR process, and most recently the Living Well Tool is an exploration of patient beliefs and revelations about the meaning of living well with hearing loss.. A visit to the Ida Institute Web site (http://www.idainstitue.com) will introduce the audiologist to concepts and tools that can easily be incorporated in daily practice, and allow for a further exchange of ideas with audiologists around the world through participation in their interactive forums.

PUT THE AUDIOGRAM AWAY

The audiogram seems to have become a security blanket for most audiologists. The results are clear to us, we have identified the hearing loss, and we will base many of our decisions on these findings. We place it on a table before a patient and begin to explain the meaning of the O's and X's . . . for a sloping loss we can fit this hearing aid and for a severe loss that one, associating the hearing aid directly to the results on the audiogram. Ask most people with a hearing loss and they will tell you they don't understand their audiogram anyway. Yet, we tend to focus our counseling on degree and nature of hearing loss, perhaps because it is easier to talk about test results than the impact of the hearing loss itself. Are we afraid to veer away from the audiogram into the gray world of emotions and self-adjustment? Do we feel we are not trained adequately to engage in affective discussion with our patient? But then who is? Who better than the audiologist, with a keen understanding of hearing loss and its impact on communication and psychosocial functioning? Who better than the audiologist to address the feelings associated with hearing loss and relate supportively to those who are suffering? The bond between patient and audiologist can result in shared decisions regarding rehabilitation and support throughout the process. The audiologist can lead the person with hearing loss through the obstacles by providing a supporting hand.

People typically live many years with hearing loss before seeking help. Even when they are ready to seek help, they might not be ready for hearing aids, the help that we are always quick to offer. We talk to patients with varying degrees of hearing loss and expect a certain type of reaction to a specific audiogram. If they present with a moderate level of loss, we expect they will complain about trouble communicating. But what if they say, "I don't have any problem?" What is our typical reaction? We claim they are in denial or haven't come to terms with the fact they have hearing loss. We are too quick to judge, too quick to let the audiogram sway our impressions. But, perhaps, they are not yet ready? Perhaps, they need more time, more communication failure, more nudging, or perhaps more counseling? Engaging patients in dialog about hearing loss, encouraging participation of communication partners, accepting decisions about hearing loss are all ways that can help build successful therapeutic relationships. We do not have to teach our patients about their hearing loss; they have plenty of knowledge on their own. Embrace their knowledge and let them move at their own pace toward whatever rehabilitation becomes appropriate.

It is important as audiologists that we remember the journey that led our patients to us. We need to take time and listen. Stop talking. Let this individual with hearing loss share his journey, his life with hearing loss and the people who make up his world. Work together to identify areas of difficulty, and share the goal of improving communication. Put the audiogram down and interact. Embrace our role as counselors and provide a person-centered service that will allow a shared partnership between you, the patient, and, yes in many circumstances, technology. However, instead of having technology at the center of this relationship, let's make sure it is the person with hearing loss at the core.

REFERENCES

ASHA. (2001). Knowledge and skills required for the practice of audiologic/aural rehabilitation. *ASHA desk reference* (Vol. 4). Rockville, MD: Author.

Duchan, J. F. (2004). Maybe audiologists are too attached to the medical model. *Seminars in Hearing, 25,* 347–354.

Erdman, S. A. (2009). Audiologic counseling: A biopsychosocial approach. In J. Montano & J. Spitzer (Eds.), *Adult audiologic rehabilitation* (pp. 171–216). San Diego, CA: Plural.

Erdman, S. A., Wark, D., & Montano, J. J. (1994). Implications of service delivery models in audiology. *Journal of the Academy of Rehabilitative Audiology, 27,* 45–60.

Gagne, J. P., & Jennings, M. B. (2011, July 5). Incorporating a client-centered approach to audiologic rehabilitation. *ASHA Leader.*

Hochberg, M. (2007, April). The doctor's white coat—an historical perspective. *Virtual Mentor, 9*(4), 310–314. Retrieved from Virtualmentor.ama-assn.org/2007/04/mhst1-0704.html

Ida Institute. (2011) *Living well with hearing loss.* Presentation at the Hearing Loss Association of America Annual Meeting. June 16, 2011, Arlington, VA.

Kochkin, S. (2009, October). MarkeTrak VIII: 25 year trends in the hearing health market. *Hearing Review*, 12–30.

Montano, J. (2009). Defining audiologic rehabilitation. In J. Montano & J. Spitzer (Eds.), *Adult audiologic rehabilitation* (pp. 25–38). San Diego, CA: Plural.

Montano, J. (2011). Building relationships: An important component to the aural rehabilitation process. *ENT and Audiology, 20*(4), 91–92.

Ross, M. (1997). A retrospective look at the future of aural rehabilitation. *Journal of the Academy of Rehabilitative Audiology, 30,* 11–28.

Steering Committee ASHA Special Interest Division 7. (1992, August). Spotlight on Special Interest Division 7: Audiologic rehabilitation. *ASHA,* 18.

Ventry, I. M., & Weinstein, B. E. (1982). The hearing handicap inventory for the elderly: A new tool. *Ear and Hearing, 3*(3), 128–134.

ESSAY 15

Noise Exposure and the ❧ Potential Impact on Hearing in ❧ the Pediatric Population

Yula C. Serpanos and Abbey L. Berg

It is an honor and privilege to be asked to contribute this chapter in the memory of Dr. Sadanand Singh. There is not a person in the communication sciences and disorders profession who is unfamiliar with his name and publishing company. Always gracious and a true gentleman, Dr. Singh greeted everyone who came in contact with him with warmth and a smile. Although you may not have been ready to write a book he was encouraging and supportive to everyone in the field. He touched people both personally and on the more public level, a legacy not many achieve. There are few individuals who are irreplaceable; Dr. Sadanand Singh is one of those. The profession mourns our loss and is grateful for his support, contributions, and friendship.

BACKGROUND AND CONCERNS

A key role in audiologic scope of practice, in addition to the identification, assessment, and rehabilitation of auditory/vestibular disorders, is the promotion of hearing wellness, hear-ing loss prevention, and protection (American Speech-Language-Hearing Association [ASHA], 2004). Increases in noise exposures that are part of the social environment and unrelated to occupational exposure or physiologic changes due to age and/or disease have heightened the need to educate the public on the hazards of noise-related hearing loss. Depending on sound level and duration of exposure, noise-related hearing impairment is associated with tinnitus and sensorineural high frequency hearing loss (HFHL), typically in the 3000 to 6000 Hz region. After age, excessive exposure to noise is the most common cause of acquired sensorineural HFHL (Royster, 1996).

The impact of noise on hearing in the pediatric population warrants attention. The resiliency of the auditory system due to noise exposure in children is unknown and may be different than adults (Niskar, Kieszak, Holmes, Esteban, Rubin, & Brody, 2001). Factors such as individual variation in the anatomical structures of the external auditory canal and middle ear structures, exposure to ototoxic drugs, and genetics affect suscepti-bility (National Institutes of Health [NIH], 1990). High-frequency hearing loss affects speech recognition particularly in background noise, and can compromise academic perfor-mance as well as social relationships in young individuals (Niskar, Kieszak, Holmes, Este-ban, Rubin, & Brody, 1998). Children with noise-related hearing loss are at further risk for greater levels of hearing loss in adulthood (Brookhouser, 1992).

There are societal costs to hearing loss as well. Ruben (2000) calculated the economic effect of communication disorders and found considerably higher unemployment rates and lower income; reported income for the hearing-impaired population was 40 to 45% of that of the non-hearing-impaired. Of note, communication disorders were more prevalent in individuals of lower socioeconomic status (SES) than individuals of mid- to high-SES (Ruben, 2000).

An increase in hearing loss in the pediat-ric and adolescent populations has been well documented over the past two decades, espe-cially in the high frequency regions. The most recent National Health and Nutrition Exami-nation Survey (NHANES) reports that 1 in 5 adolescents presents with hearing loss, most commonly in the high frequencies, a one-third increase in prevalence within the decade (Shar-gorodsky, Curhan, Curhan, & Eavey, 2010). Berg and Serpanos (2011) found that HFHL doubled over a 24-year period, from 1985 to 2008, in a group of adolescent females from an urban residential foster care facility. Niskar and colleagues (1998) reported that 13% of a cross-sectional American population of chil-dren age 12 to 19 years had HFHL ≥16 dB HL in at least one ear. In addition, an even higher prevalence of HFHL has been observed in children of low-SES (Erlandsson, Holmes, Widén, & Bohlin, 2008; Niskar et al., 2001), supporting Ruben's (2000) findings.

NOISE EXPOSURE IN THE PEDIATRIC POPULATION

Numerous sources of noise can affect the pedi-atric population from infancy to adolescence. It is well documented that excessive noise, such as is present in neonatal intensive care units (NICU), affects the overall health and development of premature infants (Ameri-can Academy of Pediatrics [AAP, 1997]). As vulnerable infants may spend many weeks or months in the NICU environment, the AAP (1997) recommends noise levels <50 dBA. In a recent study, Berg, Chavez, and Serpa-nos (2010) found noise often exceeded those levels in a newly designed NICU, suggestive of perhaps a more pervasive indication of existing noise levels in NICU environments. Modest modifications to the physical environ-ment and the routine and periodic education of medical personnel and family members to monitor conversational levels were effective in reducing excessive noise and brought noise levels within acceptable levels, that is, below 50 dBA (Berg et al., 2010).

Throughout childhood, exposures to numerous sources of excessive noise such as toys that emit intense sounds, firecrackers, and firearms may occur. Adolescents may operate or be in very close proximity to machinery that includes power tools, snowmobiles, tractors, vacuums, and lawn care devices. In addition, exposure to music, specifically, the playing of musical instruments in bands, concert atten-dance, and car-stereo listening contributes to potentially toxic levels (Brookhouser, 1992).

Among the many contributing factors of noise exposure, increasingly common is the recreational use of personal listening devices (PLDs) such as iPods and MP3 players (Vogel, Verschuure, van der Ploeg, Brug, & Raat, 2009). In the past 5 years there has been a four-fold increase in PLD device ownership by children (ASHA, n.d.). These devices have been associated with an increased incidence of HFHL as well as reported tinnitus in the adolescent population (Berg & Serpanos, 2011). Of concern to hearing is the level and frequency of device use, as a synergistic effect between the intensity level of PLDs and duration of use has been documented (Fligor & Cox, 2004). Research has shown that with frequent PLD use, adolescents tend to listen to music at high volumes and actively avoid device noise-limiting features (Vogel et al., 2009). Measures on current PLDs suggest maximum output levels up to 125 dBA depending on earphone style, with greater output levels recorded with in-ear style than with supra-aural earphones (Keith, Michaud, & Chiu, 2008).

RESPONSE TO INCREASED PREVALENCE OF NOISE EXPOSURE AND NOISE-RELATED HEARING LOSS

Steps have been taken to address the issue of excessive noise levels and the potential effect on hearing. Federal legislation enacted by United States Environmental Protection Agency Noise Control Act 42 U.S.C. §4901 (1972) to protect and inform the public on potentially hazardous noise-emitting products, established a labeling system requiring manufacturers to provide a noise rating of the product decibel output. In 1990 the National Institutes of Health (NIH) issued a consensus statement on noise and hearing loss. Recommendations included incentives to manufacturers of occupational, medical, and recreational devices to design quieter instruments as well as to regulate product noise emission. Re-establishment of a central agency

that would regulate, govern, and coordinate efforts was urged (NIH, 1990).

Research continues to investigate safe PLD listening guidelines. Fligor (2007) recommends that use of PLDs with headphones be limited to no more than one hour per day at a maximum of 60% of the gain output, and no more than 80% for 90 minutes using in-ear style earphones. Recent effort to limit the risks of hearing loss using sound isolation devices, noise cancellation earphones, or automatic volume limiting systems programmed into PLDs has occurred (Council on Science and Public Health, 2008).

In response to the increase in noise-related hearing loss, the American Academy of Audiology (AAA) and the American Speech-Language-Hearing Association (ASHA) launched hearing health education initiatives to raise public awareness. These initiatives include a Web site, national media advertisement through radio and television, school education programs, and concerts promoting safe listening practice with PLDs. The "Turn It to the Left" campaign by AAA provides fact sheets as well as a "rap" on noise-induced hearing loss (AAA, n.d.). In 2006, ASHA launched "America: Tuned In Today . . . But Tuned Out Tomorrow?" to promote safe listening practice with PLD use (ASHA, n.d.). The "Listen to Your Buds" campaign is geared to young children, and provides a source of information to parents and educators about the risk of hearing loss with PLD misuse (ASHA, n.d.).

These aggressive public health campaigns regarding the hazards of excessive noise, however, are not reaching the populations most in need, adolescents and particularly at-risk adolescents. It has been reported that adolescents often do not respond to educational efforts (Fligor & Cox, 2004). Florentine, Hunter, Robinson, Ballou, and Buss (1998) found that detrimental listening behaviors persisted in some adolescents despite evidence that cochlear damage occurred. Furthermore, Olsen Widén and Erlandsson (2004) determined that adolescents of lower-SES exhibited more risk-taking behaviors and used hearing protection less frequently than children of higher-SES. Listening to music at levels intense enough to cause hearing loss is an example of risk-taking behavior (Erlandsson et al., 2008).

Despite the rising and consistent body of evidence that confirms increased HFHL in the pediatric population, the most current AAA and ASHA hearing screening guidelines recommend hearing screening at octave intervals of 1000 to 4000 Hz, missing potentially disabling hearing loss at 3000 Hz and 6000 Hz (AAA, 1997; ASHA, 1997). In contrast, ASHA (2005) revised diagnostic test criteria for pure tone hearing threshold to include the routine testing of 3000 Hz and 6000 Hz, in addition to octave frequencies of 250 to 8000 Hz.

FUTURE DIRECTIONS

A challenge for the health and medical disciplines and governing agencies is to disseminate findings and recommendations with consensus and make accessible to the profession and general population the information gleaned from research on noise-related hearing loss, the various causes, and its prevention. The following recommendations are suggested:

1. Regular and periodic education of NICU personnel regarding noise-reduction practices, along with routine monitoring of noise levels in newborn nurseries, particularly neonatal intensive care units where infants may spend several weeks and months. This must be seen as a responsibility of audiologists.
2. Guidelines from AAA and ASHA need to reflect current knowledge; that is, the inclusion of the interoctave frequencies of 3000 to 6000 Hz in a hearing screening protocol to identify earlier HFHL.
3. Continued research to determine specific guidelines for safe listening with PLDs, toys, and other noise-emitting devices. Consensus among the hearing science and medical disciplines and governing agencies must be reached. Only then can public health campaigns on the health hazards of noise be effective.
4. Continued research and development of sound isolation devices, noise cancellation earphones, and automatic volume limiting systems, which must be programmed into toys, PLDs, and other noise-emitting products. Hearing protection devices must be comfortable, and provide natural-sounding auditory experiences for individuals to use them. Attenuation of the device must be accurately labeled (NIH, 1990).
5. Legislation to limit excessive noise levels and to require disclaimers on toys, PLDs, and other mainstream noise-emitting products. A joint committee made up of experts from various disciplines in the hearing sciences and audiology, medical, public health, and governing agencies, similar in structure to the Joint Committee on Infant Hearing, should be established. This committee would periodically review current practices and research, modifying recommendations as deemed necessary.
6. Development of effective hearing conservation campaigns that target: (a) children at young ages, beginning at preschool, and throughout the elementary years; and (b) adolescents, particularly from at-risk populations (e.g., low SES). Hearing conservation programs and campaigns must show effectiveness. These public health campaigns to raise public awareness exist for dangers and risks associated

with drug and alcohol abuse, smoking, and exposure to ultraviolet rays. Similar to other health hazards, updated hearing screening guidelines and noise education and prevention should be endorsed by the American Academy of Pediatrics.

REFERENCES

American Academy of Audiology. (n.d.). *Turn it to the left*. Retrieved June 24, 2011, from http://www.turnittotheleft.com

American Academy of Audiology. (1997). Identification of hearing loss and middle-ear dysfunction in preschool and school-age children. Retrieved June 29, 2011, from http://www.audiology.org/resources/documentlibrary/Pages/HearingLossChildren.aspx

American Academy of Pediatrics (Committee on Environmental Health). (1997). Noise: A hazard for the fetus and newborn. *Pediatrics, 100*, 724–727.

American Medical Association. (2008). Portable listening devices and noise-induced hearing loss. *Council on science and public health report 6-A-08.* Retrieved July 5, 2011, from http://www.ama-assn.org/resources/doc/csaph/csaph6a08.pdf

American Speech-Language-Hearing Association. (n.d.). Listen to your buds. Retrieved July 5, 2011, from http://www.listentoyourbuds.org/learn

American Speech-Language-Hearing Association. (1997). Guidelines for audiologic screening. Retrieved June 24, 2011, from http://www.asha.org/docs/html/GL1997-00199.html

American Speech-Language-Hearing Association. (2004). Scope of practice in audiology. Retrieved June 22, 2011, from http://www.asha.org/policy. doi:10.1044/policy.SP2004-00192

American Speech-Language-Hearing Association. (2005). Guidelines for manual pure-tone threshold audiometry. Retrieved June 22, 2011, from http://www.asha.org/policy. doi:10.1044/policy.GL2005-00014

Berg, A., Chavez, C., & Serpanos, Y. C. (2010). Noise levels in a tertiary neonatal intensive care unit. *Contemporary Issues in Communication Science and Disorders, 37*, 70–73.

Berg, A., & Serpanos, Y. C. (2011). High frequency hearing sensitivity in adolescent females of lower socioeconomic status over a 24-year period (1985–2008). *Journal of Adolescent Health, 48*(2), 203–208.

Brookhouser P. E., Worthington, D. W., & Kelly, W. J. (1992). Noise-induced hearing loss in children. *Laryngoscope, 102*, 645–655.

Erlandsson, S. I., Holmes A., Widén S.E., & Bohlin, M. (2008). Cultural and social perspectives on attitudes, noise, and risk behavior in children and young adults. *Seminars in Hearing, 29*(1), 29–41.

Fligor, B. J. (2007). Hearing loss and iPods: What happens when you turn them to 11? *Hearing Journal, 60*(10), 10–16.

Fligor, B. J., & Cox, L. C. (2004). Output levels of commercially available portable compact disc players and the potential risk to hearing. *Ear and Hearing, 25*, 513–527.

Florentine, M., Hunter, W., Robinson, M., Ballou, M., & Buus, S. (1998). On the behavioral characteristics of loud-music listening. *Ear and Hearing, 19*, 420–428.

Keith, S. E., Michaud, D. S., & Chiu, V. (2008). Evaluating the maximum playback sound levels from portable digital audio players. *Journal of the Acoustical Society of America, 123*(6), 4227–4237.

National Institutes of Health. (1990). Consensus conference: Noise and hearing loss. *Journal of the American Medical Association, 263*(23), 3185–3190.

Niskar, A. S., Kieszak, S. M., Holmes, A. E., Esteban, E., Rubin, C., & Brody, D. J. (1998). Prevalence of hearing loss among children 6 to 19 years of age: The third national health and nutrition examination survey. *Journal of the American Medical Association, 279*(14), 1071–1075.

Niskar, A. S., Kieszak, S. M., Holmes, A. E., Esteban, E., Rubin, C., & Brody, D. J. (2001). Estimated prevalence of noise-induced threshold shifts among children 6 to 19 years of age: The third national health and nutrition examination survey, 1988–1994, United States. *Pediatrics, 25*, 4–9.

Olsen Widén, S. E., & Erlandsson, S. I. (2004). The influence of socioeconomic status on adolescent attitude to social noise and hearing protection. *Noise Health, 25*, 59–70.

Royster, J. D. (1996). Noise-induced hearing loss. In J. Northern (Ed.), *Hearing disorders* (3rd ed., pp. 177–189). Needham Heights, MA: Allyn & Bacon.

Ruben, R. J. (2000). Redefining the survival of the fittest: Communication disorders in the 21st century. *Laryngoscope, 110*(2), 241–245. doi: 10.1097/00005537-200002010-00010

Shargorodsky, J., Curhan, S. G., Curhan, G. C., & Eavey, R. (2010). Change in prevalence of hearing loss in U.S. adolescents. *Journal of the American Medical Association, 304*(7), 772–778. doi: 10.1001/jama.2010.1124

United States Environmental Protection Agency Noise Control Act, 42 U.S.C. §4901. (1972).

Vogel, I., Verschuure, H., van der Ploeg, C. P., Brug, J., & Raat, H. (2009). Adolescents and MP3 players: Too many risks, too few precautions. *Pediatrics, 123*(6),e953–e958. doi: 10.1542/peds.2008-3179

ESSAY 16

Off-Label Use of ❧ Norm-Referenced Tests in ❧ Speech-Language Pathology

Insights Gained from Children With Hearing Impairment

Peter Flipsen Jr.

I did not know Dr Singh personally for very long. Thus, I cannot be certain that he had a major impact on my own career. He did, however, have some influence. I first met Dr. Singh in Boston at the 2007 ASHA convention when he agreed to publish a book dedicated to my doctoral mentor. Although he stated up front that the book we were proposing had limited appeal, he felt strongly that publishing a work honoring the career of a valued researcher in the discipline was simply the right thing to do. Of course I was pleased by his reaction, but I was also not totally surprised. Over the years I had heard many stories about him from former professors and colleagues. It had long been clear that few could match Dr. Singh's dedication to publishing in the field of communication disorders whether or not there was much profit in it. I believe that he received ASHA's Honors of the Association in 2006 largely because of this. The reaction of many in our discipline to the passing of Dr. Singh only served to reinforce my first impressions. We have lost an incredible asset to the discipline, and his impact will clearly be missed.

The use of a procedure or treatment in a way for which it was not originally intended and particularly for which it was not specifically approved is often referred to as *off-label* use. In medicine such use is not uncommon. Bradley, Finkelstein, and Stafford (2006), for example, estimated that 21% of prescriptions given out by physicians in 2001 appeared to have been for applications not specifically approved by the Food and Drug Administration. Such applications are legal and not necessarily a bad thing. They offer patients new options that may be the ultimate solution to their problem. On the other hand, they rely heavily on physician judgment about the quality and strength of often limited evidence. They also rely heavily on physician judgment about the relative and somewhat unknown risks and benefits to types of patients who have not been exposed to that treatment.

In the field of speech-language pathology one analog to such off-label use is the application of norm-referenced tests to populations for which they were not originally intended. As with off-label use by physicians, such uses in our field also rely heavily on the judgment of the practitioner, in this case the speech-language pathologist (SLP). In this particular case, that judgment tends to be guided largely by some basic principles. First, as standardized procedures, norm-referenced tests must be administered in specific ways. Changes to how a test is administered (beyond any variation specified by the test manual) would mean that the norms could not be used. For example, if the stimuli are to be presented orally, presenting them manually (e.g., using signs) would not be appropriate. Likewise the examinee must fully understand the tasks involved (i.e., know what they are being asked to do), or use of the test norms would also not be appropriate.

A second principle guiding off-label use of norm-referenced tests is that the examinee must be able to perform the tasks (i.e., understanding what is expected is not enough). Individuals with motor impairments in particular might be very challenged to perform timed tasks. As well, those with visual impairments would have trouble with a picture-pointing task, such as that used in the popular *Peabody Picture Vocabulary Test-Fourth Edition* (PPVT-4; Dunn & Dunn, 2007).

Applying both of these first two principles is usually straightforward with the most severely involved examinees. Individuals with the most severe cognitive impairments may never understand how to perform some tasks, and individuals with the most severe physical impairments may never be physically able to carry them out. It is in the case of mild and moderate impairments where clinician judgment comes into play. Our experience with particular populations may allow us to see whether use of a particular test is appropriate. Even with experience we may occasionally doubt our decisions in this regard, however.

Of course, neither of these first two principles would preclude use of norm-referenced test tasks and stimuli in alternative ways, such as using the test as a criterion measure. For example, the test stimuli could be presented in some consistent fashion that fits the examinee's situation, and raw scores could then be used to track progress in therapy (something we wouldn't, of course, do with standard scores; McCauley & Swisher, 1984). Dunn and Dunn (2007), for example, support such a criterion approach with second language learners when using their PPVT-4.

A third principle guiding off-label use of norm-referenced tests is the question of whether the examinee is similar enough to the test normative population for the norms to apply. Here we have to recall that the goal is to determine how an examinee is doing relative to *normal*, and clearly there are different senses of normal. We need to have the appropriate comparison group. Here we can take two different perspectives. First, we could be asking about cultural or linguistic similarity. If the examinees are from a nonmainstream culture, the testing process may be quite unfamiliar to them, putting them at a significant disadvantage when asked to respond to the test tasks. For example, parents of white, European background routinely engage their children in question-and-answer routines in which the adult already knows the answer to the question. In many Native American cultures, such routines rarely occur, as they may be viewed as wasting the limited breaths many native cultures assume we are born with (Harris, 1998). Another example is the inner-city African-American child whose dialect (e.g., African-American Vernacular English) has an adult target which is quite different from the mainstream English target that is assumed by most of tests we use. Some test manuals do offer guidance for adjusting for such dialect differences, whereas many do not. Without such adjustments, speakers of nonstandard dialects may be inadvertently labeled as having a language disorder, when no such disorder exists.

Such potential confusions were a major motivation for the development of the *Diagnostic Evaluation of Language Variation* (DELV; Seymour, Roeper, de Villiers, & de Villiers, 2003).

The second perspective on similarity to the normative population (assuming cultural and linguistic similarity) is the degree to which the examinee has been represented in the normative population. This is the ultimate question of who we are to compare our clients against. According to Hutchinson (1996), it depends on our goal. Hutchinson noted that comparing an individual with a traumatic brain injury to a population of others with similar injuries may be crucial to planning treatment and/or accommodations while comparing them to those without such injury may be crucial to determining school and/or grade placement. Similar arguments could readily be made for other populations such as those who have cognitive or hearing impairments.

NEW INSIGHTS FROM STUDYING CHILDREN WITH HEARING IMPAIRMENT

SLPs working with individuals with hearing impairment have long resisted the temptation to use most norm-referenced tests with children with hearing impairment (the exception being use of the few such tests that have been specifically normed on this population). In the era of stand-alone schools for the deaf the basic argument was that the most appropriate comparison group was peers from the same population. Recent trends to downsize or close such schools in favor of mainstreaming have muted the validity of such arguments. However, two reasons for avoidance of such tests continue to be voiced. First, ensuring comprehension of the instructions may be a problem, since these tests must almost always be presented orally. Except for those with

milder hearing losses and/or those with better amplified hearing acuity, using these tests violates the first principle described above. Second, there is a practical reason. If such tests are used, the resulting standard scores are often below the lowest limits of the norms. We commonly see *floor effects* with reports such as "below 40." Such scores are essentially meaningless, as they offer minimal insight into how far below normal the performance was. This very poor performance at least suggests that children with significant hearing impairment are a qualitatively different population, compared to children with normal hearing. This would then also constitute a violation of the third principle described above.

Some recent developments suggest that it might be acceptable to engage in some type of off-label use with this particular population. The first relates specifically to children with severe or profound hearing loss who receive cochlear implants. Clinicians with limited experience with this population may assume that because of their hearing loss, the use of norm-referenced tests would still be inappropriate. Clinicians with more experience, however, appreciate that aided thresholds with a cochlear implant elevate these children from a severe or profound loss to a very mild or mild loss. Even with such knowledge, clinicians might still hesitate to apply such tests. Two recent studies suggest that such hesitation is unwarranted. Baldassari et al. (2009) evaluated a group of 36 children who had been fitted with cochlear implants at an average age of 33 months. The children's performance on the *Test of Auditory Comprehension* (TAC; Southwest School, 1981), which is a test normed on children with hearing impairment who used hearing aids, was examined. Results showed significantly better performance by the children with implants. At the same time, comparison against children with normal hearing using both the *Test of Auditory Comprehension of Language* (TACL; Carrow-Woolfolk, 1999) and the *Bracken Basic Concept Scale-Revised* (BBCS-R; Bracken, 1998) indicated average performance within one standard deviation of their age group mean. Note that no actual control groups were used in that study; the comparisons were against the test norms only. A study by Flipsen (2011) looked at speech production performance of 15 children with cochlear implants with an average age of implantation of 42 months. Results from the *Goldman-Fristoe Test of Articulation* (GFTA-2; Goldman & Fristoe, 2000) indicated only one floor effect score. When amount of implant experience (what might be called *hearing age*) was used for the comparisons instead of chronological age, 14 of 15 children performed within 1.5 standard deviations of their age group mean. Again, this was relative to the norms for children with normal hearing; there was no control group in the study. Together, these two studies suggest that meaningful results can be obtained for these children with tests normed on the normal-hearing population. Perhaps most importantly, these findings highlight the fact that clinicians should be regularly revisiting their assumptions about their assessment practices.

Another development in this area relates to obtaining meaningful test scores with individuals with hearing impairment, but without cochlear implants. As noted above, scores of "below 40" are not very informative. Vaden (2001) studied 11 children age 6 to 11 years with bilateral hearing loss, who used hearing aids and primarily spoken language to communicate. The goal of the study was to examine the role of spoken language skills in problem-solving abilities in this population. Initial test results indicated several floor effect scores. In trying to examine the relationship between the two types of skills, such floor effect scores could not reasonably be used. In order to obtain more precise and thus more meaningful standard scores, Vaden chose to mathematically extrapolate the values in the normative tables downward. Doing so provided more specific standard scores and allowed her to show that language skills significantly predicted problem solving skills. Although the validity of such an extrapolation approach has not been established, findings from that study motivated Flipsen, Thelin, and Thelin (2002) to revisit the question of how to deal with floor effects. In addition to the possibility of extrapolating the normative tables downward, two other solutions were suggested by Flipsen et al. (2002). First, many clinicians may not be aware that some test authors and publishers actually have and will make available, on request, what are sometimes called *extended norms tables*. These represent additional data that are usually based on smaller samples that were not included in the published norms. Rather than pure extrapolations, these represent a combination of data on real children who exhibited very low performance, combined with some amount of extrapolation.

The second solution for dealing with floor effect scores that was proposed by Flipsen et al. (2002), was to use mean and standard deviation values provided in many test manuals to compute *z*-scores, which indicate the number of standard deviations from the mean. For example, using Table 4.18 on p. 51 of the PPVT-4 test manual, a child age 5 years, 2 months who achieved a raw score of 13 would have scored at 3 standard deviations below the mean. The calculation goes like this: examinee's raw score (13) – age group raw score mean (82.2), divided by age group raw score standard deviation (23.1). For tests that count errors rather than number of items correct, such as the GFTA-2, a raw score of 34 for the same child would yield a score of 2.5 standard deviations from the mean. This was calculated using data in Table 6.5 on p. 55 of the GFTA-2 manual, as: age group raw score mean (8.6) – examinee's raw score (34), divided by age group raw standard deviation (10.8).

CONCLUSION

We have many reasons to avoid off-label use of norm-referenced tests. However, new developments can alter our sense of when to do so. Recent performance by children with cochlear implants suggests that it may be appropriate to use such tests with these children. Likewise, despite a tendency to avoid these tests because of floor effects, there appear to be ways to turn such effects into meaningful test scores.

REFERENCES

Baldassari, C. M., Schmidt, C., Schubert, C. M., Srinivasan, P., Dodson, K. M., & Sismanis, A. (2009). Receptive language outcomes in children after cochlear implantation. *Otolaryngology-Head and Neck Surgery, 140,* 114–119.

Bracken, B. (1998). *Bracken basic concept scale-revised.* San Antonio, TX: Psychological Corporation.

Bradley, D. C., Finkelstein, S. N., & Stafford, R.S. (2006). Off-label prescribing among office-based physicians. *Archives of Internal Medicine, 166,* 1021–1026.

Carrow-Woolfolk, E. (1999). *Test for auditory comprehension of language.* Austin, TX: Pro-Ed.

Dunn, L. M., & Dunn, D. M. (2007). *Peabody Picture Vocabulary Test-Fourth Edition.* Minneapolis, MN: NCS Pearson.

Flipsen, P., Jr. (2011). Examining speech sound acquisition for children with cochlear implants using the GFTA-2. *Volta Review, 111*(1), 25–37.

Flipsen, P., Jr., Thelin, J. W., & Thelin, S. J. (2002, July). *Very low test scores: Some issues and solutions.* Poster presented at the 23rd annual Symposium on Research in Child Language Disorders (SRCLD), Madison, WI.

Goldman, R., & Fristoe, M. (2000). *Goldman-Fristoe Test of Articulation-Second Edition.* Minneapolis, MN: NCS Pearson.

Harris, G. A. (1998). American Indian cultures: A lesson in diversity. In D. E. Battle (Ed.) *Communication disorders in multicultural populations-Second Edition,* (pp. 117–156). Boston, MA: Butterworth-Heinemann.

Hutchinson, T. A. (1996). What to look for in the technical manual: Twenty questions for users. *Language, Speech, and Hearing Services in Schools, 27*(2), 109–121.

McCauley, R. J., & Swisher, L. (1984). Use and misuse of norm-referenced tests in clinical assessment: A hypothetical case. *Journal of Speech and Hearing Disorders, 49,* 338–348.

Seymour, H. N., Roeper, T. W., de Villiers, J., & de Villiers, P. A. (2003). *Diagnostic evaluation of language variation.* San Antonio, TX: PsychCorp.

Southwest School for the Hearing Impaired. (1981). *Test of auditory comprehension.* North Hollywood, CA: Foreworks.

Vaden, K. A. (2001). *Language in relation to problem solving abilities in children with hearing impairment.* Unpublished master's thesis, University of Tennessee, Knoxville, TN.

PART IV

Communication Disorders and Movement Science

ESSAY 17

Collaborating With Exercise Science

Helping Older Adults Maintain Cognition and Communication

Michelle Gray, Barbara Bennett Shadden, Melissa Powers, and Ro DiBrezzo

Within the year after Dr. Singh created Plural Publishing, he sent me an email saying several colleagues had suggested I might be a good person to write an aphasia textbook. In our subsequent phone conversation, I said I had nothing new to add to the typical textbook market. Dr. Singh then asked what I would like to write about. I hesitantly shared my explorations of the impact of acquired neurogenic communication disorders on a person's sense of self, on their ability to share their life story. I talked about how closely I was working with sociology and psychology colleagues Pat Koski and Fran Hagstrom as we tried to understand this idea of narrative self. Dr. Singh essentially said, "Go for it," and we did! It is that kind of vision, that openness to new ideas and to interdisciplinary perspectives that made Dr. Singh a leader. Without him, our work probably would not have appeared in book form. Most research and publication is in part just plain work. For me that one book was more a labor of love because it was personal as well as professional . . . and Dr. Singh allowed it to come to life.

— BBS

It is not necessary to be a practitioner in speech-language pathology or exercise science to know that mental and physical exercise are widely praised as ways to forestall some of the less pleasant consequences of normal and pathological aging. In the movement sciences, the evidence for the health benefits of exercise is well established (Thompson, Gordon, & Pescatello, 2010), although more research is needed particularly relative to the mechanisms of exercise. In the cognitive domain, numerous programs have been created to explore the efficacy of different cognitive interventions on specific cognitive behaviors and overall cognitive functioning in normally aging persons, as well as those with mild cognitive impairment (MCI) and/or dementia. Benefits have been identified, although many questions remain regarding the breadth of benefits as well as their generalizability.

The vast majority of studies of the benefits of mental and physical exercise for aging individuals are prime examples of translational research, in that the intervention is designed to be as close as possible to any practical application of the program, should the outcomes prove efficacious. One of the hallmarks of translational work is the fact that it typically involves interdisciplinary initiatives. A particularly intriguing line of research and potential preventive intervention for speech-language pathologists (SLPs) is the effects of physical exercise (with and without cognitive exercise) on cognitive/linguistic functions. Both cognitive and physical exercise programs have been shown to prevent cognitive decline or promote cognitive functions in the aging. With the appropriate translational research, such programs could make a difference in the lives of aging Baby Boomers.

The idea of preventing cognitive decline and more importantly preventing/delaying the onset of conditions like Alzheimer's disease is consistent with the scope of practice of SLPs (Schreck, 2010). In the American Speech-Language Hearing Association's (ASHA) 1988 position statement on prevention, prevention activities are defined as those that work toward elimination of the onset of disorders or that promote maintenance of optimal communication. ASHA's recognition of the unique needs of aging individuals can be seen in its commitment to the national Partnerships for Health in Aging initiative sponsored by the American Geriatrics Society (AGS).

SLPs are comfortable with the idea of exercise in a number of arenas (e.g., oral sensorimotor function in dysarthria or swallowing), and it has been suggested that we apply principles of exercise science to disorders such as dysphagia (Burkhead, Lazarus, Robbins, & Steele, 2008). However, partnerships with exercise scientists and involvement in exercise programs are the exception, not the rule. At the University of Arkansas, through the Office for Studies on Aging and the Human Performance Laboratory, one such partnership has continued over more than a decade, leading to multiple research projects and community exercise programs involving cognitive/linguis-

tic outcome measures. The collaboration has been a rich one, resulting in additional data on the effects of exercise participation on memory, mood, executive function, and language behaviors (Powers, Fort, Di Brezzo, & Shadden, 2008; Powers, Gray, Shadden, & Di Brezzo, 2007; Shadden, Powers, Di Brezzo, & Gray, 2008). Our experiences make clear that there are numerous opportunities for additional collaborations between communication disorders professionals and exercise scientists.

There is extensive literature on the effects of cognitive training on the functioning of both normally aging adults and those with or at risk for cognitive impairments. However, this essay focuses primarily on what is known about the impact of physical activity and exercise on cognition in aging individuals. The brief literature review is used to encourage speech-language pathologists as clinicians and researchers to become more involved in collaborative endeavors with those in the movement sciences. The essay concludes with recommendations for both translational research and clinical initiatives.

EXERCISE, FUNCTIONAL PERFORMANCE, AND COGNITIVE HEALTH AMONG OLDER ADULTS

It has long been recommended that all individuals, regardless of age, participate in regular, moderate to vigorous intensity activity most days of the week (Thompson et al., 2010). Participation in such activities reduces risk of illness, disease, and cognitive impairment and increases executive control, especially in late life (Chodzko-Zajko et al., 2009). The latter is an important consideration given consistent evidence that there are age-related decrements in executive functions. Cross-sectional studies suggest that higher levels of physical activity result in lower incidence of cognitive impairment and dementia (Laurin, Verreault, Lindsay, MacPherson, & Rockwood, 2001). More specifically, walking speed has been given greater attention of late, due to its negative association with overall mortality (Studenski et al., 2011) and positive association with cognitive ability (Marquis et al., 2002).

Even with the large body of evidence for the benefits of exercise participation, older adults remain less physically active than their younger counterparts (Pleis, Ward, & Lucas, 2010). In addition, these physical activities are generally less intense (Rafferty, Reeves, McGee, & Pivarnik, 2002). Although physical activity at any intensity has been shown to be efficacious for older adults, elevated cardiorespiratory fitness has also been linked to reduced cognitive decline over time among older adults (Barnes, Yaafe, Satariano, & Tager, 2003). Participating in regular exercise three or more days per week was associated with a reduction in the incidence of Alzheimer disease (Larson et al., 2006). Similarly, total distance walked, regardless of intensity, was positively related to performance on the Mini Mental State Examination (MMSE; Yaffe, Barnes, Nevitt, Lui, & Covinsky, 2001), a screening measure of current cognitive impairment. These studies suggest that regular physical activity at any intensity is directly related to cognitive function among older adults.

Cognition has been linked to functional fitness among older adults. Functional fitness is defined as having adequate muscular strength, endurance, and flexibility to perform activities of daily living. Cognitive speed-tasks are especially good predictors of functional performance, although non-speeded and sensory tasks are also predictive of functional performance (Wood et al., 2005). Bell-McGinty and colleagues (2002) have reported that tests of executive function account for 54% of the variance in functional status, even after accounting for age, sex, and education. Cognitive performance, rather than cognitive impairment, has also been associated with

increased rate of falls in an 8-year prospective study of adults over the age of 70 years (Anstey, von Sanden, & Luszcz, 2006). Participants scoring one point higher on the MMSE at baseline experienced 10% fewer falls over 8 years and change in performance on the MMSE was positively associated with number of falls experienced. In unpublished work by our group (Gray & Powers, 2011), the 8-foot up-and-go, a measure of dynamic balance and speed, has been positively correlated to Trail Making performance ($r = .653$). Also, the short physical performance battery, a measure of functional fitness among older adults, has been significantly correlated with better scores on the Trail Making test as well as fewer depressive symptoms (CES-D). In many of these studies, it can be difficult to determine whether cognitive functioning is influencing physical performance, or vice versa.

Recently, a new body of literature has emerged on the effects of regular exercise in protection against cognitive decline. Effects of interventions can be determined using change in indices of cognitive functions or measures of neural structure or function, such as atrophy of the hippocampus and total brain volume. However, given the cross-sectional nature of many studies, it can be difficult to discern cause-effect relationships. To explore such causal relationships, Colcombe and colleagues (2006) performed a longitudinal study of the impact of aerobic exercise over a six-month interval. The authors found increases in brain volume after the exercise program among a group of previously sedentary older adults. In a similar study, activity of the frontal and parietal lobes was increased after six months of a walking program in a group of community dwelling older adults (Colcombe et al., 2004).

In a meta-analysis of all randomized controlled trials between 1966 and 2001, Colcombe and Kramer (2003) report a greater effect on cognition for studies utilizing a combination of aerobic and resistance training when compared to aerobic-only interventions. This meta-analysis also established that the greatest effects of exercise interventions occurred in executive functions, although there were also significant effects for controlled processing, spatial tasks, and speeded tasks. Although the supporting evidence is limited, resistance training alone has also resulted in improvements in performance of cognitive tasks (Cassilhas et al., 2007; Lachman, Neupert, Bertrans, & Jette, 2006).

UNDERLYING PHYSIOLOGIC MECHANISMS

The specific mechanisms for the relationship between physical activity participation, physical function, and reduced cognitive impairment have not been definitively identified. In a recent review, Ratey and Loehr (2011) suggest that these mechanisms may be systemic (i.e., brain volume and electrocortical activity), molecular (i.e., brain-derived neurotrophic factor and insulin-like growth factor-1), and cellular (i.e., synaptic plasticity, neurogenesis, and vascular function). These pathways likely intersect with each other as increased synaptic plasticity may be due to increased activity of brain-derived neurotrophic factor and insulin-like growth factor-1. Most studies examining the mechanism linking physical activity and cognition use aerobic activities such as walking and jogging. Further study is needed to explain the mechanist link between resistance training and cognition.

THE BOTTOM LINE

It is hardly surprising to find that cognition and physical activity are linked in the elderly, given the underlying neural bases for such behaviors. Although there is no clear-cut exercise

prescription for increasing cognitive ability or maintaining cognition throughout life, there does seem to be a common theme across the reviewed literature. Any exercise, even at a low intensity and less than the recommended allotment, is better than being completely sedentary. Longitudinal studies suggest that participating in moderate activity for a lifetime protects individuals against cognitive impairment even when genetically predisposed for diseases such as Alzheimer disease (Larson et al., 2006). Furthermore, it is never too late to increase physical fitness and/or cognition. Longitudinal studies have shown exercise to be a beneficial and safe means of increasing cognition even at advanced ages (Colcombe & Kramer, 2003).

The American College of Sports Medicine, the primary national organization for exercise scientists, has developed recommendations for health and functional fitness for older adults (Thompson et al., 2010). As these guidelines are not specific for improvements in cognitive ability, we must rely on the limited literature that has linked physical activity and improvement and/or maintenance of cognitive ability. The majority of the studies reviewed used aerobic-type exercises. These types of activities are known to increase blood flow to the brain and have been postulated to increase cognition. However, resistance-type exercise has also been found to increase cognition among community-dwelling older adults.

RECOMMENDATIONS FOR COMMUNICATION SCIENCES AND DISORDERS

So what does the link between cognition and exercise among older adults mean for clinicians and researchers in speech-language pathology? First, as noted earlier, part of the scope of practice in our discipline involves prevention. Schreck (2010) has described an emerging role for SLPs in screening and prevention of cognitive deficits associated with aging. Key preventive elements she targets include: exercise, daily living activities, stress reduction, emotional stability, and general cognitive training. Thus, given the increasing number of older Americans and their desire to stay physically and mentally active, SLPs can facilitate maintenance of cognition and prevention of decline by: supporting older clients and their significant others in efforts to maintain appropriate levels of physical activity; encouraging older adults to engage in supervised exercise programs; and offering input and guidance to those conducting exercise programs in the community regarding the introduction of cognitive activities along with the physical components

Second, although SLPs do not routinely think of exercise programs as playing a role in treatment for clients with cognitive-communicative disorders, there is some evidence to suggest the collaboration between the two professions is beneficial. Lorenzen and Murray (2008) have encouraged clinicians to explore the benefits of a combination of physical fitness training and speech-language treatment. They discuss positive outcomes of such combined programs for both normally aging adults and those with specific communication disorders secondary to stroke, multiple sclerosis, and traumatic brain injury. Certainly, more research is needed in this area, and the work would require the alliance between an exercise scientist and an SLP. Considering the many neurological benefits attributed to exercise, it is reasonable to explore its role in combination with cognitive-communicative treatment specifically.

Finally, there clearly are many unanswered questions about the basic relationships between exercise and cognitive functioning as individuals age. In the research conducted to date, communication disorders professionals have played a limited role. Once again, there is a need for much stronger interdisciplin-

ary research partnerships between speech-language scientists and exercise scientists, as well as those in related disciplines. Only through such partnerships can appropriate physical and cognitive variables be targeted and systematically manipulated (including attention to the linguistic domain where the least work has been done). As the majority of exercise programs are conducted in groups, the role of group involvement as a social and communicative variable that provides additional framework for enhanced self-esteem and self-efficacy. These interactions should be explored and systematically studied, as it may play a role in promoting both physical and cognitive functioning.

What is important in this brief overview is the concept that interdisciplinary partnerships linking cognitive and physical functioning should be embraced by communication disorders professionals as we prepare for the Baby Boomers in our clinical caseloads and our research populations. As exercise scientists and SLPs share knowledge of the physical and cognitive domains, it will be possible to understand better the underlying mechanisms contributing to both normal changes in cognitive functioning and recovery from specific communication impairments. Translational research lies at the heart of such endeavors.

REFERENCES

American Speech-Language-Hearing Association. (1988). *Prevention of communication disorders* [Position statement]. Available from http://www.asha.org/policy. doi: 10.1044/policy. PS 1988-00228

Anstey, K. J., von Sanden, C., & Luszcz, M. A. (2006). An 8-year prospective study of the relationship between cognitive performance and falling in very old adults. *Journal of the American Geriatrics Society, 54,* 1169–1176.

Barnes, D. E., Yaffe, K., Satariano, W. A., & Tager, I. B. (2003). A longitudinal study of cardio-respiratory fitness and cognitive function in healthy older adults. *Journal of the American Geriatrics Society, 51,* 459–465.

Bell-McGinty, S., Podell, K., Franzen, M., Baird, A. D., & Williams, M. J. (2002). Standard measures of executive function in predicting instrumental activities of daily living in older adults. *International Journal of Geriatric Psychiatry, 17,* 828–834.

Burkhead, L., Lazarus, C., Robbins, J., & Steele, C. (2008, November). *The application of principles of exercise physiology to dysphagia rehabilitation.* Short course presented at the Annual Convention of the American Speech-Language-Hearing Association, Chicago, IL.

Cassilhas, R. C., Viana, V. A. R., Grassmann, V., Santos, R. T., Santos, R. F., Tufik, S., & Mello, M. T. (2007). The impact of resistance exercise on the cognitive function of the elderly. *Medicine & Science in Sports & Exercise, 39*(8), 1401–1407.

Chodzko-Zajko, W. J., Proctor, D. N., Fiatarone-Singh, M. A., Minson, C. T., Nigg, C. R., Salem, G. J., & Skinner, J. S. (2009). Position stand: Exercise and physical activity for older adults. *Medicine & Science in Sports & Exercise, 41*(7), 1510–1530. doi: 10.1249/MSS.0b013e3181a0c95c

Colcombe, S. J., Erickson, K. I., Scalf, P. E., Kim, J. S., Prakash, R., McAuley, E, . . . Kramer, A. F. (2006). Exercise: An active route to healthy aging: Aerobic exercise training increases brain volume in aging humans. *Journal of Gerontology: Medical Sciences, 61A*(11), 1166–1170.

Colcombe, S., & Kramer, A. F. (2003). Fitness effects on the cognitive function of older adults: A meta-analytic study. *Psychological Science, 14*(2), 125–130.

Colcombe, S. J., Kramer, A. F., Erickson, K. I., Scalf, P., McAuley, E. Cohen, N. J., . . . Elavsky, S. (2004). Cardiovascular fitness, cortical plasticity, and aging. *Proceedings of the National Academy of Sciences, 101*(9), 3316–3321.

Gray, M., & Powers, M. (2011). *Relationships between physical functioning outcomes and measures of cognitive function.* Unpublished raw data.

Lachman, M. E., Neupert, S. D., Bertrand, R., & Jette, A. M. (2006). The effects of strength training on memory in older adults. *Journal of Aging and Physical Activity, 14,* 59–73.

Larson, E. B., Wang, L., Bowen, J. D., McCormick, W. C., Teri, L., Crane, P., & Kukull, W. (2006). Exercise is associated with reduced risk for incident dementia among persons 65 years of age and older. *Annals of Internal Medicine, 144,* 73–81.

Laurin, D., Verreault, R., Lindsay, J., MacPherson, K., & Rockwood, K. (2001). Physical activity and risk of cognitive impairment and dementia in elderly persons. *Archives of Neurology, 58,* 498–504.

Lorenzen, B., & Murray, L. L. (2008). Benefits of physical fitness training in healthy aging and neurogenic patient populations. *Perspectives on Neurophysiology and Neurogenic Speech and Language Disorders, 18,* 99–106.

Marquis, S., Moore, M., Howeison, D. B., Sexton, G., Payami, H., Kaye, J. A., & Camicioli, R. (2002). Independent predictors of cognitive decline in healthy elderly persons. *Archives of Neurology, 59,* 601–606.

Pleis, J. R., Ward, B. W., & Lucas, J. W. (2010). Summary health statistics for U.S. adults: National health interview survey, 2009. *National Center for Health Statistics, Vital Health Statistics, 10*(249), 1–206.

Powers, M., Fort, I., Di Brezzo, R., & Shadden, B. B. (2008, November). *Effect of resistance training on cognitive function in older women.* Program No. 295-5. 2008 Abstract Viewer. National Harbor, MD: The Gerontological Society of America.

Powers, M., Gray, M., Shadden, B. B., & Di Brezzo, R. (2007). Mood and memory changes following exercise in older adults [Abstract]. *Gerontologist, 47* (II), 615.

Rafferty, A. P., Reeves, M. J., McGee, H. B., & Pivarnik, J. M. (2002). Physical activity patterns among walkers and compliance with public health recommendations. *Medicine & Science in Sports & Exercise, 34*(8), 1255–1261.

Ratey, J. J., & Loehr, J. E. (2011). The positive impact of physical activity on cognition during adulthood: A review of underlying mechanisms, evidence and recommendations. *Reviews in the Neurosciences, 22*(2), 171–185.

Schreck, J. S. (2010, November). *The impact of "normal" aging on cognitive-communication skills.* Short course presented at the Annual Convention of the American Speech-Language-Hearing Association, Philadelphia, PA.

Shadden, B. B., Powers, M., DiBrezzo, R., & Gray, M. (2008, November). *Influence of mood, memory, and health status on Cookie Theft picture description performance.* Poster session presented at the Annual Convention of the American Speech-Language-Hearing Association, Chicago, IL.

Studenski, S., Perera, S., Patel, K., Rosano, C., Faulkner, K., Inzitari, M., . . . Guralnik, J. (2011).

Gait speed and survival in older adults. *Journal of the American Medical Association, 305*(1), 50–58. doi: 10.1001/jama.2010.1923

Thompson, W. R., Gordon, N. F., & Pescatello, L. S. (Eds.). (2010). *ACSM's guidelines for exercise testing and prescription* (8th ed.). Philadelphia, PA: Lippincott Williams & Wilkins.

Wood, K. M., Edwards, J. D., Clay, O. J., Wadley, V. G., Roenker, D. L., & Ball, K. K. (2005). Sensory and cognitive factors influencing functional ability in older adults. *Gerontology, 51,* 131–141.

Yaffe, K., Barnes, D., Nevitt, M., Lui, L., & Covinsky, K. (2001). A prospective study of physical activity and cognitive decline in elderly women. *Archives of Internal Medicine, 161,* 1703–1708.

ESSAY 18

❧ Movement Science for the SLP ❧

Fran Redstone

Although I did not have the pleasure of know-ing Dr. Singh well, I greatly respected his appreciation for both the research and clinical aspects of our field. Moreover, he consistently provided support for new ideas and encour-agement to new authors. As a newly-minted academic, I remember being introduced to him at an ASHA convention. I was grateful for his sincere interest and enthusiasm for my work. And as a long-time therapist-turned-researcher, I appreciate the clinical practicality of Plural's available titles, an embodiment of Dr. Singh's commitment to the highest level of client care.

Personally, I was brought up in the Bronx, in New York. Professionally, I was brought up on children with cerebral palsy. It is somewhat disconcerting that so much of what happened to me professionally was a matter of being in the right place at the right time. For example, my first job was with three classes of children with cerebral palsy and "other orthopedically handicapped" children. Times have changed! I got this job because a supervisor overheard me mention that I was interested in working with neurologically impaired children. Little did she know that I knew nothing about neurologic impairment. While in this job, I shared a space with a physical therapist and noted that when she treated the same children I worked with, she did a much better job get-ting sound out of them than I did. The PT was totally unaware of this because it was not her goal. This observation changed the nature of how I worked with children for the next 40 years.

I was lucky enough to work with, and learn from, some extraordinarily talented SLPs as well as gifted therapists from other disciplines. The concept of a multidisciplinary approach is ideal for children with cerebral palsy. Each individual discipline has its unique contribution for improving the child's func-tioning. For example, PTs deal with the move-ments of ambulation, OTs the movements of the upper extremities for reaching and manip-ulation, and SLPs the movements of the oral area for speech and swallowing. The field of movement science is the unifying concept that makes us realize that movement is movement.

According to Palisano (2004), the field of movement science allows us to understand human motion that involves many disciplines. Speech is perhaps the most refined and highly developed set of movement behaviors that humans produce. It is the acoustic output of a series of complex movements that reflects a cognitive-linguistic goal. Speech will develop when all systems: cognitive, motor, linguistic, and sensory are well integrated. The speech-language pathologist's work begins when these systems are not fully integrated and affect the areas of swallowing or language. This often occurs in children with neuromotor disorders such as cerebral palsy. This paper will address some basic principles of movement that are important for the SLP working with children who have disorders such as cerebral palsy with swallowing/feeding and speech issues. In addition, the importance of this knowledge for SLPs working with children who have more subtle speech problems such as those with articulation disorders will be considered.

Cerebral palsy is an aggregate of developmental disorders of movement and posture that result in varied clinical manifestations and activity limitations (Bax, Goldstein, Rosenbaum, Leviton, & Paneth, 2005; Reddy, 2005). It is described as the "most common developmental disability with associated motor impairment" (Treviranus & Roberts, 2003, p. 203). As speech and swallowing both depend on an intact motor system, SLPs who are committed to working with children diagnosed with a neuromotor disorder need to be attuned to the principles of movement science. This understanding can significantly improve the resulting provision of care for these children.

Although both researchers and practitioners in our discipline acknowledge that feeding and swallowing depend on normal muscle tone and posture, especially for the neurologically impaired client, it is also imperative to recognize that the movements of speech do so as well. For speech to be possible the subsystems of the speech production system: respiration, phonation, and articulation need to be working effectively and efficiently. Therefore, SLPs need to know the implications of muscle tone, posture, and movement on the development of communication skills for speech. Researchers such as Ballard (2001) and Kamm, Thelen, and Jensen (1990) note this. They state that the field of motor learning and control can aid the SLP when presented with a client with speech motor control issues. This

knowledge will enable SLPs to provide more holistic intervention. It is interesting that practitioners of other disciplines are educated in movement science throughout their graduate careers. SLPs are often at a disadvantage since they generally learn these principles only after graduation.

Cerebral palsy is the model of how a motor impairment can affect the speech production/swallowing system and its development. Accordingly, researchers (Ruscello, 2008) acknowledge the importance of movement principles for children with developmental dysarthria. However, Bleile (1995) notes that children with articulation disorders may be considered children with specific motor impairments although no physical damage is apparent. There may be something inherent in their system that does not allow their tongues to hit the intended target. According to Bliele (1995), 92% of SLPs treat children within this group. It, therefore, is important for SLPs working with this larger group of children to have the knowledge of movement science.

We make speech movements extremely rapidly, and we can approach an intended target many ways. Speech movements are considered both fast and flexible. This is why so many children have difficulty with speech. It is hypothesized that the speed and flexibility occurs because of the interaction of our feedforward and feedback systems. The feedforward aspect provides the triggering of internalized programs that provide the speed, and feedback lets us change our movements when needed. However, this is based on "normal." The underlying assumption is an intact neuromotor system. Therefore, when working with a child with a known disorder, certain principles should be addressed in order to provide the most effective and efficient intervention.

Several fundamentals of motor control for speech/swallow development include reduction of the degrees of freedom, the provision of postural stability and alignment, and the delivery of appropriate sensory input. The mastering of these principles and the employment of the therapeutic techniques to achieve them will lead to improved oral movements for feeding and speech, as well as enhanced movements for manipulation of objects needed for linguistic/concept development and efficient AAC use.

According to Bernstein (1967), simplifying motor control for a function such as speech or feeding occurs by reducing the elements or degrees of freedom within a function, so that each muscle does not need to be individually controlled. Typical infants may stabilize parts of their body, thereby reducing the degrees of freedom, in order to function within any new task. In the area of speech development, it has been hypothesized that the speech sounds that develop early (stops) are those whose total constriction controls the degrees of freedom (Green, Moore, Higashikawa, & Steeve, 2000). Additionally, the concept of "fixing" describes the way in which a child with cerebral palsy may attempt to control the degrees-of-freedom (Howle, 2002). Bly (1983) states that the child with hypotonia lacks stability from which to move and learns to "hold himself artificially" (p. 42). This child may continue with the "rigid" movement which interferes with the development of higher level skills as the nervous system may not allow the flexibility and variety of movement selection that are available to a physically typical child. This lack of flexibility may also account for the oral movements during speech of the child with a residual articulation disorder (Preston & Edwards, 2009). The principle of controlling the degrees-of-freedom is also used during practice in intervention to increase the consistency of a response (Duffy, 2005).

Providing postural stability through positioning is another therapy technique that is appropriate for the SLP as it will increase movement possibilities by decreasing the child's

need to fix. Most important to the SLP is that postural stability allows for the alignment of oral structures for feeding and speech. It is related to head and trunk stability (Bosma, 1972, 1986; Langley & Thomas, 1991; Robbins, 1992). The recommended head posture is upright with neutral head position or neck flexion. Head and trunk alignment through postural stability is even more important to facilitate the coordination of phonation and articulation for well-produced speech in the child with cerebral palsy. For example, if the child's head is hyperextended, a typical position for both hypo- and hypertonic children, resting tongue position and tongue movement will be more negatively influenced by gravity than if a neutral head flexed position had been attained prior to initiation of speech. In addition, a hyperextended head is more likely to produce hypertonicity (Nwaobi, 1986) in a child with cerebral palsy leading to an inability to produce phonation or make a subtle tongue movement for a /t/, /d/, and /n/.

Head and trunk alignment also allows the proper alignment of the articulators for accurate and efficient speech production for children with more restricted speech motor problems such as an articulation disorder. For example, I remember supervising a clinician who was working with a physically typical child with a lateral lisp. I observed a difference between the child's head position during rest and speech. When the child initiated speech he hyperextended his neck just slightly. This threw his oral structures out of alignment leading to protracted jaw and lateral emission of air. Working on head position and jaw position was the answer to this child's problem, not years in therapy fighting gravity.

However, in the same way the child's tongue position noted in the last example was dependent on jaw and head position, head position is dependent on trunk control (Herman & Lange, 1999; Langley & Thomas, 1991; Seikel, King, & Drumwright, 2005).

This is especially important for children with muscle tone problems. To achieve alignment of the head with the trunk, the pelvis should be well stabilized. This has been researched more extensively for the process of swallowing than for speech. If the head is not stable, then the fine movements of the jaw and tongue needed for feeding will be impaired (Jones-Owens, 1991; Ottenbacher, Hicks, Roark & Swinea, 1983; Redstone & West, 2004; Seikel et al., 2005; West & Redstone, 2004). Although less research is available investigating alignment and sound production, one good example is the study (Hulme, Bain, Hardin, McKinnon, & Waldron, 1989) using adaptive equipment that targeted pelvic stability and head/trunk alignment. It found that upright positioning with stability and a neutral pelvic tilt led to increased frequency and variety of early vocalizations for children with cerebral palsy. Thus, it appears that a structure such as the pelvis, which is significantly distal to the oral area, influences the movements of both swallowing and speech.

Experiences providing varied sensory information are considered "an integral part of movement control and coordination" (Van Der Merwe, 1997, p. 5). This is emphasized in the Neuronal Group Selection Theory (NGST), which states that neural diversity allows a child to select a movement that matches the needs of a task (Sporns & Edelman, 1993). Selection of neuronal groups is based on the varied sensory information that results from a child's experiences. The movements repeated during these early experiences strengthen the synaptic connections (Hadders-Algra, 2000). In fact, it is believed that the "role of sensory information in motor development is larger than previously presumed" (Hadders-Algra, 2000, p. 570), but children with neuromotor impairments typically have impaired sensory systems (Nashner et al.,1983; Neilson & O'Dwyer, 1984). There are many sensory treatment programs available to improve oral

sensitivity for speech but little research to support them.

Netsell (1982) noted that the sensory information used for normal speech control arises from posture and movement. This again supports the need for SLPs working with children with cerebral palsy and other neuromotor disorders to understand the principles of movement science. Additionally, Redstone and Kowalski (2011) found that typical young adults with a history of speech therapy had poorer balance reactions when compared to those with no history of previous speech therapy. We may consider including balance exercises for improved postural control for children with more subtle motor disturbances, such as those with articulation disorders, along with their speech therapy.

Sensory input in disabled populations to improve feeding has been studied (Arvedson & Brodsky, 2002; Gosa & McMillan, 2006; Wolf & Glass, 1992). All agree that determination of a sensory problem through a thorough assessment is imperative, and individualization of each program is critical.

Other principles of motor learning that have been widely addressed include the need for practice and saliency. SLPs need to provide many opportunities for a client to practice. Therefore, when writing a goal, the 80% should be 40 of 50 opportunities instead of the more typical 4 of 5. Drill work is always easier with adults than with children. Adults know the value of drills but children just find them tedious. SLPs must strive to be creative clinicians and find ways to make this important practice fun. For example, the child who really likes Sponge Bob, Spiderman, or Dora the Explorer, will be motivated to reach and attain better head/trunk alignment. Or the SLP can hold the stimulus below eye-level to induce a desirable chin-tuck or chin-neutral position.

Another motor principle is saliency of the exercise. If a goal is improved speech, your treatment must focus on speech. If lack of strength is impeding the improvement of speech/feeding, the strength training must address the specific movement or muscles needed for that movement. Then these muscles must immediately be put to work in a functional context. Therefore, an SLP should know specifically what is being addressed by a certain exercise and specifically why it is being addressed to improve that client's oral functioning.

As SLPs we also need to be aware of prerequisites of motor learning. However, I have always thought of these as precursors to learning any task. For a client, child or adult, to improve, there must be motivation and attention to a task. The reduction of degrees-of-freedom mentioned previously allows practice to be more consistent, because it limits the scope of movement and attention (Duffy, 2005). Again, it is our creativity as therapists that makes the difference. We may use the best evidence-based techniques in the world and still not achieve progress if a child is not motivated or attentive.

Although I have primarily addressed movement science as it applies to children with a diagnosed movement disorder, I have also stressed that speech is a motor skill and that SLPs should understand the principles of movement science when planning intervention, even for a child with an articulation disorder. Although improving posture, alignment, and stability is imperative when addressing the oral movements of a child with cerebral palsy, adherence to these principles will enhance, facilitate, accelerate, and generally improve the progress of a typical child who is in a speech program as well. In addition, the observance of motor learning principles, such as providing many repetitions and opportunities for the movement, will increase the likelihood of a positive outcome for anyone.

As Kamhi (2006) states in relation to speech disturbances, there are many techniques available to clinicians. It is the task of the SLP to decide which will be most effective for each child. There is no protocol that will work for all children. We need to remember that each client has "unique characteristics and circumstances" (Kamhi, 2006, p. 271). Everything must be individualized. The Dynamic Systems Theory of motor learning states that muscles are functionally organized (Sporns & Edelman, 1993) and depend on the task, the constraints of the body, and the environment (Mathiowetz & Haugen, 1994). The task may be talking or eating, walking, or reaching. The constraints may be structural, neurologic, or, even more typically, height or obesity. The environment may be enriched, impoverished, or somewhere in between. No two children are the same. Therefore, our treatment should not be the same.

There is a plethora of therapeutic products commercially available to the SLP. One can open a catalog and find aids for positioning, sensory stimulation, and speech facilitation. We can find books/programs that tell us to begin at step one and continue through to step eight. However, without knowledge of the underlying theoretical bases and motor principles these tools may be useless. Or worse, they can be counterproductive.

REFERENCES

Arvedson, J. C., & Brodsky, I. (2002). *Pediatric swallowing and feeding: Assessment and management* (2nd ed.). San Diego, CA: Singular.

Ballard, K. J. (2001). Principles of motor learning and treatment for AOS. *Perspectives on Neurophysiology and Neurogenic Speech and Language Disorders, 11*, 13–18.

Bax, M., Goldstein, M., Rosenbaum, P., Leviton, A., & Paneth, N. (2005). Proposed definition and classification of cerebral palsy. *Developmental Medicine and Child Neurology, 47*, 571–576.

Bernstein, N. A. (1967). *The co-ordination and regulation of movements.* Oxford, UK: Pergamon Press.

Bleile, K. M. (1995). *Manual of articulation and phonological disorders.* San Diego, CA: Singular.

Bly, L. (1983). *The components of normal movement during the first year of life.* Oak Park, IL: Neurodevelopmental Treatment Association.

Bosma, J. F. (1972). *Oral sensation and perception: The mouth of the infant.* Springfield, IL: Charles C. Thomas.

Bosma , J. F. (1986). Development of feeding. *Clinical Nutrition, 5,* 210–218.

Duffy, J. R, (2005). *Motor speech disorders: Substrates, differential diagnosis, and management* (2nd ed). St Louis, MO: Elsevier Mosby.

Gosa, M., & McMillan, L. (2006). Therapeutic considerations for children and infants with feeding tubes. *Perspectives in Swallowing and Swallowing Disorders, 15,* 15–20.

Green, J. R., Moore, C. A, Higashikawa, M., & Steeve, R. W. (2000). The physiologic development of speech motor control: Lip and jaw coordination. *Journal of Speech, Language, and Hearing Research, 43,* 239–255.

Hadders-Algra, M. (2000). The neuronal group selection theory: A framework to explain variation in normal motor development. *Developmental Medicine and Child Neurology, 42,* 566–572.

Herman, J. H., & Lange, M. L. (1999). Seating and positioning to manage spasticity after brain injury. *NeuroRehabilitation, 12,* 105–117.

Howle, J. M. (2002). *Neurodevelopmental treatment approach: Theoretical foundations and principles of clinical practice.* Laguna Beach, CA: NDTA.

Hulme, J. B., Bain, B., Hardin, M., McKinnon, A., & Waldron, D., (1989). The influence of adaptive seating devices on vocalization. *Journal of Communication Disorders, 22,* 137–145.

Jones-Owens, J. L. (1991). Prespeech assessment and treatment strategies. In M. B. Langley & L. J. Lombardino (Eds.), *Neurodevelopmental strategies for managing communication disorders in children with severe motor dysfunction* (pp. 49–80). Austin, TX: Pro-Ed.

Kamhi, A. G. (2006). Treatment decisions for children with speech–sound disorders. *Language, Speech, and Hearing Services in Schools, 37,* 271–279.

Kamm, K., Thelen, E., & Jensen, J. L. (1990). A dynamical systems approach to motor development. *Physical Therapy, 70,* 763–775.

Langley, M. B., & Thomas, C. (1991). Introduction to the neurodevelopmental approach. In M. B. Langley & L. J. Lombardino (Eds.), *Neurodevelopmental strategies for managing communication disorders in children with severe motor dysfunction* (pp. 1–28). Austin, TX: Pro-Ed.

Mathiowetz, V., & Haugen, J. (1994). Motor behavior research: Implications for therapeutic approaches to CNS dysfunction. *American Journal of Occupational Therapy, 48,* 733–745.

Nashner, L. M., Shumway-Cook, A., & Marin, O. (1983). Stance posture control in select groups of children with cerebral palsy: Deficits in sensory organization and muscular coordination. *Experimental Brain Research, 49,* 393–409.

Neilson, P. D., & O'Dwyer, N. J. (1984). Reproducibility and variability of speech muscle activity in athetoid dysarthria of cerebral palsy. *Journal of Speech and Hearing Research, 27,* 502–517.

Netsell, R. (1982). Speech motor control and selected neurologic disorders. In S. Grillner, B. Lindblom, J. Lubker, & A. Persson (Eds.), *Speech motor control* (pp. 247–261). New York, NY: Pergamon Press.

Nwaobi, O. M. (1986). Effects of body orientation in space on tonic muscle activity of patients with cerebral palsy. *Developmental Medicine and Child Neurology, 28,* 41–44.

Ottenbacher, K., Hicks, J., Roark, A., & Swiena, J. (1983). Oral sensory motor therapy in the developmentally disabled: A multiple-baseline study. *American Journal of Occupational Therapy, 37,* 541–547.

Palisano. R. J. (2004). *Physical and occupational therapy in pediatrics.* Binghamton, NY: Haworth Press.

Preston, J. L., & Edwards, M. L. (2009). Speed and accuracy of rapid speech output by adolescents with residual speech sound errors including rhotics. *Clinical Linguistics & Phonetics, 23,* 301–318.

Reddy, S. K. (2005). Commentary on definition and classification of cerebral palsy. *Developmental Medicine and Child Neurology, 47,* 508–509.

Redstone, F. (2004). The effects of seating position on the respiratory patterns of preschoolers with cerebral palsy. *International Journal of Rehabilitation Research, 27,* 283–288.

Redstone, F. (2005). Seating position and length of utterance of preschoolers with cerebral palsy. *Perceptual and Motor Skills, 101,* 961–962.

Redstone, F., & Kowalski, E. (2011). The effect of balance on speech production. *Perceptual and Motor Skills, 112,* 749–760.

Redstone, F., & West, J. (2004). The importance of postural control for feeding. *Pediatric Nursing, 30,* 97–100.

Robbins, J. (1992). The impact of oral motor dysfunction on swallowing: From beginning to end. *Seminars in Speech and Language, 13,* 55–69.

Ruscello, D. M. (2008) *Treating articulation and phonological disorders in children.* St. Louis, MO: Mosby.

Seikel, J. A., King, D. W., & Drumwight, D. G. (2005). *Anatomy and physiology for speech, language, and hearing* (3rd ed.). Clifton Park, NY: Thomson Delmar.

Sporns, O., & Edelman, G. M. (1993). Solving Bernstein's problem: A proposal for the development of coordinated movement by selection. *Child Development, 64,* 960–981.

Treviranus, J., & Roberts, V. (2003). Supporting competent motor control of AAC systems. In J. C. Light, D. R. Beukelman, & J. Reichle (Eds.), *Communicative competence for individuals who use AAC: From research to effective practice* (pp. 199–240). Baltimore, MD: Paul H. Brookes.

Van Der Merwe, A. (1997). A theoretical framework for the characterization of pathological speech sensorimotor control. In M. R. McNeil (Ed.), *Clinical management of sensorimotor speech disorders* (pp. 1–26). New York, NY: Thieme.

West, J., & Redstone, F. (2004). Alignment during feeding and swallowing: Does it matter? A review. *Perceptual and Motor Skills, 98,* 349–358.

Wolf, L. S., & Glass, R. P. (1992). *Feeding and swallowing disorders in infancy.* San Antonio, TX: Therapy Skill Builders.

ESSAY 19

ꙮ Verbotonal Body Movements ꙮ

Carl W. Asp, Madeline Kline, and Kazunari J. Koike

With warm affection, the first author acknowledges the inspiration and friendship of the late Dr. Sadanand Singh.

INTRODUCTION

In 1939, Petar Guberina established in his dissertation how vocal-pitch change (intonation) adds meaning (language) to conversational speech. He applied this strategy for teaching normal-hearing people to speak before reading a foreign language and called it Structural-Global-Audio-Visual (SGAV). During 1954 to 1957, he began applying this strategy to hearing impairment; however, he felt that more effective treatment tools were needed when using the application to the hearing impaired because of the severity of their speech errors (Guberina, 1972).

Based on findings from movement researchers such as Piaget (1973), Laban (1974), Jaques-Dalcroze (1930), and Luria (1976), Guberina proposed the use of body movements for correction of those speech errors. By using body movements, he created pro-

prioceptive stimulation to both hemispheres of the listener's brain. The ability of the human brain to change with optimal stimulation is called neuroplasticity. Body movements also facilitate this neuroplasticity. At five years or younger, the child easily learns to speak two different languages simultaneously with *optimal stimulation* (Piaget, 1973). Use of body movements makes it easier for the young child's brain to lock onto the speech rhythms, which are the same rhythms he experiences in his mother's womb. The baby first experiences the movements, then internalizes them as rhythm and intonation (R/I) patterns. Thus, body movements are scientifically based to create *optimal learning* for the listener's brain.

This essay explains in detail how body movements are used as a treatment tool for the hearing impaired, primarily young children, and how seven perceptual parameters for correcting R/I and phoneme errors are used in conjunction with body movements. Essay 42 further describes five areas of applications and five basic Verbotonal principles (Asp, 2006, revised 2011; Asp, Guberina, & Pansini, 1981, revised 2011).

BODY MOVEMENTS

Figure 19–1 shows a parent phonating /i/ with an upward body-movement, while her son wears a speech wrist-vibrator and sits on a speech vibrating board. Though proprioceptive and tactile feedback, the child feels his mother's speech rhythms.

Figure 19–2 shows the first author phonating /a/ with an open body movement with three children, each wearing a speech wrist-vibrator and a headphone. All three children feel and hear what they are imitating. Body movements are natural and simple to use once a few basics are understood.

Figure 19–3 shows the Verbotonal Training Unit (VTU) with a microphone, a speech vibrator, and a headphone. The unit is adjusted to the Optimal Frequency Response (OFR) for each client.

Figure 19–4 shows a 2-year-old speaking into the microphone, while wearing the speech wrist-vibrator and the headset, both set for her OFR. She feels and hears her voice, which brings a big smile. She likes feeling and hearing her voice.

Based on muscular generalization, body movements are a powerful treatment tool for indirectly teaching R/I patterns of conversational speech. Children love to *move while vocalizing,* as it comes naturally. For them,

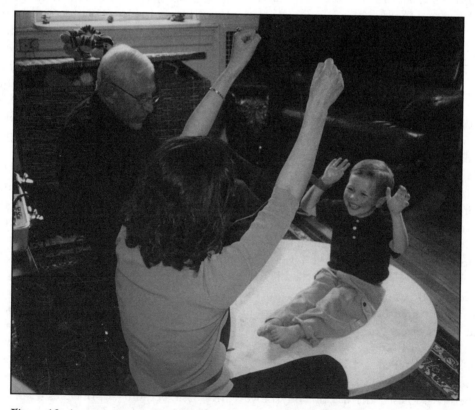

Figure 19–1. *A parent says /i/ accompanied by an upward body movement while her young son is seated on a speech-vibrating board and wears a wrist vibrator.*

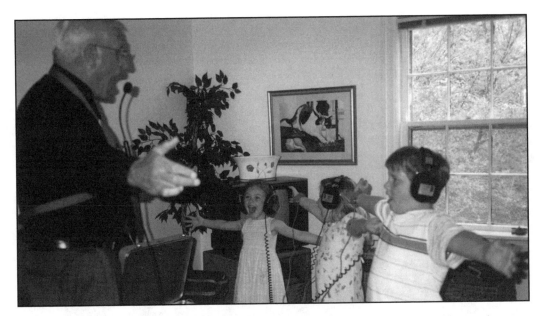

Figure 19–2. *The first author says /a/ with an open body movement for three older children, each wears a wrist vibrator and a headphone.*

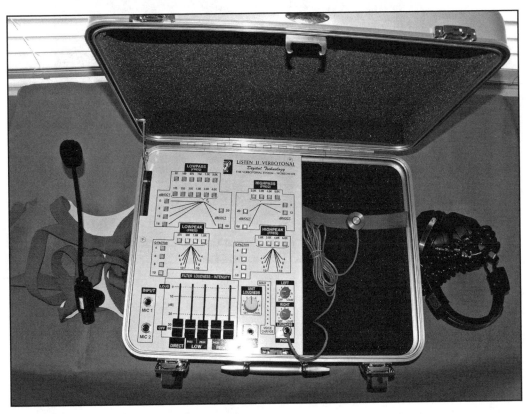

Figure 19–3. *Verbotonal Training Unit (VTU) with a microphone, a speech vibrator, and a headphone. casp@utk.edu.*

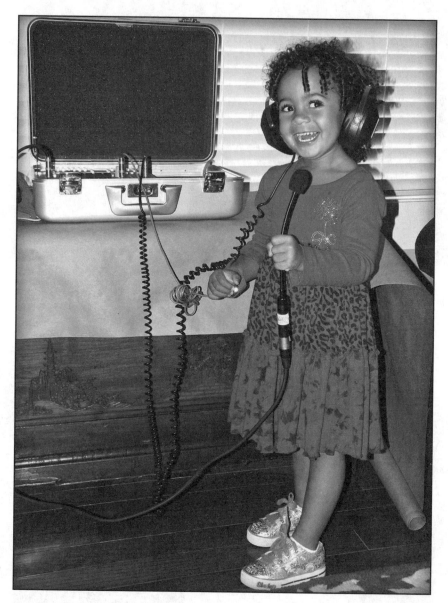

Figure 19–4. *A 2-year-old speaking into the microphone, while wearing the speech wrist-vibrator and the headset, both set for her OFR.*

dynamic emotional exchanges simulate meaningful real spoken language situations. Children need natural learning situations, which body movements provide.

Body and speech movements are three dimensional. They include forward-backward, side-to-side, up-down, and inward-outward movement. Crossing the midline to train laterality stimulates both hemispheres of the brain.

Table 19–1 illustrates the use of body movements and speech modifications, based on the seven perceptual parameters.

Table 19–1. Body Movement and Speech Modification Input Based on the Seven Perceptual Parameters

Parameters	Degree	Speech Modification	Body Movement
Rhythm	Less	Less stress and loudness Monotone, flat quality Less vocal pitch	Actions are away from body center Beat defines body action (less space) Rock, swing, bounce, turn/all directions
	More	Stressed syllables (more vocal pitch) Increase loudness Increase vocal pitch, short rhymes	Repeat movement sequences Step/kick, bounce, swing with rhythm Elevate moves to emphasize stress
Intonation (vocal pitch)	Less	Unstressed, flat, monotone Less pitch change, less loudness Shorten rate	Alternate direction, relaxed, less direct Level plane, less dynamic, less gesture Shorter, give in to gravity
	More	Stressed syllables (more vocal pitch) Longer voicing of vowels and words Raise or lower vocal pitch for meaning	Dynamic whole body use (reach, bend) Rising, falling, with arms to emphasize Diagonal, upward/downward
Tension	Less	Open vowels, simple melodic rhythms Nursery rhyme rhythm patterns Use relaxed sounds with melody	Light-tense, fast (flick, touch) Indirect space (curve, twist, bend) Body expression directs flow
	More	Increase vocal pitch and rate Pause, build anticipation Lengthen, sustain sounds	Strong-tense (pull, press, strike) Direct space (long, strong, quick) Alternate large to small, small to large
Tonality (spectral pitch)	Less	Less tense phonemes Open vowels Lower space	Lower space, downward releasing Action with sound play (BA/bear walk) Body expressions, movement situations
	More	Higher tonality Tense vowels Higher space with most tense phonemes	Higher space Vary degree of tension, size, strength Various forms of whole body actions

continues

141

Table 19–1. *continued*

Parameters	Degree	Speech Modification	Body Movement
Duration (tempo)	Less	Less loudness	Shorter, slower, unidirectional
		Slow, relaxed tempo with pause	Consistent, repeating rhythm
		Singing sounds and words	Direct space, focus with direction
	More	Faster articulations	Stronger, fast/slow (glide, shake)
		Start slow and increase speed	Dynamic whole-body rhythmic moves
		Control vocal pitch, vary intonation	Side to side (beat), circular (rhythm)
Pause	Less	Shorten rate	Fast, quick, with rhythm
		Faster tempo with melodic phrasing	Direct space, consistent flow
		Simple short rhythm patterns	One direction at a time
	More	Longer pause between syllables	Whole body expression (go/stop)
		Slow rate (voice, no voice)	Stop, use visual focus between moves
		Longer, louder vowels	Increase size, lengthen with pause
Loudness	Less	Voiceless sounds	Wavy, zig-zag, gliding actions
		Short, less intonation	Free-flowing body parts, indirect space
		Less vocal pitch	Whole body, sideways, forward/back
	More	Louder vs. softer	Small increasing to large use of space
		Stressed sounds, longer voicing	Exaggerated whole-body expressions
		Demonstrative, exclamatory sounds	Direct, strong, large (all body parts)

SPEECH RHYME

Body movements are used with speech rhymes (also called nursery rhymes or musical stimulation). Speech rhymes are preferred because tonality (see detail in Essay 42) is utilized. For example, a low-tonality rhyme is: "Ah-Boo, Ba-Boo, Boo-Boo, Baa." A high-tonality speech rhyme is: "Shower-Shower, Take-a-Shower, Wash-Your-Shoulders, Take-A-Shower." The first rhyme has seven syllables and the second 16 syllables. The low tonalities are used with preschool children, working toward the high tonalities with older children, following normal developmental patterns of speech sounds. The clinician uses her natural movements, as a band leader by following the speech rhythm and stressing some syllables/words. The goal is to emphasize the rhythms to lengthen memory span, and not to correct phonemes. At first some children will hum the rhythm as do all children with normal hearing. Daily practice with speech rhythms is fun. Children like repeating until they master a rhythm. The clinician also uses published nursery rhymes, with mixed tonalities including "Humpty-Dumpty," "Twinkle-Twinkle," "Five-Little-Monkey-Jumping-On-The-Bed," and so forth. All speech rhymes with body movements are effective for lengthening the child's memory span.

SITUATIONAL TEACHING: PRAGMATICS

To maximize learning, the clinician creates short, meaningful stories that draw the children into the situation. The following five levels are used for both individual and group therapy:

Level 1: the conversation is: "Hi, Mama, Hi Baby, Let's Walk, Walk-Walk-Walk." A toy mama and a toy baby are characters that make the situation real. Later, other characters are added: "Daddy," "Puppy," and so forth. The young child observes only the situation.

Level 2: the child is drawn into the situation and participates.

Level 3: all conversation is from the children's memory; he has internalized the story.

Level 4: for older children, the children act out the story as a play.

Level 5: the clinician writes the story to teach reading and writing.

Situational teaching turns speech into spoken language. Each situation has meaning (language). The clinician uses body movements to stimulate, dramatize, and correct spoken language.

PERCEPTUAL PARAMAMETERS FOR CORRECTING R/I AND PHONEME ERRORS

All infants and children learn spoken language and acceptable behavior by imitating what they see, hear, and feel from those close to them. This *imitation phase* is a powerful early learning tool. The Verbotonal clinician has the child imitate what she says. Seven perceptual parameters are used to analyze and correct the child's listening errors in conjunction with body movements and other individual or group training sessions.

The seven speech parameters are: (1) rhythm, (2) intonation (vocal-pitch change), (3) tension, (4) tonality (spectral pitch of each phoneme), (5) duration, (6) pause, and (7) loudness. The parameters occur simultaneously in all speech utterances. A skilled clinician may hear the errors in many parameters. After analyzing the child's imitation, however, she selects one or more parameters to modify and to correct his imitation. Later, the child answers rather than imitates.

Stages of correction start with developing normal rhythm and intonation (R/I) with at least an eight-syllable memory span in binaural listening. The expression of emotions is used regularly, because emotions develop memory. Once R/I muscle memory is automatic, the child doesn't forget; it's like running, riding a bicycle, swimming, and so forth.

Rhythm

Conversational speech is very fast; the rate is five syllables or twelve phonemes per second. In a *conversational minute* there are 300 syllables or 720 phonemes. Both the speaker and the listener lock on to the syllabic rhythm of 5/second. At first, the young child repeats the last syllable like it came first, because the rate is too fast for his memory. How can a clinician quicken his listening?

The Verbotonal clinician places the infant on a sounding board and attaches a wrist vibrator, so he can feel the fast speech rhythm as he did in the mother's womb. She gently guides him from involuntary reflex phonation to voluntary babbling and then on to normal R/I pattern. She teaches him a many-to-one speech rhythm, for example, /ma-ma-ma/ (pause) /ma/. When the young child can pause and produce one /ma/, he demonstrates control of his speech rhythm. Body movements using the infant's arms or legs activate proprioception, allowing internalization of the speech rhythm. The clinician begins with 2/4 and 4/4 patterns, and then the more difficult 3/4 rhythms.

As the child advances, he is able to voluntarily produce a two-syllable pattern. This rhythm can be trochaic, iambic, or spondee. Common trochaic rhythms (stressed-unstressed) are: "mommy, daddy, baby, doggie, and so forth." A stressed syllable emphasizes the meaning (language) in the R/I pattern. The R/I pattern is used for listening through spoken language. Spoken language is the basis for higher brain levels, like writing, reading, spelling, and analytic skills. All adult listeners anticipate the speech rhythms of a talker. This anticipation is taught early to our children.

Intonation (Vocal Pitch Change)

Speech is an expression of our emotions. Human vocal-pitch changes (intonation) accompanied by human facial changes are an expression of our emotions. They result in our vocal pitch changing one or more octaves higher or lower than our average vocal pitch. Intonation humanizes our speech. Researchers have identified over 40 positive and 40 negative emotions. Most people consider happy,

angry, loving, confident, anxious, stressed, and relaxed as being the most common.

The average vocal pitch of adult males is 125 Hz; adult females are one octave higher at 250 Hz; young children are higher depending on their weight and height. When a person is depressed, vocal pitch is flat and difficult to understand. Emotions like being very happy, elated, excited, and afraid change vocal pitch an octave or more.

The clinician uses speech vibrators, headsets, and body movements, so the child can feel and hear changes in his vocal pitch. The tension changes in the body movements transfer from the child's body to his vocal pitch. The clinician uses intonation patterns with a wide emotional range. For example, giving a look of disgust and pointing while saying the vowel /u/ implies that something is not desirable and should be avoided. Body language in practical situations helps children internalize the pragmatics of their pre-word language.

Tension

Muscular generalization describes how increased tension in an arm-reaching body movement generalizes to the speech movement, and results in a higher vocal-tension with higher vocal-pitch.

The clinician expresses tension changes by increasing and decreasing muscle tension in her body movements and her vocal patterns. These tension changes stimulate proprioceptive feedback.

Each phoneme has an optimal tension. On a 10-point scale, the vowel /a/ at a value of 1 is less tense than the vowels /u/ and /i/ with a value of 2. All consonants have more tension than vowels. The voiceless consonants /p/, /t/, /k/, have a value of 10, whereas the voiced /b/, /d/, /g/ are less tense with a value of 9. Tension affects how phonemes are perceived.

When the tension of /m/ is increased, it is perceived as /b/, and when /b/ is increased /p/ is perceived. Thus, the degree of tension is the perceptual difference in the /m/→/b/→/p/ phonemes. This may explain how children who are deaf with high body tension, hear the word /mama/ as /baba/ or /papa/. Body tension affects perception. Many clinicians may not be aware of the tension parameter; however, it is a very effective and important treatment tool for correcting phoneme and R/I errors.

Tonality (Spectral Pitch)

The clinician begins with homogenous low-tonality syllables, such as /m/, /b/, /u/. Then she moves to the mid-tonality category /t/, /d/, /k/, /g/, /a/, and so forth. The homogenous tonality of syllables follows the phonemic development order of normal-hearing children. The tonality categories are based on the child's listening skills. Tonality correction through listening develops intelligible speech.

Tonality categories are used for error analysis and correction. For example, if /s/ is substituted for /t/, the clinician adds more low frequency energy and/or cuts high frequency energy on a Verbotonal training unit. She also uses a quick tense body movement so the child will both feel and hear the quickness (plosive) of the /t/ vs the longer duration of the error /s/. The Verbotonal clinician follows the scientific observation "all phonemes are contained in one phoneme" (see Essay 42), so any error is possible. With regular correction in a variety of coarticulation contexts, the child hears and feels the correct motor patterns of a correct /t/. Optimal correction is within the child's auditory memory span.

In diagnostic individual therapy, the clinician evaluates the child's speech perception (listening) in all tonality categories. For example, /mu-mu/, /la-la/, /si-si/ used separately or together is a Six Syllable Sound Test. At a higher developmental level, the clinician use words, for example, "move-cat-cease" in the same tonality categories as the nonsense syllables. Using words introduces the *guessing factor*, which may not be a true assessment of the child's listening skills. If more tonality syllables are needed, all 8-logatomes are used: / bru-bru/, /mu-mu/, /bu-bu/, /vo-vo/, /la-la/, /ke-ke/, /shi-shi/, /si-si/. Listening helps the child self-correct his errors and establish carryover. If not corrected early, lifelong permanent errors are established.

Duration (Tempo)

Along with body movements, the clinician changes speech tempo from slow (two syllables/second) to normal (five syllables per second) to fast (eight syllables per second). The child simultaneously imitates her movements and vocalizations, using the same speech tempo. This helps the child vary speech tempo. In the beginning, the clinician uses a slow tempo, which is an optimal condition. Later, a quicker vocal tempo with quicker body movements expands the child's capacity for listening. As the child's optimal tempo quickens, his auditory memory span lengthens.

Pause

Most speech rhythms have pauses (the absence of speech). In the 1940s, AT&T Laboratory determined that a pause was critical in remembering a phone number. A telephone number contained seven numbers and one pause. For example, 523-0996 is easy to remember because the pause separates 523 and 0996 into two groups. If the area code is added, for example, 1-423-523-0996, it is too long for the listener memory span. An eight-digit memory span should be the minimum memory span for everyone, including our children.

Most pauses increase body and vocal tension; it signals there is more to come. A pause is like a written sentence using a semicolon: I cannot go out; it's raining. The semicolon replaces the conjunction *because*. The pause with increased tension separates the 3-numbers (pause) and the 4-numbers. The child's auditory memory span will be expanded with a pause.

At a lower development level, infants babble and don't stop until they are out of breath. The clinician uses body movements to illustrate the *many-to-one* principle of speech control. She voices /ma-ma-ma-ma/ (pause) /ma/. Then, she follows with one controlled /ma/. When the child produces a one controlled /ma/, he controls his babbling and his speech.

Loudness

How do we know how loudly to speak? Normal hearing individuals can naturally monitor their own voice level; however, people of severe to profound hearing loss, including children, cannot self-monitor their voice and tend to speak louder. To help the hearing-impaired child, the clinician changes loudness with body movements so that the child can feel and hear very loud in contrast to very soft. The child imitates loudness, and uses body movement to vary his loudness. These changes develop proprioceptive feedback to feel the loudness control needed. This teaches self-control and pleasant voice quality. The clinician also alters the distance from the child so that he can learn to use the optimal voice level at all distances.

VIBROTACTILE PHASE FOR LISTENING

Verbotonal uses a multisensory, five channel input: (1) vestibular, (2) tactile, (3) proprioceptive, (4) auditory, and (5) visual. The clinician regularly checks the client's binaural listening by covering her face. Body movements especially help to activate proprioceptive and tactile stimulation for the awareness of body and limbs as the infant vocalizes and moves in space. The vestibular organ and cochlea anatomically are side by side in direct connection. The vestibular system controls speech rhythms for listening, muscle tone, balance, and the body in space. The vestibular organ responds to sound/vibrations from 2 to 1000 Hz. A speech vibrator used with body movements helps the 0- to 2-year-old infant feel/hear the rhythm and intonation (R/I) of spoken language. Sensorimotor intelligence (Piaget, 1973) or normal space perception is needed for all phases of learning. This helps the infant's speech to change from involuntary reflex movements to voluntary babbling, speech awareness, and R/I patterns. It prepares the infant for effective hearing aid(s) and/or cochlear implant(s).

Young normal-hearing children vocalize while moving. For example, the clinician has a group of children imitate her heavy-slow-walking steps while producing /ba/ with each step. Then, she changes to /pa/ with light pointed steps. Therefore, body movements become vestibular exercises to help the child organize his body and speech in space.

SUMMARY

This essay described body movements as one of the Verbotonal treatment tools to restructure the child's brain. Body movements based on the seven parameters can both stimulate and correct errors of listening through spoken language, and can be applied to all communication problems.

Acknowledgments. The authors thank Mary Koike, Wayne Kline, and Jan Asp for editing this text.

REFERENCES

Asp, C. W. (2006, rev. 2011) (casp@utk.edu). *Verbotonal speech treatment*. San Diego, CA: Plural.

Asp, C. W., Guberina, P., & Pansini, M. (1981, rev. 2011) (casp@utk.edu). *Verbotonal method for rehabilitating people with communication problems*. New York, NY: World Rehabilitation Fund.

Guberina, P. (1939). *Speech intonation and language*. Unpublished PhD dissertation, Sorbonne University, Paris, France.

Guberina, P. (1972). *Case studies in restricted bands of frequencies in auditory rehabilitation of deaf*. U.S. Office of vocational rehabilitation, OVR-YUGO-2-63.

Jaques-Dalcroze, E. (1930). *Eurhythmics: Art and education*. Salem, NH: Ayer.

Laban, R. (1974). *The language of movement*. Boston, MA: Play.

Luria, A. R. (1976). *The cognitive development: Its cultural and social foundations*. Cambridge, MA: Harvard University Press.

Piaget, J. (1973). *The child and reality*. New York, NY: Grossman.

ESSAY 20

The Martial Arts of Communication

Dana Battaglia

Although I never had the honor of meeting Dr. Singh, his work has certainly had positive effects on my academic career and professional development. To say that he was accomplished during his lifetime is an understatement, and both researchers and clinicians have benefited from the fruits of his labor. The opportunity to contribute to this work as a tribute to Dr. Sigh is the smallest note of thanks I can write. I am grateful for his contributions to the field, trailblazing efforts to support young academics, and generosity not only to the profession, but also to humanity.

INTRODUCTION

The practice of martial arts is essentially a way of life, attempting to maintain peace over aggression above all else. There is a further etiquette of social behavior in martial arts, in which one gives what one puts out into the world. Effective application of the philosophy of martial arts can lead to a positive quality of life. As such, most martial artists are accomplished not only in the martial arts, but in other areas of life (e.g., speech-language pathology, philosophy, business, acting).

As both a martial artist and a speech-language pathologist, it is immediately apparent to me how the strategies employed in martial arts training are parallel to those in communication intervention. The structure and sequential nature of a martial arts curriculum is similar to that of communication training for individuals with pragmatic deficits. More specifically, martial arts practice lies within the framework of applied behavior analysis (ABA). Procedures such as shaping, prompting and fading, as well as reinforcement, are also systematically employed in an effort to increase effective communication in individuals with autism spectrum disorders (ASD).

Given that individuals with ASD do not naturally acquire language from the environment, they require specific instruction using systematic task analysis to target specific skills. Martial arts instruction is remarkably parallel in instructional style. This essay proposes that participation in martial arts can address communication deficits commonly identified in individuals with ASD, using similar strategies employed in ABA.

MARTIAL ARTS

"Martial arts" is a western term which is used to describe a system of self-defense, combat, and sport derived from Asia (Morgan, 1992). Martial arts may be categorized according to several different taxonomies; level of contemporary style (e.g., traditional, modern), geographical origin (e.g., India, China), and technique (e.g., open fist, closed fist), with several hybrid forms between these.

The term "kata" is used to describe patterns of movement, in which one who is training in martial arts practices stances, punches, and kicks in an organized manner, and with repetition (Morgan, 1992). In a typical kata, there is an opening salutation, a sequence of maneuvers, and then a closing salutation, indicating that the form is complete. It is a well-choreographed sequence of movement, designed to hone one's skills, and advance toward multiple attackers. In several dojos throughout the world, kata are practiced in unison. Such practice facilitates a sense of unity, as well as observational learning from peers.

During martial arts training, the value of instructional feedback and positive reinforcement has been established as a method to generalize self-defense and combative skills (Harding, Wacker, Berg, Rick, & Lee, 2004). Using two conditions: drilling, then drilling plus feedback, progress in 28 punching techniques and 26 kicking techniques was investigated (Harding et al., 2004). Results revealed that reinforcement and extinction procedures increased response variability. Such findings clearly demonstrated the effects of planning for generalization during training.

Martial arts may be considered a game of strategy. It is a way of conquering the enemy without aggression (Tzu, 2002). Ultimately, the practice of martial arts is a way of life, a zen practice (Lee, 1975; Musashi, 1982; Tzu, 2002). One assumes a position in the world,

both physical and spiritual, and measures relationships according to physical proximity to others. Tzu (2002) discussed this in terms of shifting patterns of influence upon one another. How one manages this dynamic interrelationship in the world was first described the notion of "shih," in the context of war and conquest. Shih, which emphasizes timing, is essentially the appropriate time to engage, attack, and ultimately subdue the enemy (Tzu, 2002). According to Samurai tradition, it is the "spirit of direct communication" where one is enlightened, and therefore becomes a flawless fighter (Musashi, 1982, p. 56). Such skills may be generalized to a large number of scenarios (Stokes & Baer, 1977).

AUTISM SPECTRUM DISORDERS

The term "autism" was first coined by Paul Eugen Bleuler (Donnellan, 1985), a Swiss scientist seeking to describe schizophrenia. The term stemmed from the Greek word "autos" meaning "self." Autism was more thoroughly described by Leo Kanner (1943). According to the fourth edition of the *Diagnostic Statistical Manual-Revised* (American Psychiatric Association, 2000), the diagnosis of autism falls under the larger umbrella term of pervasive developmental disorders. Within this term, there are five sub-diagnoses: autistic disorder, Rett disorder, childhood disintegrative disorder, Asperger disorder, and pervasive developmental disorder not otherwise specified. Autistic disorder, synonymous with autism or classic autism, is diagnosed according to a collection of deficit areas. An individual must present with a minimum of six deficits (American Psychiatric Association, 2000). Two deficits must be in the area of social interaction (e.g., impairments in eye contact and/or failure to develop appropriate relationships with peer), and a minimum of one deficit in the area of communication (e.g., delay or total absence in development of spoken language). The third area of deficit consists of restricted and repetitive patterns of behavior (e.g., obsessive preoccupations).

COMMON CHARACTERISTICS OF COMMUNICATION IN INDIVIDUALS WITH ASD

As per the diagnostic process (e.g., collection of deficits in three major areas), compounded with the five disorders encompassed under the umbrella of ASD, the impact of language skills on autism is highly variable. However, there are common threads in communication that are inherent to the diagnosis that fall within social, communication, and behavioral-sensory domains. A majority of individuals later diagnosed with ASD will have experienced some sort of delay in language development, excluding individuals with Asperger syndrome (Tager-Flusberg, Paul, & Lord, 2005).

For the purposes of this essay, discussion of communication deficits will be restricted to pragmatic skills, defined as the use of language in social contexts to affect others (Owens, 2008; Prelock, 2006). In terms of pragmatic skills in early childhood development, individuals on the autism spectrum have been reported to be less responsive to their own name being called (Lord, 1995; Osterling & Dawson, 1994). Joint attention has been reported to be compromised as well (Jones & Carr, 2004). Although individuals with ASD may use their language skills to communicate, these attempts are qualitatively different. They tend to direct their interactions more toward adults than peers (McHale, Marcus & Olley, 1980). Significantly fewer communicative acts are observed, when compared to typical peers in a classroom setting (Stone & Caro-Martinez, 1990). Although children with

ASD may respond to peer interactions, they may demonstrate persistent difficulty in initiating interactions, expansion of conversational topic, and/or maintaining an exchange (Janzen, 2003).

Paralinguistic, extralinguistic, linguistic, and conversational features of pragmatic skills are often compromised in individuals with ASD. More specifically, paralinguistic features such as pitch, intensity, and intonation during conversation are inappropriate (Fay & Schuler, 1980; Lord & Paul, 1997). Extralinguistic features include use of body language and gesture to enhance meaningful communication. Such features of pragmatic skills are frequently stilted or absent (Prelock, 2006). Linguistic features, such as the ability to attend to a communicative partner, respond in kind, and disengage appropriately are compromised (Prelock, 2006). Finally, two important conversational features of pragmatic skills that are limited or absent in individuals with ASD are appropriate eye gaze and use of proximity during social interaction (Prelock, 2006).

These challenges, superimposed with idiosyncratic behavioral sensory interests, may result in conversations which are stilted and perseverative in nature. Individuals with ASD may be rigid in conversational style and unaware of subtle suggestions to topic shift. Shic and colleagues (2011) conducted an eye tracking study which indicated that individuals with ASD as early as 20 months of age demonstrate qualitative differences in their activity monitoring of others. The inability to learn via observation can pose challenges with making judgments relative to the appropriateness of both verbal and nonverbal interaction.

To summarize, individuals with ASD will have difficulty with making inferences, learning through observation, and transitioning within and between tasks. These individuals will ultimately experience difficulties in flexibility of language use, as well as integration of information and derivation of meaning from context (Williams, 2010). Ultimately, these communicative challenges highlight deficits in both verbal and nonverbal communication, which will inevitably impact quality of life. With respect to treatment in pragmatic skills, successful procedures utilized within the frameworks of both speech-language pathology and ABA are shaping, prompting, and fading.

APPLIED BEHAVIOR ANALYSIS

Children with ASD do not acquire language, nor learn from the environment in ways similar to their typically developing peers. They can, however, learn new skills using a carefully structured environment. Applied behavior analysis (ABA) is defined as a systematic study of socially significant human behavior, involving scientific investigation of environmental variables (Cooper, Heron, & Heward, 2007). ABA is a scientifically driven discipline with a substantial body of literature supporting its effectiveness as an intervention for individuals with ASD. Within the framework of ABA, instruction is broken down into discrete, measurable units, to successively approximate a given end target. Prompting procedures may be employed, and once an individual achieves mastery, these prompts are faded. Necessary considerations within the framework of ABA are intensity, duration, quality, and setting (Maurice, Green, & Luce, 1996). Teaching is employed consistently and with repetition, to afford the learner multiple opportunities for practice. Once a skill is mastered, it is maintained and generalized, while new skills are continually being introduced (Maurice et al., 1996). With respect to the domain of language and communication, discrete trial instruction and the replacement of challenging behavior with more appropriate social interactions have been supported (Goldstein, 2002).

Shaping is a procedure where a new target behavior is taught in small, sequential units (Hegde, 1998). Shaping is synonymous with the term successive approximation, and is used to help an individual move toward completion of a desired objective (Cooper et al., 2007; Hegde, 1998). For individuals with ASD, communication can be considered a socially driven behavior, which frequently requires shaping toward the ultimate end goal of effective communication. Prompts include stimuli, added to the request for an individual to perform a desired behavior, to increase the likelihood that the desired behavior will occur (Hegde, 1998). Prompts may be in the form of verbal instruction, modeling, or physical guidance (Cooper et al., 2007). Prompting may be provided in any combination of these three forms, as well as to varying degrees (e.g., phonemic cue, video model, partial physical). Finally, prompt fading is a procedure in which prompting is systematically reduced (Hegde, 1998). Fading is used to facilitate independence toward a desired goal, and is accomplished successfully when one obtains the same result as when presented with a prompt previously (Cooper et al., 2007).

CONCLUSION

Musashi (1982) defines zen as both a discipline and an approach to daily life. Zen is a necessary daily practice, as is effective communication, which impacts one's quality of life. As such, one may equate effective communication among individuals to be a zen practice. In martial arts, the path to enlightenment is the ability to share one's thoughts with others. In speech-language pathology, such ability is the core of communication. For individuals with ASD, communication is the core of the deficit area. When viewed from a frame of reference of martial arts, "the enemy" is the inability to communicate effectively.

In traditional curricula for martial arts training, techniques are systematically taught for purposes of acquisition of a skill set (Harding et al., 2004). Such skills are prompted and shaped, and then reinforcement is faded. One must be strongly rooted in the earth with solid punches, kicks, and blocks prior to combining and embellishing these basic foundations. Many individuals with ASD demonstrate splinter skills, resulting in gaping holes in their linguistic foundation. The same principle of successive approximation holds true for developing language and ultimately effective communication. In typical language development, children first acquire single words, then move on to two- and three-word utterances. As this occurs, the expansion of different forms of grammar (e.g., nouns, verbs) and syntax (e.g., subject-verb-object) occur simultaneously.

Individuals who are effective at communication learn one phrase in one context (e.g., with a caregiver at home), then generalize to different scenarios (e.g., school, community) and across different people (e.g., relatives, friends). Individuals who are developing language in a typical fashion are also able to learn by observation (e.g., navigating entry to a game on the playground during recess).

Similar to language acquisition, learning martial arts techniques requires learning one technique in context, (e.g., drills in the dojo), generalization to multiple scenarios, (e.g., self-defense on the street), and across different individuals (e.g., attackers of different size, strength, and skill). Performing techniques in a group affords martial artists opportunities for observational learning (e.g., katas).

For individuals with ASD, there is a lack of generalization of communication skills. An understanding of the ever-evolving communication patterns and nuances between two individuals is equivalent to the notion of shih

in the martial arts. When one has not only acquired skills, but generalized them for effective and independent use, then true mastery has been achieved. This is the martial arts of communication.

REFERENCES

American Psychiatric Association. (2000). *Diagnostic and statistical manual of mental disorders: DSM-IV-TR* (4th ed., text revised). Washington, DC: Author.

Cooper, J. O., Heron, T. E., & Heward, W. L. (2007). *Applied behavior analysis* (2nd ed.). Upper Saddle Hill, NJ: Pearson Education.

Donnellan, A. (Ed.). (1985). *Classic readings in autism*. New York, NY: Teachers College Press.

Fay, W., & Schuler, A. L. (1980). *Emerging language in autistic children*. Baltimore, MD: University Park Press.

Goldstein, H. (2002). Communication intervention for children with autism: A review of treatment efficacy. *Journal of Autism and Developmental Disorders, 32*(5), 373–396.

Harding, J. W., Wacker, D. W., Berg, W. K., Rick, G., & Lee, J. F. (2004). Promoting response variability and stimulus generation in martial arts training. *Journal of Applied Behavior Analysis, 3*(2), 185–195.

Hegde, M. N. (1998). *Treatment procedures in communication disorders* (3rd ed.). Austin, TX: Pro-Ed.

Janzen, J. E. (2003). *Understanding the nature of autism: A guide to the autism spectrum disorders* (2nd ed.). San Antonio, TX: Therapy Skill Builders.

Jones, E., & Carr, E. (2004). Joint attention in children with autism: Theory and intervention. *Focus on Autism and Other Developmental Disabilities, 19*(1), 13–26.

Kanner, L. (1943). Autistic disturbances of affective contact. *Nervous Child, 2*, 217–250.

Lee, B. (1975). *Tao of jeet kune do*. Valencia, CA: Ohara.

Lord, C. (1995). Follow-up of two year olds referred for possible autism. *Journal of Psychology and Psychiatry, 36*(8), 1365–1382.

Lord, C., & Paul, R. (1997). Language and communication in autism. In D. Cohen & F. Volmar (Eds.), *Handbook of autism and pervasive developmental disorders* (2nd ed., pp. 195–225). Hoboken, NJ: John Wiley & Sons.

Maurice, C. Green, G., & Luce, S. C. (Eds.). *Behavioral intervention for young children with autism: A manual for parents and professionals* (pp. 29–44). Austin, TX: Pro-Ed.

McHale, S., Marcus, L., & Olley, J. (1980). The social and syntactic quality of autistic children's communications. *Journal of Autism and Developmental Disorders, 10*, 299–314.

Morgan, F. E. (1992). *Living the martial way. How to develop attitudes based on the ancient Asian martial arts.* Fort Lee, NJ: Barricade Books.

Musashi, M. (1982). *The book of five rings. Gorin no sho.* New York, NY: Bantam Books.

Osterling, J., & Dawson, G. (1994). Early recognition of children with autism: A study of first birthday video tapes. *Journal of Autism and Developmental Disorders, 24*(3), 247–258.

Owens, R. E. (2008). *Language development. An introduction* (7th ed.). Boston, MA: Pearson.

Prelock, P. (2006). *Autism Spectrum Disorders. Issues and assessment intervention.* Austin, TX: Pro-Ed.

Shic, F., Bradshaw, J., Klin, A., Scassellati, B., & Chawarska, K. (2011). Limited activity monitoring in toddlers with autism spectrum disorder. *Brain Research, 1380,* 246–254.

Stokes, T. F., & Baer, D. M. (1977). An implicit technology of generalization. *Journal of Applied Behavior Analysis, 10*(2), 349–367.

Stone, W. L., & Caro-Martinez, L. M. (1990). Naturalistic observations of spontaneous communication in autistic children. *Journal of Autism and Developmental Disorders, 20,* 437–453.

Tager-Flusberg, H., Paul, R., & Lord, C. (2005). Language and communication in autism. In F. R. Volkmar, R. Paul, A. Klin, & D, Cohen (Eds.), *Handbook of autism and pervasive developmental disorders, Volume 1* (pp 335–364). Hoboken, NJ: John Wiley & Sons.

Tzu, S. (2002). *The art of war. The Denma translation.* Boston, MA: Shambala.

Williams, D. (2010). *Developmental language disorders. Learning, language, and the brain.* San Diego, CA: Plural.

ESSAY 21

❧ Storybook Yoga ❧

Integrating Shared Book Reading and Yoga to Nurture the Whole Child

Susan Hendler Lederer

Dr. Sadanand Singh inspired us to think like translational speech-language pathologists. By publishing titles from a variety of disciplines, he encouraged us to both learn from the voices of others, as well as share our own unique perspectives. As a pediatric speech-language pathologist with expertise in child language acquisition and disorders, I, too, have been inspired to make connections across disciplines. The results have included the publication of children's books, music, and innovative programs designed to help professionals and parents support the development of all children. StoryBook Yoga is one such program.

A famous Indian legend tells of six blind men who, for the first time, encounter an elephant. One comes upon the tusk and concludes the elephant is like a spear; another explores the trunk and believes the elephant is like a snake; a third likens the elephant to a fan as he strokes the ear (Saxe, 1872). Of course, none truly understands the elephant as he has not considered the whole animal.

Considering the whole child, like the whole elephant, is best practice according to the National Association for the Education of Young Children (NAEYC). In their 2009 position paper NAEYC states, "All the domains of development and learning—physical, social and emotional, and cognitive—are important, and they are closely interrelated. Children's development and learning in one domain influence and are influenced by what takes place in other domains" (NAEYC, 2009, p. 11). Therefore, NAEYC concludes early childhood educators must create active and engaging experiences within and across the four major developmental domains.

As speech-language pathologists (SLPs) working with young children, we, too, must consider the needs of the whole child within and across domains. Creating learning experiences within the cognitive domains of language and literacy is our specialty. For example, we use shared book reading to foster language skills such as vocabulary development and story comprehension, as well as emergent literacy skills such as phonological awareness and book concepts. We incorporate other developmental domains by creating extension activities such as bookmaking, which also fosters fine motor skills, or story re-enactments to encourage social development among the "actors" and cognitive/pretend play skills. However, these activities are still primarily designed to address the language and literacy goals.

How do we more fully embrace NAEYC's position and better address development of the whole child within our language/literacy activities? More specifically, how can we reconceptualize shared book reading to integrate cognitive (linguistic, literacy, pretend play), motor, social, and emotional goals? Translational speech-language pathology challenges us to look outside our discipline for answers. In this essay, we will look way beyond speech-language pathology and early childhood education. We look to the east and yoga for innovation. By integrating shared book reading and yoga, we can create an active and engaging, transdisciplinary experience, as recommended by NAEYC and inspired by translational speech-language pathology.

WHY YOGA?

Yoga is an ancient system of exercise and philosophy of living first practiced in India over 5000 years ago. In Sanskrit, "yoga" means "union"; the union of body, mind, and spirit. Yoga includes a physical practice of poses (in Sanskrit called "asanas"), breathing exercises (called "pranayamas"), and meditation (called "dhyana'). The benefits of yoga are vast and anecdotal reports are now being supported by systematic research studies, including specific research on children (for reviews, see Birdee et al., 2009; Galantino, Galbavy, & Quinn, 2008; Kaley-Isley, Peterson, Fischer, & Peterson, 2010). Perhaps this is why, in a 2007 Centers for Disease Control (CDC) survey, there were over 1.5 million children practicing yoga in the United States (Barnes, Bloom, & Nahin, 2008).

YOGA AND PHYSICAL DEVELOPMENT AND HEALTH

For the body, yoga promotes strength, flexibility, and balance. Health benefits include improved cardiopulmonary function, increased blood flow and oxygenation through massage to internal organs, a healthy brain, and a good night's sleep (Khalsa, 2002; McCall, 2007). Developmentally, yoga facilitates fine and gross motor development; eye-hand coordination; motor planning; coordination of the central nervous system through midline movements/balanced activity of opposing muscle groups; and body awareness, respect, and confidence (Galantino, Galbavy, & Quinn, 2008). To illustrate some of these benefits, consider the following poses. The dog pose (http://www.yoga-training-you.com/yoga-for-beginners.html) promotes strength in the arms and legs whereas the cat-cow sequence (http://www.yoga-training-you.com/free-yoga-moves.html) promotes flexibility of the spine. The tree pose (http://www.yoga-training-you.com/online-yoga-instruction.html) fosters balance whereas the sun salutation (http://www.yoga-training-you.com/surya-namaskar.html) (often modified for children) links poses to improve cardiopulmonary function and motor planning.

YOGA AND COGNITIVE DEVELOPMENT

For the mind, yoga improves attention, concentration, and memory necessary for listening and learning. Yoga has been shown to decrease the stress hormone cortisol and increase serotonin which is responsible for attention and memory, as well as increase activity in the orbitofrontal cortex, and parietal and temporal regions also associated with attention

(Khalsa, 2002; McCall, 2007). Research on children with Attention Deficit/Hyperactivity Disorder (ADHD) has demonstrated overall reduction in symptoms and increased time on task (for review, see Birdee et al., 2009; Kaley-Isley, Peterson, Fischer, & Peterson, 2010). As attention can be practiced, it is posited that attention to breathing and poses (especially balance poses) builds attention skills necessary for learning.

In addition to attention, yoga can be used to facilitate cognitive development in the areas of pretend play, language, and literacy. As children practice different yoga poses, many named for animals, they rehearse decentration (an important pretend play skill) by assuming the roles of the animals. Children in the downward facing dog pose can bark, pant, and wag their tails. In the cat pose, children can meow and lick their paws. Language/vocabulary can be facilitated by teaching children more sophisticated animal names such as "cobra," (as opposed to "snake") (http://www.yoga-training-you.com/surya-namaskar.html) or "pigeon" (as opposed to "bird") (http://www.yoga-training-you.com/pigeon-pose.html). Finally, by framing a children's yoga class with a storybook, a variety of language and emergent literacy skills can be targeted.

YOGA AND EMOTIONAL AND SOCIAL DEVELOPMENT

Yoga supports the development of emotional skills such as self-esteem and self-regulation, and social skills such as building community, kindness, and respect. Yoga is considered a practice, which gives children permission to be less than perfect. But it also offers challenges which provide opportunities to take pride in "trying" and "succeeding" thus helping children develop self-esteem (Powell, Gilchrist, & Stapley, 2008).

Self-regulation (i.e., inhibiting impulsive behaviors/engaging in planned behaviors) is possible when there is a balanced emotional state. Yoga has been shown to decrease the sympathetic nervous system's "fight or flight" stress reactions while increasing the parasympathetic's calm (Khalsa, 2002; McCall, 2007). Yoga fosters a balanced emotional state in a variety of ways including deep, rhythmical breathing; reciprocal, rhythmical chanting (e.g., call and response monkey noises); and alternating calming poses (e.g., forward bends such as "child's resting pose") (http://www.yoga-training-you.com/hatha-yoga-pose.html) with energizing poses (e.g., back bending heart openers such as "bridge") (http://www.yoga-training-you.com/yoga-poses.html). When in a calm, even state, children are more able to make thoughtful, socially appropriate behavior choices.

Social skills can be addressed using yoga in three unique ways. First, by practicing together and adding some partner or group poses (e.g., while doing the tree pose, all hold hands in a circle to form a "forest"), social skills are addressed. Children can be taught to drop their hands if they are about to fall and bring down the rest of the forest! Second, developing an appreciation for nature through the poses can support development of kindness and respect for all. Finally, children can be taught to acknowledge each other with the traditional Sanskrit greeting, "Namaste," which I translate as, "We are all special." Ending each class with simultaneous chanting of "om" (i.e., the universal sound of peace and harmony) and "Namaste" is a reminder that we are one community.

STORYBOOK YOGA

You do not have to have your own yoga practice or any special materials to introduce StoryBook Yoga (Lederer, 2008) to children.

Start by picking a book off your shelf that contains animals (e.g., dog, cat, snake) and/or natural wonders (e.g., tree, sun, star) for which there are yoga poses. In Appendix 21–A, there is a list of children's books that I have used to create successful StoryBook Yoga lessons. If you are new to yoga, I recommend Baron Baptiste's *My Daddy Is a Pretzel* (Baptiste, 2004), a children's book in which poses are illustrated and explained. To learn other child-friendly poses, try *The Complete Idiot's Guide to Yoga for Kids* (Komitor & Adamson, 2000).

In general, look for short books, one to two lines per page. See-saw books or list books work well (especially those with predictable and repetitive schemes or phrases such as *Dear Zoo* (Campbell, 1999); *Brown Bear; Brown Bear* (Martin, 1992); or *It Looked Like Spilt Milk* (Shaw, 1947). Illustrated songs, such as *Old MacDonald* (Pearson, 1984), often work well. Make sure each book contains mention or pictures of animals/natural wonders to practice at least one strength (e.g., dog), one flexibility (e.g., cat), one balance (e.g., tree), and one pose sequence (e.g., sun). Incorporate deep breathing before and after poses, plus other breathing inspired by book characters (e.g., lion, bunny). Finally, I recommend books with universal themes such as peace (e.g., *The Peace Book*, Parr, 2004) and tolerance (e.g., *It's Okay to Be Different*, Parr, 2001).

To begin, sit together comfortably and quietly get ready with closed eyes and some slow, deep, rhythmic breathing in and out through the nose for three rounds. Introduce the story of the day followed by the "book" poses (e.g., butterfly pose and twists to simulate opening/closing the book and turning the pages) (See http://www.yoga-training-you.com/different-yoga-positions.html). Begin to read and stop when you come to a yoga opportunity. Put the book down and practice the yoga pose. After the pose, return to sitting, and with eyes closed, slowly and deeply breathe in and out through the nose again for two to three rounds. Resume reading, stopping again for a pose and again, slow, deep breathing. When the book is finished, instruct the children to lie down for rest which allows the body to integrate the yoga movement and breathing experiences. Offer back massages to further enhance the resting pose. At the end of relaxation, all return to sitting. You may choose to chant "om" together. To close, children place their palms together, thumbs to their hearts and with eye contact, acknowledge each other with "Namaste; we are all special."

To further bring your StoryBook Yoga lesson to life, add music. Before you begin reading, move through Berkner's "These Are My Glasses" (Berkner, 2001) or Mar's "It's Time to Read" (Harman, 2005). As you read, use other animal-related songs such as "Who Let the Dogs Out" (Douglas, 1998) or "The Goldfish" (Berkner, 2001). At the end of your StoryBook Yoga lesson, play some relaxing music for the final resting pose such as Kermit the Frog's "Rainbow Connection" (Williams & Ascher, 1979) or any other soothing music. The StoryBook Yoga CD (Lederer, 2008) has yoga instructions narrated before, during, and after each of the 11 songs including a book song, a relaxation song, and nine animal/natural wonder songs.

ADAPTATIONS FOR CHILDREN WITH SPECIAL NEEDS

The two main objectives of children's yoga are to practice safely and have fun. As yoga is a personal practice, there is no need to expect children's expressions of traditional poses to look like the ones in pictures. We can help our children who are ambulatory, by physically assisting them into a pose or inviting them to use a wall for support. Partner poses and group poses, such as holding hands in a circle in a ring of trees, can also be helpful. For nonambulatory children, poses can be adapted to be practiced while seated in their chairs. For high energy children, challenging poses, balance poses, and games in which poses are held and timed can increase engagement. Deep breathing after each pose with eyes softly closed or backrubs in child's resting pose can calm and refocus children when needed. For additional information about yoga for children with disabilities, the reader is referred to Erwin and Lederer's (2010) "Let's Practice Yoga" from http://www.pbs.org/parents/inclusivecommunities/yoga.html

CONCLUSION

Translational speech-language pathology suggests that we are better able to serve our clients when we communicate across disciplines and even across continents! StoryBook Yoga, a transdisciplinary approach to shared book reading, meets this challenge. By integrating shared book reading with yoga and music, we can foster development simultaneously in the cognitive, physical, emotional, and social domains. Namaste!

REFERENCES

Barnes, P.M., Bloom, B., & Nahin, R. (2008, December 10). *National health statistics reports: Complementary and alternative medicine use among adults and children: United States, 2007.* Retrieved from http://www.cdc.gov/nchs/data/nhsr/nhsr012.pdf.

Birdee, G., Yeh, G., Wayne, P., Phillips, R., Davis, R., & Gardiner, P. (2009). Clinical applications of yoga for the pediatric population: A systematic review. *Academy of Pediatrics, 9*(4), 212–220.

Coleman, S. (n.d.) *Yoga and massage training.* Retrieved from http://www.yoga-training-you.com/index.html

Erwin, E., & Lederer, S. (2010). *Let's practice yoga: The promise and practice for children with disabilities.* Retrieved from http://www.pbs.org/parents/inclusivecommunities/yoga.html

Galantino, M., Galbavy, R., & Quinn, L. (2008). Therapeutic effects of yoga for children: A systematic review of the literature. *Pediatric Physical Therapy, 20*(1), 66–80.

Kaley-Isley, L., Peterson, J., Fischer, C., & Peterson, E. (2010). Yoga as a complementary therapy for children and adolescents: A guide for clinicians. *Psychiatry, 7*(8), 20–32.

Khalsa, D. (2002). *Meditation as medicine.* New York, NY: Fireside.

Komitor, J., & Adamson, E. (2000). *The complete idiot's guide to yoga with kids.* Indianapolis, IN: Macmillan.

Lederer (2008). *StoryBook Yoga.* Baldwin, NY: Educational Activities. Retrieved from http://www.edact.com/storybook-yoga-compact-disc.html

McCall, T. (2007). *Yoga as medicine.* New York, NY: Bantam.

National Association for the Education of Young Children (NAEYC). (2009). Position statement on developmentally appropriate practice. Retrieved from http://www.naeyc.org/positionstatements/dap

Powell, L., Gilchrist, M., & Stapley, J. (2008). A journey of self-discovery: An intervention involving massage, yoga and relaxation for children with emotional and behavioural difficulties attending primary schools. *European Journal of Special Needs Education, 23*(4), 403–412.

Saxe, G. (1872). *The blind men and the elephant.* Retrieved from http://en.wikisource.org/wiki/The_Blindmen_and_the_Elephant

APPENDIX 21–A

Recommended Children's Books and Music

RECOMMENDED CHILDREN'S BOOKS

Baptiste, B. (2004). *My daddy is a pretzel: Yoga for parents and kids.* Cambridge, MA: Barefoot Books.

Brett, J. (2003). *On Noah's ark.* New York, NY: G. P. Putnam's Sons.

Cabrera, J. (2000). *Over in the meadow.* New York, NY: Holiday House.

Campbell, R. (1999). *Dear zoo.* New York, NY: Little, Simon.

Carle, E. (1984). *The very busy spider.* New York, NY: Philomel Books.

Carle, E. (1993). *Today is Monday.* New York, NY: Philomel Books.

Carle, E. (2007). *From head to toe.* New York, NY: Harper Festival.

Martin, B. (1992). *Brown bear, brown bear, what do you see.* New York, NY: Henry Holt & Company.

Parr, T. (2001). *It's okay to be different.* New York, NY: Little, Brown & Company.

Parr, T. (2004). *The peace book.* New York, NY: Little, Brown & Company.

Parr, T. (2005). *Reading makes you feel good.* New York, NY: Little, Brown & Company.

Parr, T. (2009). *The feel good book.* New York, NY: Little Brown, Brown & Company.

Pearson, T. C. (1984). *Old MacDonald had a farm.* New York, NY: Dial Books for Young Readers.

Sendak, M. (1962). *Chicken soup with rice: A book of months.* New York, NY: HarperCollins.

Shaw, C. G. (1947). *It looked like spilt milk.* New York, NY: HarperCollins Children's Books.

Westcott, N. B. (2003). *I know an old lady who swallowed a fly.* Boston, MA: Little, Brown Children's Books.

Williams, S. (1990). *I went walking.* San Diego, CA: Gulliver Books.

RECOMMENDED CHILDREN'S MUSIC

Berkner, L. (2001). The goldfish. [Recorded by L. Berkner] on *Victor Vito* [CD]. New York, NY: Two Tomatoes Records (2001).

Berkner, L. (2001). These are my glasses. [Recorded by L. Berkner] on *Whaddya think of that* [CD]. New York, NY: Two Tomatoes Records (2001).

Douglas, A. (1998). Who let the dogs out. [Recorded by Baha Men] on *Rugrats in Paris: The movie* [CD]. New York, NY: Maverick Records (2000).

Harman, M. (2005). It's time to read. [Recorded by M. Harman] on *StoryBook Yoga* [CD]. Baldwin, NY: Educational Activities.

Lederer, S. (2008). *StoryBook Yoga* [CD]. Baldwin, NY: Educational Activities.

Williams, P., & Ascher, K. (1979). Rainbow connection. [Recorded by Kermit the Frog] on *The Muppet Movie.* [CD]. New York, NY: Muppet Music, Inc. (1993).

PART V

❦ Audiology and Hearing Science ❦

ESSAY 22

Reflections on ❧ Translational Research in ❧ Tinnitus and Hyperacusis

David M. Baguley

It is a pleasure and a privilege to contribute to this volume of essays in honor of Dr. Singh. I knew him for many years, and would seek him out at American Academy of Audiology (AAA) conventions where we would talk about international audiology matters, and specifically the situation in the United Kingdom. In 2007 Plural Publishing agreed to publish the book Hyperacusis: Mechanisms, Diagnosis and Therapies *by myself and Professor Gerhard Andersson (from Sweden). This was an example of the support Plural, and specifically Dr. Singh, gave to fringe topics, as at the time there was little interest in decreased sound tolerance. Since then hyperacusis has entered the mainstream of clinical audiology, included in both Featured Sessions and Keynote talks at recent AAA conventions. There are many other such examples where the work of Dr. Singh through both Singular and Plural Publishers supported the development of audiology, and facilitated teaching and research across the breadth of the discipline. This strong legacy is a testament to the giftedness and commitment of Dr. Singh, and his involvement in audiology enriched both the clinical discipline, and also the lives of those who knew him.*

INTRODUCTION

In this essay my aim is to reflect on translational research regarding tinnitus and hyperacusis. I will ask some searching questions about the applicability of basic science to these symptoms, and about the insights that the clinical situation might give to the basic scientists. In concluding I will indicate that significant treatment uncertainties presently exist, and how research might seek to resolve these.

DEFINITIONS AND EPIDEMIOLOGY

The experience of tinnitus may be complex (Andersson et al., 2005), involving several (sometimes many) different sounds which may vary over time in tone, intensity, and perceived point of origin. Modulating factors may include emotional state, the auditory environment, and muscle tension in the head and neck. Despite this complexity, it is interesting to note that the descriptors used by persons with tinnitus (hiss, buzz, sizzle, ring, for example) are almost invariably indicative of a simple or unformed perception, and also that a good proportion of people are unable to describe their sound at all (Andersson et al., 2005). Definitions of tinnitus can be lengthy, but essentially describe a perception of sound that is not evoked by external stimulation. The distinction has been made between *subjective* tinnitus, which can only be heard by the individual, and *objective* tinnitus, which can be heard or measured by an external observer. An example of an objective tinnitus would be spontaneous otoacoustic emissions (SOAE), though the majority of persons with SOAE are unaware of them and do not report them as tinnitus. A subcategorization of some forms of tinnitus as *somatosounds* can be useful, indicating those sounds produced by bodily processes, but which may not be audible to an external observer. Some forms of pulsatile tinnitus and middle ear myoclonus can be categorized as somatosounds.

Considering hyperacusis, this does not refer to Superman's ability to hear a telephone ringing several blocks away, but to the experience of sound in the environment as intense and uncomfortable (Baguley & McFerran, 2011). For some individuals this can be all sound, even when of modest intensity, but for others it can be specific sounds. This latter situation has been described as *phonophobia*, but the use of the suffix *phobia* is not necessarily correct or helpful, implying an essentially psychological mechanism. Some (Jastreboff & Hazell, 2004) use the term *misophonia* (dislike of sound) to capture the aversion aspect of the symptom, but again an emotional mechanism is implied that may not be suitable.

Epidemiologic data regarding tinnitus are complex (Moller, 2011). Prevalence rates are influenced by definitions, and by the dura-

tion and severity of the reported sensation. Incidence rates are influenced by the ease of access to tinnitus services in a particular health economy, and by help-seeking behaviors in particular cultures. The ground is firmest beneath us when we ask about experiences of any tinnitus at all, and about clinically significant (hence severe) tinnitus. In the former case, studies indicate that up to 30% of adult persons in the general population in the Western world have experienced tinnitus at some time or other, and that 0.5% of the population have tinnitus that they report as severe (Moller, 2011). The situation regarding tinnitus in childhood is less clear, but seems broadly similar (Baguley & McFerran, 2002).

Information regarding the epidemiology of hyperacusis is sparse (Baguley & McFerran, 2011). A postal questionnaire in Sweden (Andersson et al., 2002) indicated a point prevalence (that is experience of everyday sound being uncomfortably loud on the day of questioning) of 9%, but this is felt to be unrepresentative of the clinical situation. An estimated 2% of the adult population with clinically significant issues with reduced sound tolerance has been proposed (Baguley & Andersson, 2007), but this is inferential and not yet supported with empirical evidence. Firm information regarding sound tolerance in childhood is not yet available, and reports of associations between hyperacusis and autistic spectrum disorder, and with attention deficit hyperactivity disorder, await systematic investigation.

PRESENTLY AVAILABLE TREATMENTS

Truly effective treatments for tinnitus and hyperacusis continue to elude us. Presently available treatments are largely composed of information and/or counseling, sound therapy (hearing aid or wide-band sound generator), and relaxation techniques. Tinnitus therapy can be delivered on a self-help basis (McKenna et al., 2010). The aim of tinnitus therapy is to promote habituation to the perceived stimulus, and to limit the impact. The differences between the various treatment protocols in use, Tinnitus Retraining Therapy (TRT) (Jastreboff & Hazell, 2004) and Cognitive Behavioral Therapy (CBT) (Andersson et al., 2005, Hesser et al., 2011) for example, firstly are in large part differences in emphasis rather than substantial variance, and secondly in the philosophical underpinning of the technique. For instance, proponents of TRT adhere to a view that tinnitus distress develops due to classical conditioning, whereas a CBT clinician would use the language of evaluative conditioning and selective attention.

Recent systematic reviews should allow the clinician to form a view as to the efficacy of interventions for tinnitus. Considering CBT (Hesser et al., 2011; Martinez-Devesa et al., 2010), the indications are that it can be effective at reducing tinnitus related distress, but does not alter the perceived intensity of the tinnitus. The quality of evidence regarding sound therapy for tinnitus is too poor for firm conclusions to be drawn (Hobson et al., 2010), and the number of papers investigating TRT that are of sufficiently robust experimental design is very low (Phillips et al., 2010). One should note, however, that there are significant challenges in trial design for tinnitus interventions. A placebo version of masking sound may be possible, but blinded placebo versions of counseling are not. Although no excuse for the shortcomings of the tinnitus literature, this does help one understand that context.

Developments are underway. These involve both the evolution of presently existing techniques, and the formulation of novel interventions for tinnitus and hyperacusis. Regarding the former, the investigation of the latest psychotherapy techniques, specifically Acceptance Based Therapy, represents a third wave of CBT (Westin et al., 2011). The implementation of novel sound therapy strategies include the use of music, filtered either to increase (Davis et al., 2007) or decrease (Wilson et al., 2010) activity at the frequency region of the tinnitus. Novel interventions include transcranial magnetic stimulation (Meng et al., 2011), and the development of new drugs to inhibit tinnitus (Langguth & Elgoyhen, 2011). A cautious optimism is appropriate regarding such work.

It would seem that tinnitus and hyperacusis would be a fertile field for translational research. What, then, is the reality of the situation?

TRANSLATIONAL RESEARCH IN TINNITUS AND HYPERACUSIS

By translational research, I mean that endeavor to take basic research findings and apply them to a specific clinical sensation. In my opinion and that of others (Bauer, 2011) regarding tinnitus, this is a two-way process, in that findings within and reflections on clinical scenarios can also inform and guide basic research. For this to be truly effective, a collaborative and multidisciplinary ethos is required.

There are indications that in the field of tinnitus and hyperacusis there is a move away from a previous emphasis on the expertise and experience (and hence opinion) of a small number of senior researchers and clinicians, toward a community approach, characterized by collaboration. This is multidisciplinary in nature, and Table 22–1 details the disciplines that are presently engaged in tinnitus research, although the list is not exhaustive. There are indications also that this community aspires to high quality research, especially with regard to experimental design. As mentioned above, there are challenges in the application of double-blind randomized placebo-controlled trial

Table 22–1. The Disciplines Involved in Tinnitus and Hyperacusis Research

- Audiology
- Otology
- Neurology
- Auditory Neuroscience
- Psychology
- Psychiatry
- Radiology
- Epidemiology
- Pharmacology
- Genetics

(RCT) experimental design to tinnitus and hyperacusis, but this is by no means unique to these symptoms, and there is much to learn from other research areas, such as chronic pain. In no small part, the efforts of the Tinnitus Research Initiative (http://www.tinnitus research.org) have either instigated or built upon such developments, and this has been warmly welcomed by many in the field.

There is a long journey ahead, however, and research into tinnitus and hyperacusis has generally been of low quality, and often performed by busy clinicians who have not been encouraged to apply rigor to their experimental designs, hence the many observational studies in this area rather than RCT.

Let us now examine the challenges evident in translational research for tinnitus and hyperacusis, asking the following questions:

What are the barriers to translational research in tinnitus and hyperacusis?

Why has the involvement of pharmacology been so late in contributing to tinnitus and hyperacusis?

What questions do the experience of patients with tinnitus and hyperacusis raise about our understanding of human hearing?

WHAT ARE THE BARRIERS TO TRANSLATIONAL RESEARCH IN TINNITUS AND HYPERACUSIS?

There are a number of substantial challenges to translational research in this area. One major issue is the complexity of the experience of severe, distressing tinnitus. Let us consider a young adult male who develops a mild noise induced hearing loss, and severe debilitating tinnitus, following a visit to a night club, during which he became mildly intoxicated. There is self-blame, and this patient has broken sleep, and is struggling to concentrate at work. The issues that are likely to arise in a clinical appointment, and the clinical/research perspectives that might underpin our understanding, are indicated in Table 22–2.

It can be seen that even in a fairly simple clinical scenario, a variety of perspectives need to be brought to bear. A number of reflections can be made. The first is that whatever clinician(s) are involved with this patient, a combination of strategies is indicated. Whatever the "home" discipline of the lead clinician for this patient, be they psychology or audiology based, an understanding of other perspectives is needed: they must at least be literate in and sympathetic to other perspectives. Second, although basic science models such as animal models of NIHL and tinnitus may help us determine the physiological substrate of the auditory dysfunction, they do not, and cannot, shed light on the complex emotional context in such a patient. Jean Marc Gaspard Itard (1774–1838) was an historical figure involved with tinnitus. Itard was a physician, and an early proponent of otology, and

Table 22–2. Issues Arising from Patient Experiences

Issue	Relevant Clinical/Research Perspectives
Cochlear dysfunction and NIHL	Basic cochlear science Animal models of NIHL
Metabolic mechanisms of NIHL and relationship to intoxication	Basic cochlear science
Central reorganization as a consequence of cochlear dysfunction	Auditory neuroscience
Where is the ignition site of the tinnitus?	Auditory neuroscience
Self-blame	Psychotherapy
Sleep management	Audiology (use of bedside sound) Psychology (sleep hygiene)
Concentration	Psychology
Use of hearing aids and/or ear level sound generator?	Audiology
Hearing protection in future	Audiology

wrote on the subjects of tinnitus and deafness. Itard described tinnitus as, "an extremely irksome discomfort which leads to a profound sadness in affected individuals" (cited in Stephens, 2000), and it is difficult to see how these aspects of tinnitus experience could be captured within an animal model.

Another significant barrier is that of funding. It has been estimated that if one were to calculate all the research funding awarded worldwide for tinnitus in any given year, then the resulting figure would be less than the cost of a single armored tank (Salvi, personal communication). A compelling case needs to be made for funding streams for tinnitus and hyperacusis research, though the global financial situation is not promising in that regard. Such a case would need to build upon the data regarding the extent of the tinnitus problem, and the significant progress that is now being made. In times of limited resources, it is even

more important that colleagues work together for maximum benefit from funding, and that results are shared in a timely fashion.

WHY HAS THE INVOLVEMENT OF PHARMACOLOGY BEEN SO LATE IN CONTRIBUTING TO TINNITUS AND HYPERACUSIS?

Many tinnitus experts have had repeated requests from big pharmaceutical companies to talk about tinnitus. That industry is interested in tinnitus as the market is potentially very large indeed, and there is no truly effective treatment at present. In my experience the initial enthusiasm of the companies is moderated when they hear of what is known about potential sites at which drugs might inhibit tinnitus. They then realize that although there is much speculation, there remains little by the way of fact. There are indications that this too is changing, however, with several compounds under active investigation. A drug called Vestipitant, which has positive effects on some anxiety types, was recently shown not to be effective in tinnitus and hyperacusis in a trial involving GlaxoSmithKlein and clinical colleagues in Cambridge and in Colchester, UK (Roberts et al., 2011). The compounds AM101 (Muehlmeier et al., 2011) and Neramexane (Suckfull et al., 2011), both of which are thought to have a glutamate antagonist action, have recently undergone Phase II trials, with some promising proof of concept and safety data. The interested reader is directed to http://www.clinicaltrials.gov for information about ongoing studies.

This level of activity is heartening, as it represents a source of revenue for tinnitus research outside the academic/philanthropic streams, and research by the pharmaceutical industry is presumably of robust experimental design. Where opportunities present for clinical audiologists to be involved, they should be grasped. Even though pharmacology is rarely part of our initial training, collaborative work can allow us to represent our distinctive understanding of the tinnitus and hyperacusis situations.

WHAT QUESTIONS DO THE EXPERIENCE OF PATIENTS WITH TINNITUS AND HYPERACUSIS RAISE ABOUT OUR UNDERSTANDING OF HUMAN HEARING?

If translational research really is a two-way process, then reflections upon the experiences of people with tinnitus and hyperacusis should raise questions about our understanding of human hearing, and thus guide basic science research. In this section I venture some personal observations, in the hope that they might provoke some further thought.

The first regards the primitive nature of tinnitus, in that the descriptors used are, as mentioned above, very simple. Is this an indication that the sites of interest for a tinnitus researcher might not be in the cortex, but within the brainstem? Further signposts in that direction might be the propensity for tinnitus to be modulated by somatic input from the jaw and neck muscles (Sanchez & Rocha, 2011). If correct, then that might mean that the chances of success for novel intervention strategies that target the auditory cortex, such as transcranial magnetic stimulation, might not be high, and indeed the initial promise of that particular technique has not yet been borne out (Meng et al., 2011).

A question deriving from hyperacusis experiences concerns the perception of auditory intensity. The auditory neuroscience literature (Florentine, 2011) is open about the fact that there is much yet to be known in this regard, and the ways in which midbrain auditory structures are able to encode intensity over a relatively small range, but a range that can move dependent on the auditory environment, is of great interest in that regard.

Another set of questions concerns the relationship between hearing and emotion. The deep distress evoked by either severe tinnitus or hyperacusis indicate to the clinician that strong functional associations exist between the auditory system and the limbic system. Whether tinnitus and hyperacusis distress represent dysfunction of such associations is yet to be explored. This is potentially of some clinical importance, as once the development of such a relationship is understood, one can start to consider how it might be effectively undone. In the Tinnitus Clinic the interventions of counseling and relaxation therapy may be poor tools for the size of the task.

TREATMENT UNCERTAINTIES

In closing, I acknowledge the significant treatment uncertainties that exist for tinnitus and hyperacusis. These include (among many others) the ignition site of tinnitus in any specific patient, the extent to which personality affects treatment outcomes, and the optimal treatment for a particular individual. Well-designed research is needed to consider the many issues that arise in clinical work with tinnitus and hyperacusis, and at times the amount of work that is yet to be done is daunting. Despite, and perhaps because of this, tinnitus and hyperacusis remain fascinating, and a compelling source of translational research.

Acknowledgment. David M. Baguley's research is supported by an NHS East of England Senior Clinical Academic Fellowship.

REFERENCES

Andersson, G., Baguley, D. M., McKenna, L., & McFerran, D. (2005). *Tinnitus: A multidisciplinary approach*. London, UK: Whurr.

Andersson, G., Lindvall, N., Hursti, T., & Carlbring, P. (2002). Hypersensitivity to sound (hyperacusis): A prevalence study conducted via the Internet and post. *International Journal of Audiology, 41*, 545–554.

Baguley, D. M., & Andersson, G. A. (2007). *Hyperacusis*. San Diego, CA: Plural.

Baguley, D. M., & McFerran, D. J. (2002). Current perspectives on tinnitus. *Archives of Disorders in Children, 86*, 141–143.

Baguley, D. M., & McFerran, D. J. (2011). Hyperacusis and disorders of loudness perception. In A. R. Moller, B. Langguth, D. DeRidder, & T. Kleinjung (Eds.), *Textbook of tinnitus* (pp. 13–24). New York, NY: Springer.

Bauer, C. (2011). Translational tinnitus research. *Audiology Today, 23*, 62–63.

Davis, P. B., Paki, B., & Hanley, P. J. (2007). Neuromonics tinnitus treatment: Third clinical trial. *Ear and Hearing, 28,* 242–259.

Florentine, M. (2011). Loudness. In M. Florentine, A. N. Popper, & R. R. Fay (Eds.), *Loudness* (pp. 1–16). New York, NY: Springer.

Hesser, H., Weise, C., Westin, V. Z., & Andersson, G. (2011). A systematic review and meta-analysis of randomized controlled trials of cognitive-behavioral therapy for tinnitus distress. *Clinical Psychology Review, 31*, 545–553.

Hobson, J., Chisholm, E., & El Refaie, A. (2010). Sound therapy (masking) in the management of tinnitus in adults. *Cochrane Database Systematic Reviews, 8*.

Jastreboff, P. J., & Hazell, J. W. P. H. (2004). *Tinnitus retraining therapy: Implementing the neurophysiological model*. Cambridge, UK: Cambridge University Press.

Langguth, B., & Elgoyhen, A. B. (2011) Emerging pharmacotherapy of tinnitus. *Expert Opinion on Emerging Drugs*, Dec 8. [Epub ahead of print].

Martinez-Devesa, P., Perera, R., Theodoulou, M., & Waddell, A. (2010). Cognitive behavioural therapy for tinnitus. *Cochrane Database Systematic Reviews, 8*.

McKenna, L., Baguley, D. M., & McFerran, D. (2010). *Living with tinnitus and hyperacusis*. London, UK: Sheldon Press.

Meng, Z., Liu, S., Zheng, Y., & Phillips, J. S. (2011). Repetitive transcranial magnetic stimulation for tinnitus. *Cochrane Database Systematic Reviews, 5*.

Moller, A. R. (2011). Epidemiology of tinnitus in adults. In A. R. Moller, B. Langguth, D. DeRidder, & T. Klienjung (Eds.), *Textbook of tinnitus* (pp. 29–38). New York, NY: Springer.

Muehlmeier, G., Biesinger, E., & Maier, H. (2011). Safety of intratympanic injection of AM-101 in patients with acute inner ear tinnitus. *Audiology and Neurotology, 16,* 388–397.

Roberts, C., Inamdar, A., Koch, A., Kitchiner, P., Dewit, O., Merlo-Pich, E., . . . Baguley, D. M. (2011). A randomized, controlled study comparing the effects of vestipitant or vestipitant and paroxetine combination in subjects with tinnitus. *Otology and Neurotology, 32,* 721–727.

Sanchez, T. G., & Rocha, C. B. (2011) In A. R. Moller, B. Langguth, D. DeRidder, & T. Klienjung (Eds.), *Textbook of tinnitus* (pp. 429–434). New York, NY: Springer.

Stephens, D. (2000) A history of tinnitus. In R. S. Tyler (Ed.), *Tinnitus handbook* (pp. 437–448). San Diego, CA: Singular.

Suckfüll, M., Althaus, M., Ellers-Lenz, B., Gebauer, A., Görtelmeyer, R., Jastreboff, P. J., . . . Krueger, H. (2011). A randomized, double-blind, placebo-controlled clinical trial to evaluate the efficacy and safety of neramexane in patients with moderate to severe subjective tinnitus. *BMC Ear Nose and Throat Disorders, 11,* 1.

Westin, V., Schulin, M., Hesser, H., Kaerlsson, M., Noe, R. Z., Olofsson, U., . . . Andersson, G. (2011). Acceptance and commitment therapy versus tinnitus retraining therapy in the treatment of tinnitus: A randomised controlled trial. *Behavior Research and Therapy, 49,* 737–747.

Wilson, E. C., Schlaug, G., & Pantev, C. (2010). Listening to filtered music as a treatment option for tinnitus: A review. *Music Perception, 27,* 327–330.

ESSAY 23

❧ What Is Auditory Neuropathy? ❧
Translational Studies That Distinguish Inner Hair Cell (IHC) from Auditory-Nerve (AN) Dysfunction

Anthony T. Cacace and Robert F. Burkard

In the book Controversies in Central Auditory Processing Disorder, *edited by Cacace and McFarland and published by Plural (2009), Cacace and Burkard discuss auditory neuropathy (AN) in the chapter, "Auditory Neuropathy: Bridging the Gap Between Basic Science and Current Clinical Concerns." Dr. Sadanand Singh endorsed publication of the book and encouraged the authors to write on topics that would bring controversial issues to the forefront. It was his belief that education and discussion would help to resolve difficult issues in the fields of audiology and speech-language pathology so that the science in this area would advance and ultimately, society at large would benefit. In keeping with this tradition, we explicate on the subject of AN and attempt to further clarify issues relevant to this topic. In so doing, we honor the memory of Dr. Singh for his philosophical insights, encouragement, and long-time support.*

BACKGROUND

Although a substantial number of papers have been published on this topic, there continues to be confusion concerning *what is* and *what is not* auditory neuropathy (AN). This concern has been voiced repeatedly (e.g., Cacace & Burkard, 2009; Cacace & Pinheiro, 2011; Loundon et al., 2005; Marsh & Kazahaya, 2009; Rapin & Gravel, 2006) and at the heart of the matter is differentiating inner hair cell (IHC) dysfunction from AN. This is not a trivial issue, as an accurate site-of-lesion assessment is key to establishing the appropriate diagnosis. Having this information will in turn enhance the utility of genotype-phenotype relationships, offer direction for rehabilitation, and perhaps provide successful treatment outcomes for some. Herein, we discuss terminology and definitions, consider appropriate tests of measurement, and provide relevant examples to elaborate on this distinction. Because of the brevity of this essay, by necessity, our coverage is representative but not exhaustive.

The hallmark features of AN are absent (desynchronized) auditory brainstem responses (ABRs), absent acoustic-stapedius reflexes, and present otoacoustic emissions (transient or distortion product) or cochlear microphonic potentials (CMs). Although AN has been the primary term used to codify this distinctive entity, others terms are also being used (e.g., auditory dys-synchrony; auditory neuropathy/auditory dys-synchrony, AN/AD; auditory neuropathy spectrum disorder, ANSD, etc.), some of which are not well defined, adding confusion and not clarity to the literature.

WHAT'S IN A NAME?

The common denominator to each of these terms is the word *neuropathy*, defined as a "disorder, often toxic, of the neuron" (e.g., Stedman, 2006, p. 1312). When applied to AN, this definition indicates that if IHCs are primarily affected and if pathology/dysfunction does not directly involve "neurons," then by definition, the condition is *not* a neuropathy. Furthermore, if one assumes that the primary dysfunction of AN is in the peripheral auditory system, then similarities to other peripheral neuropathies should be apparent. Indeed, such is the case as in known entities such as Friedreich's ataxia and the hereditary motor and sensory neuropathies (Charcot-Marie-Tooth disease), where parallels exist between degeneration of dorsal root ganglion and the spiral ganglion of the auditory nerve (Satya-Murti & Cacace, 1982). Although the term *auditory neuropathy spectrum disorder* (ANSD) appears to address the issue of degree or range of severity, this term is somewhat ambiguous. For example, if IHC dysfunction is included as part of the spectrum, then the term will obviously require refinement and updating. While the term *dys-synchrony* does not have a precise definition, the term *synchrony* does, as it is defined as "the simultaneous appearance of two separate events" (Stedman, 2006, p. 1887). Thus, if we assume that dys-synchrony refers to abnormal synchrony, then with respect to the auditory modality, it refers

to a disruption between stimulus presentation and near-simultaneous discharge of a population of auditory nerve fibers.

In human studies, neural synchrony is indexed by the ABR, an acoustically driven population response of neural activity recorded from surface electrodes on the scalp. As a physiologic measure, it is highly dependent on available populations of auditory neurons discharging synchronously in response to an abruptly gated acoustic stimulus, such as clicks or short-duration tone bursts with rapid rise/fall times. Signal averaging in the time domain is the typical computational processing strategy by which these potentials are extracted from the background neural activity. Even though there is variability or *jitter* in threshold and latency values of responses at the single-unit level due to traveling-wave delay and in the timing of the metabolic cascade leading to neural excitation, such effects are not obvious in the averaged recordings. In normal-hearing and neurologically normal individuals, the ABR is characterized by a series of temporally precise peaks occurring within the first 10 milliseconds following the stimulus, representing synchronized activity from the auditory nerve and associated generators in brainstem pathways. However, in cases of neuropathologic changes affecting the nerve (overt demyelination, segmental demyelination and re-myelination, toxicity effects, metabolic disturbances including hypoxic and ischemic effects, pressure from tumors, severe depopulation of neurons, etc.), increased temporal dispersion (jitter) of neural activity occurs. These pathologic processes affect the morphology of the ABR waveform, ranging from prolonged absolute and interpeak latencies, reductions in amplitude, broadening or absence of selected peaks, to elimination of the entire response. Such effects can occur in the presence or absence of peripheral hearing loss, based on the pure-tone audiogram. Clearly, the greater the jitter in the underlying neural activity, the more dys-synchronized the averaged ABR appears. Presently, there is no quantification metric of ABR de-synchronization and it remains as a qualitative feature of the response. Burkard and Don (2012) provide a more detailed discussion about neural synchrony. They contrast synchrony, as measured in single-unit responses (which is a measure of phase locking) to synchrony in population responses (which is an across-neuron discharge measure). They also discuss the possibility that ABR peak latencies and amplitudes provide useful information about neural synchrony and suggest the use of several stimulus and response manipulations that might be used to make the ABR a more sensitive metric of neural synchrony.

GENETIC MUTATIONS RESULTING IN IHC LOSS

Having defined fundamental response characteristics of AN, we now highlight the distinction between IHC dysfunction and AN using two genetic mutations that affect output properties of IHCs: otoferlin (OTOF) and the vesicular glutamate transporter (VGLUT3). Additionally, in the animal literature and specifically with respect to chinchilla species, IHCs can preferentially be affected by the anticancer drug, carboplatin. Depending on dose, damage to IHCs can be partial or complete but with relative sparing of the outer hair cells (OHCs). Although an in-depth review of this topic is beyond the scope of the current essay, it has been reviewed in detail elsewhere (Cacace & Burkard, 2009). In the OTOF and VGLUT3 mutations, the molecular machinery and functionality of the sensory cell is perturbed, resulting in either complete loss of *exocytosis* (neurotransmitter release) or absence of neurotransmitter loading into synaptic vesicles. Such effects predictably lead to

profound hearing loss, as most auditory nerve projections to the central auditory system are via large caliber myelinated Type I afferents (≥95%), which exclusively innervate IHCs (Spoendlin, 1985).

As relevant examples, OTOF and VGLUT3 mutations demonstrate test results that are most often *confused* with AN, *absent* acoustically evoked ABRs and *intact* OAEs. However, in these disorders the absence of acoustically evoked ABRs is not due to the prototypical desynchronization of neural activity, which is the putative hallmark of AN. The ABRs are absent because there is either a lack of excitatory neurochemical release from the ribbon synapse of the IHC or where synaptic vesicle release occurs, but without any effective excitation of primary auditory neurons. In the case of the OTOF mutation, there is a lack of calcium-dependent exocytosis in the transduction cascade. Although work in basic science has tentatively identified OTOF as the calcium sensor of the IHC (e.g., Johnson & Chapman, 2010), available evidence also indicates that its role is more complex (e.g., Reisinger et al., 2011; Zak et al., 2011). Nevertheless, this is a presynaptic sensory cell effect that should *not* be confused with or construed as a neuropathy of the auditory nerve.

In the case of the VGLUT3 mutation, whereas calcium-dependent exocytosis is unaffected, synaptic vesicles are not loaded with the excitatory neurotransmitter glutamate. Thus, when the cell is depolarized and vesicles are released from the ribbon synapse at the active zone of the IHC, neural excitation does *not* occur. The effect is equivalent to the IHC "shooting blanks" with respect to initiating the excitation cascade of the auditory nerve. Although underlying mechanisms are different for the OTOF and VGLUT3 mutations, the functional outcomes and test characteristics are quite similar; profound hearing loss with intact OAEs. However, for human studies, the story is not finished here. If we put these aforementioned results in the context of an infant being considered for cochlear implantation (CI), further tests are required to clarify the IHC versus AN site of lesion distinction. These include: (1) genetic testing to evaluate for OTO*F* or VGLUT3 mutations (the number of genetic mutations affecting IHC function will no doubt grow as the knowledge base in this area increases over time), and (2) electrically evoked ABRs (eABRs) to consider the viability the auditory nerve. If genetic testing confirms the OTO*F* or VGLUT3 mutation and if eABRs show robust responses, then the prognosis shifts from bleak to rosy. Indeed, identification of the OTO*F* mutation establishes a primary sensory cell defect and the presence of eABRs indicates that a substantial population of normally functioning auditory nerve fibers and spiral ganglion cells (neural reserve) is available for electrical stimulation, enabling the CI to operate effectively. Thus, if the following pattern of test results is manifest: profound hearing loss, *absent* acoustically evoked ABRs, normal eABRs, normal OAEs, and genetic testing confirming the OTO*F* or VGLUT3 mutation, then we can assume that IHC dysfunction is at the core of the problem. Under these conditions, animal studies and clinical data justify a favorable prognosis and provide support for the contention that a CI will have a high probability of success (e.g., Roullon et al., 2006; Roux et al., 2006; Ruel et al., 2008; Varga et al., 2003).

In the case of true neuropathies of the auditory nerve (e.g., Friedreich's ataxia, Mohr Tranbjaerg syndrome, Charcot-Marie-Tooth disease, dominant optic atrophy) (e.g., Cacace & Pinheiro, 2011; Satya-Murti & Cacace, 1982), where temporal bone histology has effectively documented a neural site of lesion (e.g., Bahmad et al., 2007; Hallpike et al., 1980; Merchant et al., 2001; Spoendlin, 1974), conventional amplification and/or use of a CI may be considered but it is doubtful

if such alternatives will be a viable long-term solution for restoring useful auditory function (e.g., Gibson & Graham, 2008). Exceptions may exist, but what is needed to resolve this issue is extensive follow-up data to provide the necessary evidence base, so that better informed decisions and counseling options can be made in the future.

In an experimental animal model, long-term low-level hypoxia has been found to differentially affect IHC versus OHC function with secondary effects from IHC damage producing glutamate excitotoxicity. The excitotoxicity serves to injure primary auditory neurons and negatively impact upon auditory-nerve function (Sawada et al., 2001). Under these conditions, test results indicate that OAEs remain intact but elevated ABR thresholds and altered ABR waveforms are manifest. Indeed, such effects can have a range of severity that may not be limited to the auditory periphery. Brainstem lesions (periventricular leukomalasia) and cortical dysfunctions (memory, language, and learning problems) can also occur, which complicates treatment (see Cacace & Burkard, 2009 for a more detailed discussion). Thus, long-term low-level hypoxia can produce sensory and neural hearing loss and central nervous system complications that often require extensive and long-term rehabilitation and educational assistance in affected individuals.

SOME OUTSTANDING ISSUES IN DELINEATING IHC DYSFUNCTION FROM AN

Apart from delineating IHC dysfunction from AN, as noted in OTO*F* and VGLUT3 mutations, other ways of making the IHC/AN distinction are evolving, albeit with many unresolved questions. On the one hand, using electrocochleography (ECoG), Gibson and

Sanli (2007) found that when CMs super-impose on large positive potentials (aka, an abnormal positive potential, APP) and when eABRs were recorded, individuals performed better with CIs than individuals having similar results but with abnormal eABRs. The implication being that this differential pattern of results may serve to distinguish IHC lesions versus those individuals with true neuropathies of the auditory nerve. It is also noteworthy that the APP has not been reported in AN with hearing loss in the mild-to-moderate or mild-to-profound range (e.g., Santarelli et al. 2008). Using ECoG to click stimuli, Santarelli and colleagues (e.g., Huang et al., 2009; Santarelli & Arslan, 2002; Santarelli et al., 2008; Santarelli et al., 2009) found that in most individuals with AN, a negative potential, often identified as the summating potential (SP) was observed or other cases where a SP with a compound action potential (CAP) was prolonged in duration in comparison to controls. In normal individuals, presenting clicks at very high rates resulted in a modest decrease in SP and CAP amplitude. This observation is predicable, as hair cell potentials show only modest adaptation but auditory nerve responses show substantial loss in amplitude at high stimulus rates due to the absolute and relative refractory periods of the Type I afferents. However, in individuals thought to have IHC loss, a low-amplitude, short-duration response, which was likely the SP, was reported. In contrast, those suspected of having an AN showed a prolonged SP/CAP at low stimulation rates, but the SP/CAP was substantially reduced in duration at high stimulation rates. The prolonged SP/CAP is thought to reflect increased CAP duration resulting from the desynchronized auditory-nerve response, that is, the CAP is temporally dispersed, but to desynchronizing factors affecting the auditory nerve. At high stimulus rates, this desynchronized response shows substantial (neural) adaptation, resulting in a decrease in SP/CAP duration. Thus, in those individuals with less than profound hearing loss and with evidence of functioning OHCs but grossly abnormal CAP/ABR, it may be possible to separate IHC loss from AN by using transtympanic promontory ECoG and evaluating SP/CAP amplitude and duration, at both low and high click stimulation rates. Last, in cases of dominant optic atrophy, Huang and colleagues (2009) reported a unique sensory-cell effect like unusually prolonged CM responses to clicks that can last for the entire epoch of the ECoG recordings. Currently, this phenomenon has no compelling explanation. Although one could imagine mechanical, hair-cell, and/or even a possible neural (efferent) basis for this effect, imagining and documenting a mechanistic explanation are two entirely different matters.

SUMMARY

Being able to counsel parents effectively regarding the devastating news of a profound hearing loss in a young child is a powerful tool for any clinician to have. In those instances where profound hearing loss is indicative of IHC dysfunction with residual neural reserve, a favorable prognosis for CI performance would be extremely welcome news for any parent to hear. In contrast, when an AN diagnosis is made, such an effect is both more difficult to explain and potentially less likely to lead to an effective long-term outcome. Indeed, being able to distinguish between sensory and neural sites of lesion and potentially being able to separate neural disorders affecting the dendritic versus axonal portion of the auditory nerve, would be invaluable for site-of-lesion detection, as well as in improving our ability to predict success with a CI.

REFERENCES

Bahmad, F. J., Merchant, S. N., Nadol, J. B. Jr., & Tranebjærg, L. (2007). Otopathology in Mohr-Tranebjærg syndrome. *Laryngoscope, 117,* 1202–1208.

Burkard, R., & Don, M. (2012). The auditory brainstem response. In K. Tremblay & R. Burkard (Eds.), *Translational perspectives in auditory neuroscience: Hearing across the life span—assessment and disorders.* San Diego, CA: Plural.

Cacace, A. T., & Burkard, R. F. (2009). Auditory neuropathy: Bridging the gap between basic science and current clinical concerns. In A. T. Cacace & D. J. McFarland (Eds.), *Controversies in central auditory processing disorder* (pp. 305–343). San Diego, CA: Plural.

Cacace, A. T., & Pinheiro, J. M. B. (2011). The mitochondrial connection in auditory neuropathy. *Audiology and Neurotology, 16,* 398–413.

Gibson, W. P. R., & Graham, J. M. (2008). Editorial: "Auditory neuropathy" and cochlear implantation—myths and facts. *Cochlear Implants International, 9,* 1–7.

Gibson, W. P. R., & Sanli, H. (2007) Auditory neuropathy: An update. *Ear and Hearing, 28,* 102S–106S.

Hallpike, C. S., Harriman, D. G., & Wells, C. E. (1980). A case of afferent neuropathy and deafness. *Journal of Laryngology and Otology, 94,* 945–964.

Huang, T., Santarelli, R., & Starr, A. (2009). Mutation of OPA1 gene causes deafness by affecting function of auditory nerve terminals. *Brain Research, 1300,* 97–104.

Johnson, C. P., & Chapman, E. R. (2010). Otoferlin is a calcium sensor that directly regulates SNARE-mediated membrane fusion. *Journal of Cell Biology, 191,* 187–197.

Loundon, N., Marcolla, A., Roux, I., Rouillon, I., Denoyelle, F., Feldman, D., . . . Garabedian, E. N. (2005). Auditory neuropathy or endocochlear hearing loss? *Otology and Neurotology, 26,* 748–754.

Marsh, R. R., & Kazahaya, K. (2009). Is auditory neuropathy an appropriate diagnosis if there is no neuropathy? In K. Kaga. & A. Starr (Eds.), *Neuropathies of the auditory and vestibular eighth cranial nerves* (pp. 149–156). Hicom, Japan: Springer.

Merchant, S. N., McKenna, M. J., Nadol, J. B., Jr., Kristiansen, A. G., Tropitzsch, A., Lindal, A., & Tranebjaerg, L. (2001). Temporal bone histopathologic and genetic studies in Mohr-Tranbjaerg syndrome (DFN-1). *Otology and Neurotology, 22,* 506–511.

Rapin, I., & Gravel, J. S. (2006). Auditory neuropathy: A biologically inappropriate label unless acoustic nerve involvement is documented. *Journal of the American Academy of Audiology, 17,* 147–150.

Reisinger, E., Bresee, C., Neef, J., Nair, R., Reuter, K., Bulankina, A., . . . Moser, T. (2011). Probing the functional equivalence of Otoferlin and Synaptotagmin 1 in exocytosis. *Journal of Neuroscience, 31,* 4886–4895.

Rouillon, I., Marcolla, A., Roux, I., Marlin, S., Feldman, S., Couderc, R., . . . Loundon, N. (2006). Results of cochlear implantation in two children with mutations in the OTOF gene. *International Journal of Pediatric Otorhinolaryngology, 70,* 689–696.

Roux, I., Safieddine, S., Nouvian, R., Grati, M., Simmler, M. C., Bahloul, A., . . . Petit, C. (2006). Otoferlin, defective in a human deafness form, is essential for exocytosis at the ribbon synapse. *Cell, 127,* 277–289.

Ruel, J., Emery, S., Nouvian, R., Bersot, T., Amilhon, B., Van Rybroek, J. M., . . . Puel, J.(2008). Impairment of SLC17A8 encoding vesicular glutamate transporter-3, VGLUT3, underlies nonsyndromic deafness DFNA25 and inner hair cell dysfunction in null mice. *American Journal of Human Genetics, 83,* 278–292.

Santarelli, R., & Arslan, E. (2002). Electrocochleography in auditory neuropathy. *Hearing Research, 170,* 32–47.

Santarelli, R., Castillo, I., Rodriguez-Ballesteros, M., Scimemi, P., Cama, E., Arslan, E., & Starr, A. (2009). Abnormal cochlear potentials from deaf patients with mutations of the otoferlin gene. *Journal of the Association for Research in Otolaryngology, 10,* 545–556.

Santarelli, R., Starr, A, Michalewski, H. J., & Arslan, E. (2008). Neural and receptor cochlear potentials obtained by transtympanic electrocochleography in auditory neuropathy. *Clinical Neurophysiology, 119,* 1028–1041.

Satya-Murti, S., & Cacace, A. T. (1982). Auditory evoked potentials in disorders of the primary sensory ganglia. In J. Courjon, F. Maurguier, & M. Revol (Eds.), *Clinical applications of evoked potentials in neurology. Advances in neurology* (Vol. 23, pp. 219–225). New York, NY: Raven Press.

Sawada, S., Mori, N., Mount, R. J., & Harrison, R. V. (2001). Differential vulnerability of inner and outer hair cell systems to chronic mild hypoxia and glutamate ototoxicity: Insights into the cause of auditory neuropathy. *Journal of Otolaryngology, 30,* 106–114.

Spoendlin, H. (1974). Optic and cochleovestibular degeneration in hereditary ataxias. 2. Temporal bone pathology in two cases of Friedreich's ataxia with vestibulo-cochlear disorders. *Brain, 97,* 41–48.

Spoendlin, H. (1985). Anatomy of cochlear innervation. *American Journal of Otolaryngology, 5,* 453–467.

Stedman, T. L. (2006). *Stedman's medical dictionary* (28th ed.). Baltimore, MD: Lippincott, Williams & Williams.

Varga, R., Kelley, P. M., Keats, B. J., Starr, A., Leal, S. M., Cohn E., & Kimberling, W. J. (2003). Non-syndromic recessive auditory neuropathy is the result of mutations in the otoferlin (*OTOF*) gene. *Journal of Medical Genetics, 40,* 45–50.

Zak, M., Pfister, M., & Blin, N. (2011). The otoferlin interactome in neurosensory hair cells: Significance of synaptic vesicle release and trans Golgi network (Review). *International Journal of Molecular Medicine, 28,* 311–314.

ESSAY 24

Single and Double Dissociations as a Frame of Reference

Application to Auditory Processing Disorders (APDs)

Anthony T. Cacace and Dennis J. McFarland

Celebrating one's life after death allows us to recall with clarity certain personal accomplishments that can become an inspiration for others to emulate. Endowed with the ability to listen to new ideas and having the intellectual skills to discuss a broad range of issues, Dr. Sadanand Singh was in the unique position to promote innovation through his role as an entrepreneur and publicist. Although this essay is neither an obituary nor a delayed eulogy, it is a celebration honoring those traits that characterize this unique individual; ones, which set him apart from others. In keeping with the literary platform of an essay, we discuss ideas that will help to advance the field of auditory processing disorders (APDs), with the hope that innovations through scientific discovery can help develop theory and also translate in a practical sense to the clinic so that more rigorous scientific methods can be applied to this area of investigation.

BACKGROUND

The area of APDs lacks a strong theoretical foundation for implementing assessments, interpreting and accounting for test results, and predicting outcomes. Although there is no gold standard at present that can be used to help resolve these deficiencies, there are ways to improve upon this untenable state of affairs and to put this area on a solid path for advancement. In Essay 25 of this book, McFarland and Cacace discuss psychometric factors, as ways to improve this area of investigation. Herein, we discuss other options to help clarify some of the outstanding issues, including making a specific diagnosis and delineating processing specializations in the auditory and visual sensory modalities.

An important first step in this process is establishing a useful definition. We define APD as "an auditory perceptual disorder that cannot be explained on the basis of peripheral hearing loss" (Cacace & McFarland, 2005; McFarland & Cacace, 1995, p. 36), with emphasis on the fact that the word *auditory*, in APD, should actually mean something. This definition has several key features; it is explicit and it is simple. There are no ambiguities in terms of *what is* and *what is not* an APD; indeed, this definition can stand alone on its own right. Furthermore, because APD is a theoretical construct, in order to conceptualize it in a meaningful way, it needs to be construed as a hypothetical disposition (McFarland & Cacace, 2009). In this regard, we can frame the assessment of APDs as a form of hypothesis testing, where the goal is to delineate a modality specific perceptual dysfunction from supramodal or polysensory dysfunctions. This view contrasts with supramodal cognitive disorders, such as those related to attention, memory, or language, where modality-specific effects would not necessarily be expected, although exceptions exist.

Thus, in current audiologic assessment for APD, two general strategies are presented, each having a different point of view. We categorize them arbitrarily into strong and weak positions/viewpoints. The *strong* viewpoint holds that modality specificity is fundamental to the diagnosis of an APD. The argument is based on the underlying tenet that if the modality specificity of the deficit cannot be demonstrated with any degree of certainty, then by definition, the diagnosis cannot be made. A necessary component in the evaluation process requires multimodal testing (e.g., use of matched tasks in multiple sensory modalities) to demonstrate the specificity of the dysfunction.

The alternative *weak* viewpoint holds that use of auditory stimuli alone is sufficient to make the diagnosis of APD. However, the argument that a diagnosis of APD can be made by use of a unimodal inclusive framework is untenable, particularly on theoretical grounds, because such an approach can lead no further than an indeterminate diagnosis. Although this position has been used for many decades, it is outdated and limited in scope; it has only produced controversy and prolonged debate. In retrospect, it has stifled the field of APDs for over 50 years. Thus, clarification between these two different positions can help drive translational studies from the laboratory to the clinic and potentially motivate others to pursue a more solid scientific path to discovery.

Indeed, by using matched tasks in multiple sensory modalities, we can evaluate simple dissociations and more complex double dissociations (DDs) that have functional value, to the extent that they can aid in the development of assessing processing specializations within and between auditory and visual cortical areas, help in identifying the modality specificity of the deficit, and thus facilitate a valid diagnosis. A functional distinction used daily in clinical audiology is the simple dissociation between conductive and sensorineural hearing loss, accomplished by comparing pure-tone air and bone-conduction thresholds at various frequencies. If hearing loss is manifest by pure-tone audiometry, and if large differences exist between air- and bone-conduction thresholds (bone-conduction thresholds being better [more sensitive] than air-conduction thresholds), then a conductive hearing loss is highly probable. However, if air- and bone-conduction thresholds are similar in the presence of elevated auditory thresholds, then a sensorineural loss is assumed. Thus, the dissociation is made between conductive and sensorineural hearing loss, and this distinction provides diagnostic specificity with respect to the site of lesion and facilitates treatment. A more complex distinction, and one that is directly related to APD, falls under the rubric of the double dissociation.

THE DOUBLE DISSOCIATION (DD)

In considering the DD, studies of brain lesions in different individuals serve as a prototypical format. Consider the scenario whereby a lesion to brain structure A impairs function X but not function Y, and a lesion to brain structure B impairs function Y but not function X. In these instances and when behavioral tests are used, one can make inferences about functions X and Y as well as their possible localization within the brain. To the extent possible in living humans, in order to produce unequivocal results in these types of studies, lesions need to be localized to specific areas and well characterized by contemporary imaging modalities. However, just like any other device applied in scientific investigations, the DD is not some magical entity without limitations (e.g., Baddeley, 2003; Dunn & Kirsner, 2003; van Orden et al., 2001). As noted by Baddeley (2003), "double dissociations are statistical tools, just like correlations and interactions. They place relatively tight constraints on attempts to provide explanations in terms of a single factor. Though less powerful than sometimes claimed, DDs remain as a useful tool in attempting to understand complex cognitive systems" (p. 131). An alternative and equally viable approach is to use reversible experimental manipulations to disable different brain areas in the same experimental subject (animal), whereby similar distinctions as noted above, can be realized. Below, we discuss both scenarios.

When the DD was formally introduced into the physiological psychology literature by Teuber (1955), it provided a conceptual framework for inferring functional characteristics and specializations of brain function in topical areas ranging from perception, to cognition, to language, to action. Although demonstrating a DD was thought to be a coup d'état for the neuropsychology and cognitive neuroscience elite, one of the more intriguing aspects of DDs not often discussed was the prospect of provoking thought and introspection of experimental outcomes, inspiring replication of experimental finding, providing alternative explanations for the results, and in retrospect, if done properly, advancing science. Historically, probably the first and most prominent example of a DD, which preceded Teuber, can be found in the early literature on aphasia secondary to brain damage (e.g., Broca, 1861; Wernicke, 1874). Broca reported patients who were *unable* to speak but could understand language (referred to as nonfluent or motor aphasia), whereas Wernicke reported patients who could produce so-called jumbled speech (referred to as fluent aphasia), but were unable to understand language. Initial postmortem analysis of individuals at the time revealed that such effects were produced by lesions in different regions of the brain. In the cases reported by Broca, damage was thought to be localized to the inferior frontal gyrus of the left hemisphere (pars opercularis and pars trangularis, now referred to as Broca's area or Brodmann's areas 44 and 45); in cases reported by Wernicke, damage was localized to the posterior aspect of the second temporal gyrus of the left hemisphere (now referred to as Wernicke's area or Brodmann's area 22). However, the viability of this DD, although undoubtedly novel at the time, has been disputed by contemporary analyses and remains controversial. A body of literature indicates that such effects cannot occur without concurrent damage to subcortical brain structures (e.g., Lieberman, 2002). This finding has been confirmed by re-imaging the famous brains of Broca's subjects (Leborgne and Lelong) using MRI, thus providing direct evidence indicating that such lesions were not localized to the classical Broca areas but extended into medial aspects of the brain which included the left basal ganglia and the entire insula (Dronkers et al., 2007).

Conceptually and practically, DDs seem to fare better in instances where modular systems are hypothesized, such as those found in the auditory and visual sensory modalities (e.g., Lomber & Malhota, 2008; Polster & Rose, 1998; Ungerleider & Mishkin, 1982) although fascinating DDs reported in Williams syndrome provide instances of modularity in cognitive systems that are considered quite provocative (see Karmiloff-Smith et al., 2003). Nevertheless, we focus on cortical streams of information processing in the auditory and visual modalities, as this framework is relevant to APDs.

The discovery, conceptualization, and dissociation of *what* and *where* processing streams within the brain including their underlying anatomical dorsal and ventral pathways can be traced to the seminal work of Ungerleider and Mishkin (1982) and Mishkin, Ungerleider, and Mako (1983) in the visual system. Based on these novel experimental findings, it was proposed that visual information processing is divided into two essential functions: assigning meaning to an object (i.e., determining *what* it is), which was shown to occur in inferotemporal cortex and accurately locating the object in space (i.e., determining *where* it is), which was shown to occur in the posterior parietal cortex. An alternate view suggests that these information processing streams mediate vision and action (Goodale & Milner, 1992). Furthermore, functional imaging data indicate that *what* and *where* processing streams also have counterparts in the human brain (e.g., Ungerleider & Haxby, 1994).

In the auditory system, similar *what* and *where* processing streams have been proposed (Rauschecker & Tian, 2000). Recent work supports this contention and indicates that these functional specializations can be doubly dissociated by using a cooling technique to deactivate the anterior and posterior auditory field to distinguish a pattern discrimination task (*what* pathway) from a spatial localization task (*where* pathway) in the same experimental animal (cat) (Lomber & Malhota, 2008). The contrasting view of *what* and *where* pathways offered by Goodale and Milner (1992) may also have a counterpart in the auditory modality, whereby a double dissociation has recently been reported in delineating *where* and *when* pathways (Lewald & Getzmann, 2011). The novelty and validity of this interesting distinction will require further scrutiny.

In humans, using functional magnetic resonance imaging (fMRI) and magneto-encephalography (MEG), Ahveninen et al. (2006) were able to show a DD between phonetic versus spatial-sound changes. The results of Ahveninen and colleagues demonstrate a localized processing stream associated with speech-sound identity (*what* pathway) localized to anterolateral Heschl's gyrus, anterior superior temporal gyrus and a posterior (*where* pathway), localized to the planum temporale and the posterior superior temporal gyrus. Because both fMRI and MEG were used in this investigation, high-resolution spatial and temporal data could be discerned. The authors showed that the *where* pathway was activated 30 ms earlier than the *what* pathway, suggesting that top-down spatial information could be used in auditory object perception.

As noted above, evidence for the modular nature of the central auditory nervous system has been reviewed by Polster and Rose (1998), who concluded that there are DDs across subjects with respect to identification of speech and nonspeech sounds. Poeppel (2001) came to a similar conclusion in his review of pure-word deafness. Individuals with pure-word deafness are impaired in the comprehension of spoken language in contrast to intact abilities to speak, read, and write. This modality-specific dissociation of language ability appears to result from bilateral damage to central auditory areas and contrasts to the primarily left-sided nature of lesions that produce supramodal language disorders. From this analysis,

Poeppel (2001) concluded that the speech code is analyzed bilaterally, and that lateralization associated with language processing occurs beyond the analysis of the input. Thus, the study of dissociations in sound and speech processing provides important insights into the modular nature of auditory processing that could potentially guide the development of improved tests of APD.

Considering a task already included in APD test batteries, Cacace et al. (1992) showed that a DD could be produced between memory spans for binary auditory sequential frequency (pitch) pattern sequences and binary sequential visual color pattern sequences in patients with partial temporal lobe extirpations for intractable epilepsy. This example demonstrates that lesions to auditory areas affect auditory but not visual tasks, and that lesions to visual areas affect visual but not auditory tasks.

Use of the DD paradigm provides support for the concept of auditory *what* and *where* processing streams. Additionally, studies of auditory agnosia and pure-word deafness support the view of the modular nature of the central auditory nervous system. They suggest that there can be both verbal and nonverbal modality-specific auditory processing disorders. The implication of these findings is that auditory processing might not be lateralized in the same way as language processing. Thus, results such as these can provide the basis for the development of new tests of auditory processing.

To date, the DD paradigm has seen limited use with traditional tests of auditory processing (e.g., Cacace et al., 1992). However, this methodology has the potential to provide insight into the nature of what these tests actually measure. We contend that this should be a priority for future evaluation of APD tests.

In summary, for perceptual studies, the DD can be a powerful approach for use in assessing APDs because it demonstrates both the *sensitivity* of the task and the *specificity* of the deficit; an approach advocated by Shallice (1988) for evaluating functional localization in the brain. Further work in this area has clear potential to advance the field of APDs.

REFERENCES

Ahveninen, J., Jääkeläinen, I. P., Raij, T., Bonmassar, G., Devore, S., Hämäläinen, M., . . . Belliveau, J. W. (2006). Task-modulated "what" and "where" pathways in human auditory cortex. *Proceedings of the National Academy of Sciences, USA, 103,* 14608–14613.

Baddeley, A. (2003). Double dissociations: Not magic, but still useful. *Cortex, 39,* 129–131.

Broca, P. (1861). Remarques sur le siège de la faculté de la parole articulé, suives d'une observation d'aphemie (perte de parole). *Bulletin for the Society of Anatomy (Paris), 36,* 330–357.

Cacace, A. T., & McFarland D. J. (2005). The importance of modality specificity in diagnosing central auditory processing disorder. *American Journal of Audiology, 4,* 112–123.

Cacace, A. T., McFarland, D. J., Emrich, J. F., & Haller, J. S. (1992). Assessing short-term recognition memory with forced choice psychophysical methods. *Journal of Neuroscience Methods, 44,* 145–155.

Dronkers, N. F., Plaisant, O., Iba-Zizen, M. T., & Cabanis, E. A. (2007). Paul Broca's historic cases: high resolution MR imaging of the brains of Leborgne and Lelong. *Brain, 130,* 1432–1441.

Dunn, J. C., & Kirsner, K. (2003). What can we infer from double dissociations? *Cortex, 29,* 1–7.

Goodale, M. A., & Milner, A. D. (1992). Separate visual pathways for perception and action. *Trends in Neuroscience, 15,* 20–25.

Karmiloff-Smith, A., Brown, J. H., Grice, S., & Paterson, S. (2003). Dethroning the myth: Cognitive dissociations and innate modularity in Williams syndrome. *Developmental Neuropsychology, 23,* 227–242.

Lewald, J., & Getzmann, S. (2011). When and where of auditory spatial processing in cortex:

A novel approach using electrotomography. *PLoS One, 9,* 1–17.

Lieberman, P. (2002). On the nature and evolution of the neural bases of human language. *Yearbook of Physical Anthropology, 45,* 36–62.

Lomber, S. G., & Malhotra, S. (2008). Double dissociation of "what" and "where" processing in auditory cortex. *Nature Neuroscience, 11,* 609–616.

McFarland, D. J., & Cacace, A. T. (1995). Modality specificity as a criterion for diagnosing central auditory processing disorders. *American Journal of Audiology, 4,* 36–48.

McFarland, D. J., & Cacace, A. T. (2009). Modality specificity and auditory processing disorders. In A. T. Cacace & D. J. McFarland (Eds.), *Controversies in central auditory processing disorder* (pp. 199–216). San Diego, CA: Plural.

Mishkin, M., Ungerleider, L. G., & Macko, K. A. (1983). Object vision and spatial vision: Two cortical pathways. *Trends in Neuroscience, 6,* 414–417.

Polster, M. R., & Rose, S. B. (2008). Disorders of auditory processing: Evidence for modularity in audition. *Cortex, 34,* 47–65.

Poeppel, D. (2001) Pure word deafness and the bilateral processing of the speech code. *Cognitive Science, 25,* 679–693.

Rauschecker, J. P., & Tian, B. (2000). Mechanisms and streams for processing of "what" and "where" in auditory cortex. *Proceedings of the National Academy of Sciences, 97,* 11800–11806.

Shallice T. (1988). *From neuropsychology to mental structure.* New York, NY: Cambridge University Press.

Teuber, H.-L. (1955). Physiological psychology. *Annual Review of Psychology, 6,* 267–296.

Ungerleider, L. G., & Haxby, J. V. (1994). "What" and "where" in the human brain. *Current Opinion in Neurobiology, 4,* 157–165.

Ungerleider, L. G., & Mishkin, M. (1982). Two cortical visual systems. In D. J. Ingle, M. A. Goodale, & R. J. W. Mansfield (Eds.), *Analysis of visual behavior* (pp. 486–549). Cambridge, MA: MIT Press.

van Orden, G. C., Pennington, B. F., & Stone, G. O. (2001). What do double dissociations prove? *Cognitive Science, 25,* 111–172.

Wernicke, C. (1874). The aphasic symptom complex: A psychological study on a neurological basis. Breslau: Kohn and Weigert. Reprinted in: R. S. Cohen & M. W. Wartofsky (Eds.), *Boston studies in the philosophy of science, Volume 4.* Boston, MA: Reidel.

Establishing the Construct Validity of the Auditory Processing Disorder (APD)

Application of Psychometric Theory to Clinical Practice

Dennis J. McFarland and Anthony T. Cacace

The legacy of Dr. Sadanand Singh is that of a respected educator, scholar, speech scientist, and successful entrepreneur. In the domain of book publishing, the library of audiology texts by Plural Publishing by itself is a noteworthy accomplishment, spanning the areas of rehabilitation, diagnostics, and basic and applied auditory processing. In this essay, we celebrate Dr. Singh's educational achievements and publishing virtuosity and add to his memory by discussing the domain of auditory processing in a meaningful way.

BACKGROUND

Concern has been expressed as to the nature of what is measured by tests of central auditory processing (Cacace & McFarland, 2005; Dawes & Bishop, 2009; Friel-Patti, 1999; Kamhi, 2011; McFarland & Cacace, 1995;

Reese, 1973). Nonetheless, these tests are used widely in clinical practice (Emanuel et al., 2011). Dawes and Bishop (2009) suggest that there is a need to improve methods for assessment and diagnosis. The present essay discusses the application of psychometric methods that may facilitate this goal.

From the perspective of psychometrics, the quality of tests can be evaluated in terms of their reliability and validity. Reliability refers to the consistency of test scores; generally indexed by use of the correlation coefficient and related to the extent to which scores on a test at one point in time correlate with scores on the same test taken at a different point in time. Validity refers to the extent to which a test measures what it is intended to measure. Although many types of validity have been enumerated in the past, this concept has evolved over the years and currently, all types of validity can be encompassed by the notion of "construct validity" (Smith, 2005). Construct validation involves the development of tests based on theory and the subsequent evaluation of theoretical expectations by empirical research. This validation research involves, in part, showing that the test relates to other measures in a theoretically meaningful manner, typically by using the correlation coefficient.

Test-retest reliability is measured over some short interval of time, such as a few days or weeks, for which any change would be due to the instability of scores rather than systematic changes in individuals, such as maturation. Use of the correlation coefficient allows for an interpretation of results in terms of the amount of variance in test scores that is due to consistent individual differences. Some researchers have evaluated whether there is a change in the group mean scores between tests as a way of evaluating reliability; for example, by using a *t*-test (e.g., Song et al., 2011). However, it is entirely possible for the ranking of individual scores to change without there being a change in group means, thus making the use of group means problematic as a metric of reliability.

The variance in test scores can be due to a variety of factors such as measurement error, short-term effects like alertness and motivation (i.e., the individual's current state), as well as to stable individual differences (i.e., traits). With large samples, measurement error and state effects will typically cancel in the group mean. However, these are important determinants of error in diagnosis (McFarland & Cacace, 2011). Although not captured by an analysis of mean differences, these sources of error are quantified by the correlation coefficient. Although analysis of group means over time provides useful information about test performance, it does not quantify the consistency of individual differences over time, and thus, should not be considered a measure of test-retest reliability.

Test-retest reliability has important implications for the accuracy of diagnosis (e.g., Cacace & McFarland, 1995; Charter & Feldt, 2001). Using cutoff scores, a high proportion of individuals will be misclassified unless reliability is high, assuming that a test measures what it is suppose to measure. For example, even with a reliability coefficient of 0.70, errors (false alarms and misses) are as likely to occur as correct detections (hits) (McFarland & Cacace, 2005). Zalewski (2005) concluded that the Staggered Spondaic Word (SSW) test was reliable based on the fact that correlations as low as 0.55 were significant. However, simply establishing that the test-retest correlation is significant is not sufficient. Small correlations can be significant with a large sample size. Rather, it is the magnitude of the consistency in test scores that is important. Often a test-retest correlation of 0.80 is considered adequate, although values in this range have been questioned (Charter & Feldt, 2001). Obviously, the higher the test-retest reliability, the lower the probability of misdiagnosis due to test score instability.

Depending on how it is used, a single test may have more than one reliability measure. For example, young children may be less consistent in their test performance than older children. Thus, reliability coefficients should be established with the population for which the test is intended. If more than one population is to be used, then more than one reliability coefficient should be evaluated. Finally, any correlation obtained from a sample is an estimate and it is important to base these estimates of reliability on an adequate sample size (e.g., Charter, 2001).

Depending on the nature of the source of instability, there are several ways in which reliability can be improved. Simply increasing the number of trials (or reversals with an adaptive psychophysical procedure) may be sufficient if instability is due to random error. Ceiling effects (i.e., performance on tests that are too easy), limit the range of scores and lower the reliability of the test measure. The design of the test can be modified to increase precision. Finally, it may be necessary to eliminate certain tests whose performance is not predominately due to a stable trait.

The concept of reliability implies that a score on a test is only an estimate of the true value of what a test measures. This means that the test is an estimate of some latent trait that is never directly observed. To reiterate, test-retest reliability is an estimate of how well test scores obtained at one point in time will generalize to scores at another point in time. Reliability sets an upper limit on validity. However, reliability does not insure that a test is valid. Validity is concerned, in part, with how well test scores will generalize to other measures of the latent construct that the test is suppose to measure. We now address this issue.

Validity is evaluated by determining whether test scores relate to other measures as expected by theory. As such, the contemporary view of validity holds that construct validation concerns the simultaneous process of measurement and theory validation (Strauss & Smith, 2009). Providing evidence for the validity of a construct and the tests that measure it, is seen as a continuing process of theory development and gathering of empirical data. Thus, a test is never validated. Rather, there is a theory and a body of data that supports the validity of a particular use of a specific test. A key element of the validation process is the use of the multitrait-multimethod matrix (Campbell & Fisk, 1959). This method makes use of correlations between multiple tests to determine the extent to which tests of the same construct correlate among themselves (convergent validity) and do not correlate with tests of other independent constructs (divergent validity). Consider an example of a matrix of correlations between several tests of auditory function and several tests of visual function. Evidence for the convergent validity of tests of auditory

processing disorder would be provided to the extent that they were all inter-correlated. Based on the theoretical criterion of modality specificity (McFarland & Cacace, 1995), evidence of divergent validity would be provided to the extent that the *auditory* test scores are not highly correlated with the *visual* test scores.

To be useful, the construct that a test is supposed to measure should explain individual differences in meaningful real-life tasks such as communication and/or educational performance (i.e., it should have *ecological validity*).)Although this might seem like an obvious requirement for a useful test, it has been asserted by the ASHA Working Group on Auditory Processing Disorders that "one-to-one correspondence between deficits in fundamental, discrete auditory processes and language, learning, and related sequelae may be difficult, if not impossible, to demonstrate across large groups of diverse subjects" (ASHA, 2005, p. 3). This position essentially insulates the construct of auditory processing from the empirical test as, when formulated in this way, the construct of auditory processing makes no predictions about real-world behavior. However, if tests are to be useful, then there should be some statistical evidence for a relationship between test scores and language, learning, and related problems. This does not mean that there needs to be a perfect relationship, but it should be possible to establish meaningful correlations in relevant populations.

Established tests of central auditory processing have become increasingly insulated from empirical tests. Although early researchers talked about specific profiles of test results associated with specific lesions of the central auditory nervous system, this approach has been abandoned, as is apparent in the current ASHA (2005) recommendations. As previously noted, statistical associations with language and learning outcomes are no longer required. For example, a failure to demonstrate modality specificity has recently been taken as evidence for problems with modality specificity, rather than limitations of "established" tests (e.g., Bellis et al., 2008). However, these developments actually represent failures to establish evidence for convergent and divergent validity. Simply stated, research has not demonstrated that these tests show the appropriate patterns of correlations with what they theoretically should and should not be related to.

One of the most basic lines of evidence for validity is provided by showing that tests measuring the same construct are correlated. In a recent study of several tests commonly used in practice, Musiek et al. (2011) report that only dichotic digit and competing sentence tests were significantly correlated. There were no significant correlations involving frequency pattern tests or tests of low-pass filtered speech. The frequent lack of concordance between various tests purported to measure APD is dealt with by postulating subtypes. However, this does not solve the problem of a lack of evidence for the validity of these constructs. Rather, it is now necessary to provide evidence for the reliability and validity of each of these subtypes. This includes showing that the tests associated with each subtype in question correlate with other measures of the subtype in question. More often than not, such information is simply lacking, thus creating further problems in this area.

Evaluation of tests of auditory processing often makes use of an analysis of sensitivity and specificity rather than reliability and validity (e.g., Musiek et al., 2011). Sensitivity is the proportion of individuals correctly diagnosed out of the total diagnosed. Specificity is the proportion of individuals not diagnosed out of the total who do not have the disorder. These measures are related to signal detection theory but, as noted by Swets (1988, page 1285), "good test data can be very difficult to obtain" owing to problems with the "truth" against which a diagnosis is made. In many cases, the "true" diagnosis is simply that the individual is "suspected" of having an APD.

In the Musiek et al. (2011) study, sensitivity and specificity were evaluated in terms of whether or not subjects had radiological confirmed lesions involving auditory cortex. Inspection of Figure 1 in Musiek et al. (2011, p. 345) indicates that there was involvement of areas outside of auditory cortex in the subjects with brain lesions, including but not limited to inferior parietal cortex, middle temporal gyrus, somatosensory, and motor cortex. On the other hand, from their Figure 1 it is not clear that patients had complete bilateral damage to all of auditory cortex. Although the lesions in this study appear to be reasonably focal, lesions restricted to only auditory cortex are rare. Thus, as discussed by McFarland and Cacace (1995), there are potential problems with using brain lesions as a gold standard for CAPD. Also lacking are the theoretical expectations of test outcomes. For example, with a lesion to the right temporal lobe, what is the expected performance for the frequency pattern test; a left ear deficit, right ear deficit, bilateral deficit? Such information is not provided.

One approach to the problem of correlating brain lesions with behavior is to quantify the extent of damage in several brain areas in each individual. These measures can then be correlated with the behaviors of interest to infer which brain regions are related to which behaviors (see Alexander et al., 2010). This brain behavior correlational analysis provides a means of determining whether a test relates to damage in brain areas it is thought to relate to (i.e., convergent validity), and is not influenced by damage in areas it is not thought to be related to (i.e., divergent validity). This analysis also allows for brain damage in a given area to be incomplete, rather than of an all-or-none manner. This is exactly the kind of analysis that provides evidence for the validity of tests by use of patients with brain lesions, and contrasts with an analysis of sensitivity and specificity that requires a level of precision generally unattainable in lesion studies.

In a simple world, it would be sufficient to give a single test to evaluate a single construct. Unfortunately, this is not the case when dealing with disorders of the central nervous system. Improving the state-of-the-art of central auditory evaluation will require relating test performance to theory in auditory anatomy/physiology, as is currently done with evaluation of the peripheral auditory system. This is in contrast to current recommendations (AAA, 2010; ASHA, 2005) that describe auditory functions in terms of the tests used clinically (e.g., temporal processing, dichotic listening, etc.). Although much remains to be learned about the central auditory nervous system, progress is being made, and there is every reason to believe that a clearer picture of how the auditory nervous system functions will emerge. Indeed, developing a science of individual differences in auditory perception represents an unique opportunity for diagnostic audiology as auditory stimuli (and to some extent central auditory anatomy) are well defined relative to many other areas of the nervous system.

In addition to reliance on theory from neuroscience, refinement of auditory processing tests will benefit from the use of modern statistical techniques that are suitable for evaluating the multitrait-multimethod matrix. Structural equation modeling (SEM) is particularly useful for evaluating theory as it allows for the comparison of alternative hypotheses (e.g., McFarland & Cacace, 2002). Examination of individual correlations is certainly necessary, but complex multivariate data require more sophisticated methods of analysis. Factor analysis has been widely applied, but there is no guarantee that the solution obtained is correct (Steiger, 1979), a fact compounded by various rotation and factor retention options. Structural equation modeling has an advantage in that the analyst can systematically evaluate alternative models and select the one that best accounts for the data.

In sum, no single test measure is a perfect index of a latent trait, as all are subject to error. Having multiple indices allows the analyst to estimate this error and provides a better estimate of the trait of interest. Consequently, the data should include several indices of each trait in question and several indices of additional traits that are of theoretical interest. Alternative hypotheses that could be evaluated with SEM include: whether there is a general central auditory ability as opposed to multiple specific central auditory abilities, whether there are central auditory abilities that are distinct from general cognitive abilities, and whether tests in an auditory battery best correlate with brain damage to auditory cortex or with polymodal areas. Obviously, the analyst's ability to evaluate these alternative hypotheses depends on the nature of the tests that are included in a given study.

CONCLUSION

To be useful, tests of central auditory functioning should be able to generalize to real-life situations (i.e., they should have ecological validity). Test results from one point in time should be able to predict results for the same test at other points in time (i.e., they should have high test-retest reliability). Moreover, test results should be able to predict scores on theoretically similar measures (i.e., convergent reliability), but not be correlated with measures of unrelated constructs (i.e., divergent validity). All of these considerations require that test construction be integrated with meaningful theory development. Available evidence indicates that current tests of auditory processing lack ecological validity in terms of predicting reading achievement and development of language skills in school-age children (grades 1–4) that are representative of national norms in terms of intelligence and socioeconomic status (Watson & Kidd, 2009). Thus, a sustained research program based on principals of modern psychometric theory could facilitate development of useful tests of auditory processing and provide better instruments for the evaluation of central auditory abilities.

REFERENCES

Alexander, L. D., Black, S. E., Goa, F., Szilagyi, G., Danells, C., & McIlroy, W. E. (2010). Correlating lesion size and location to deficits after ischemic stroke: The influence of accounting for altered peri-necrotic tissue and incidental silent infarcts. *Behavioral and Brain Functions, 6,* 6.

American Academy of Audiology. (2010). *Diagnosis, treatment and management of children and adults with central auditory processing disorder.* Available at http://www.audiology.org/resources/documentlibrary/Documents/CAPD%20Guidelines%208-2010.pdf

American Speech Hearing Association. (2005). *(Central) auditory processing disorders: Working group on auditory processing disorders.* Available at http://www.asha.org/docs/html/tr2005-00043.html

Bellis, T. J., Billet, C., & Ross, J. (2008). Hemispheric lateralization of bilaterally presented homologous visual and auditory stimuli in normal adults, normal children, and children with central auditory dysfunction. *Brain and Cognition, 66,* 280–289.

Cacace, A. T., & McFarland, D. J. (1995). Opening Pandora's box: the reliability of CAPD tests. *American Journal of Audiology, 4,* 61–62.

Cacace, A. T., & McFarland, D. J. (2005). The importance of modality specificity in diagnosing central auditory processing disorder. *American Journal of Audiology, 14,* 112–123.

Campbell, D. T., & Fisk, D. W. (1959). Convergent and discriminant validation by the multitrait-multimethod matrix. *Psychological Bulletin, 56,* 81–105.

Charter, R. A. (2001). Damn the precision, full speed ahead with the clinical interpretation. *Journal of Clinical and Experimental Neuropsychology, 23,* 692–694.

Charter, R. A., & Feldt, L. S. (2001). Meaning of reliability in terms of correct and incorrect clinical decisions: The art of decision making is still alive. *Journal of Clinical and Experimental Neuropsychology, 23,* 530–537.

Dawes, P., & Bishop, D. (2009). Auditory processing disorder in relation to developmental disorders of language, communication and attention: A review and critique. *International Journal of Language and Communication Disorders, 44,* 440–465.

Emanuel, D. C., Ficca, K. N., & Korczak, P. (2011). Survey of the diagnosis and management of auditory processing disorder. *American Journal of Audiology, 20,* 48–60.

Friel-Patti, S. (1999). Clinical decision-making in the assessment and intervention of central auditory processing disorders. *Language, Speech, and Hearing Services in the Schools, 30,* 345–352.

Kamhi, A. G. (2011). What speech-language pathologists need to know about auditory processing disorder. *Language, Speech, and Hearing Services in the Schools, 42,* 265–272.

McFarland, D. J., & Cacace, A. T. (1995). Modality specificity as a criterion for diagnosing central auditory processing disorder. *American Journal of Audiology, 4,* 36–48.

McFarland, D. J., & Cacace, A. T. (2002). Factor analysis in CAPD and the "Unimodal" test battery: Do we have a model that will satisfy? *American Journal of Audiology, 11,* 7–9.

McFarland, D. J., & Cacace, A. T. (2005). Current controversies in CAPD: From Procrustes' bed to Pandora's box. In T. K. Parthasarathy (Ed.), *An introduction to auditory processing disorders in children* (pp. 247–263). Mahwah, NJ: Lawrence Erlbaum.

McFarland, D. J., & Cacace, A. T. (2011). Covariance is the proper measure of test-retest reliability. *Clinical Neurophysiology, 122,* 1893.

Musiek, F. E., Chermak, G. D., Weihing, J., Zappulla, M., & Nagle, S. (2011). Diagnostic accuracy of established central auditory processing test batteries in patients with documented lesions. *Journal of the American Academy of Audiology, 22,* 342–358.

Rees, N. S. (1973). Auditory processing factors in language disorders: The view from Procrustes' bed. *Journal of Speech and Hearing Disorders, 38,* 304–315.

Smith, G. T. (2005). On construct validity: Issues of method and measurement *Psychological Assessment, 17,* 396–408.

Song, J. H., Nicol, T., & Kraus, N. (2011). Test-retest reliability of the speech-evoked auditory brainstem response. *Clinical Neurophysiology, 122,* 346–355.

Steiger, J. H. (1979). Factor indeterminancy in the 1930's and the 1970's: Some interesting parallels. *Psychometrika, 44,* 157–167.

Strauss, M. E., & Smith, G. T. (2009). Construct validity: Advances in theory and methodology. *Annual Review of Clinical Psychology, 27,* 1–25.

Swets, J. A. (1988). Measuring the accuracy of diagnostic systems. *Science, 240,* 1285–1293.

Watson, C. S., & Kidd, G. R. (2009). Association between auditory abilities, reading, and other language skills, in children and adults. In A. T. Cacace & D. J. McFarland (Eds.), *Controversies in central auditory processing disorder* (pp. 217–242). San Diego, CA: Plural.

Zalewski, T. R. (2005). Test-retest reliability for the SSW number of error (NOE) analysis in an adult population with hearing impairment. *Contemporary Issues in Communication Science and Disorders, 32,* 120–125.

ESSAY 26

Hearing Aid Settings for Different Languages

Marshall Chasin

Dr. Sadanand Singh was instrumental in helping me publish my first book, Musicians and the Prevention of Hearing Loss *(Chasin, 1996), through Singular Publishing. Although perhaps a decade before its time, Dr. Singh's vision was clear. His support has helped the establishment of a wide range of new areas of study in the field of audiology. A dovetail off my work with musicians is how hearing aids can be set for different languages. Although this link seems tenuous, it falls under the general category of how hearing aids respond with different inputs, whether it be music as an input to a hearing aid or Japanese. Chapters exist under his vision on music and hearing aids* (Hearing Loss in Musicians: Prevention and Management, *Chasin, 2009) through Plural Publishing and now a chapter appears in the same vein for languages and hearing aids.*

INTRODUCTION

The Speech Intelligibility Index (SII) has been used widely as a measure to evaluate optimal hearing aid performance. The SII can and does vary slightly from language to language

(Wong et al., 2007) and although this does provide some important information, especially for changes in the frequency response, it is limited. The SII is based primarily on the phoneme, or at most, short utterances (ANSI, 1997) and provides no information on the larger syntactic or morphological structures in spoken language. For example, the effect for languages that have a Subject-Object-Verb (SOV) syntactic word order has been studied (Chasin, 2008, 2011) and it has been demonstrated that those languages (e.g., Hindi-Urdu, Korean, Japanese, Turkish, Iranian) do require more hearing aid gain for softer (sentence final) level inputs than for languages such as English that possess a Subject-Verb-Object (SVO) word order. These differences would not show up on language specific measures of the SII.

Another linguistic aspect that would also not show up on an SII measure is that some languages, such as Japanese, have a rigid consonant-vowel-consonant (CVC) morphological structure. In these cases, an intense vowel can precede a relatively quiet (non-sonorant) consonant. The question arises, "Does a hearing aid require a faster release time on the compressor than would be the case in English such that the quieter consonant achieves sufficient audibility if it follows an intense vowel?" Audibility of the quieter consonants may be an important issue in languages such as Japanese. In Japanese, and some other lesser spoken languages, higher frequency consonants, typically sibilants, voiceless stops, and affricates, are of low intensity. Unless the hearing aid compression circuitry has a sufficiently quick release time after an intense vowel, the intervocalic consonant (VCV) may not have adequate gain for sufficient audibility.

It is, however, possible that with multiband compression the rigid CVC morphology is not a significant clinical issue; the vowels and intervening consonants may be in different spectral regions. Lower frequency vowels may fall within one band (below 2000 Hz), and independently the higher frequency consonants may fall within a high frequency band pass. This may be a larger clinical issue for single band hearing aids or for those hearing aids that have their band regions set to have both the low frequency vowels and higher frequency consonants handled within the same band. This issue is currently being investigated, but preliminary results do indicate that this may have been more of an issue with older style single band hearing aids than with modern multi-band compressors.

TRANSLATIONAL RESEARCH

What does this research into the study of language structure and syntax tell us about setting hearing aids for different languages? This falls into two main categories: (1) SII related static frequency response changes, and (2) non-SII related dynamic changes.

The SII related changes provide information on frequency response alterations, and are directly predictable from frequency spe-cific band importance functions. Languages that are tonal (e.g. Chinese), morae or length dependent (e.g. Japanese), or those with a phonemic proliferation of nasals (e.g. Portuguese) would require more low frequency gain than languages such as English. A mora (plural moras or morae) is a unit of sound used in phonology that determines syllable weight (which in turn determines stress or timing) in some languages. This would be observed as an increase in importance for the lower several bands on the SII measure, and although not fully researched, clinically one would begin with an increase of 5 dB in gain over a fitting for English, given similar audiometric requirements. Tones typically are on the lower frequency sonorants (i.e., vowels and nasals), and the same can be said about length related morae languages where the length of the vowels may contribute to a different meaning. Audibility of these important cues would be more important than for languages such as English which is neither tonal nor morae. Conceivably for a bilingual English/Chinese speaker, one could have program #1 set for English and program #2 set for Chinese (with about 5 dB more gain than for the English program #1). At this point in time, there is no clinical research stating that this approach would be significantly different for a tonal language versus a morae language and also that a relatively arbitrary increase of 5 dB is the ideal level. A change of 5 dB is a reasonable good clinical starting point and minimally the data do suggest that if there will be any change, it will be in the direction of improved audibility for important linguistic cues.

There are also some other mid- and high-frequency response changes that can be dependent on language. Russian (and most other Slavic languages) has both palatal and non-palatal consonants that may yield a difference in meaning. Palatalization has its spectral cue around 3000 to 3500 Hz, as does rhotacization in Chinese. An increase in gain (and perhaps output) in this frequency region for Slavic and Sinitic (e.g., Chinese) languages would be useful, but again, these would show up on the language specific SII measure. A sampling of some commonly spoken languages, along with their linguistically based frequency response changes (from English) are shown in Table 26–1.

Some hearing aid and some real ear measurement device manufacturers are beginning to incorporate language specific SII-related information into their fitting formulae, but this is only a small part of the clinical picture. These are an important first step, but will only provide frequency response information. Such frequency response changes can also be thought of as static changes that would not vary as a function of time or input level.

In contrast, there can also be dynamic non-SII related changes that are more related to the syntactic and morphological structures of a language. These changes are not currently built in to any hearing aid fitting formulae but can be. And, they are not predictable from any SII measure.

The grammatical word order in a language has some ramifications for hearing aid fittings. In English, there is a Subject-Verb-Object (SVO) word order with the final object being optional depending on the transitivity of the verb. In contrast, in other languages such as Japanese, the grammatical word order is Subject-Object-Verb (SOV). Table 26–2 shows several commonly spoken languages that possess a SOV word order.

In SOV languages, non-content words are clustered at the end of the sentence. These non-content words may be verbs, postpositions, and some adjectives. Non-content words tend to be less intense than nouns. It is a property of all human speech that given finite lung volume, as a sentence progresses, the intensity decreases: we simply run out of air. Sentence final linguistic elements are of lower intensity that sentence initial. If the sentence final element is a noun, such as an object,

Table 26–2. Some Languages That Have an SOV Word Order

Japanese	Iranian
Korean	Turkish
Hindi-Urdu	Somali*

*Somali has SOV word order but has prepositions rather than postpositions normally observed with this type of word order.

Table 26–1. A Sampling of Some Phonemic Linguistic Attributes That Would Appear on a Language Specific SII and Result in a Change in Frequency Response

Linguistic feature	Example	Difference from "English"
High-frequency consonants	Arabic	More gain above 2000 Hz
Nasals	Portuguese	More gain between 125–2000 Hz
Palatals	Russian "ch"	More gain between 3000–3500 Hz
Retroflexion	Chinese "r"	More gain between 2700–3000 Hz
Tonal	Chinese	More gain between 125–2000 Hz
Timed (morae)	Japanese	More gain between 125–2000 Hz

Source: Adapted from Chasin (2008). Used with permission of the *Hearing Review.*

there is a local increase in intensity because of the important content of the word. Sentence final nouns provide for better audibility than if they were not present. In this sense, sentence final elements are more intense in SVO languages such as English than in SOV languages such as Japanese. A stylized picture of this sentence final intensity decrease is shown in Figure 26–1.

The clinical research question that arises is whether people who speak a SOV language would require more gain for soft level inputs (e.g., sentence final) than for a SVO language such as English. If a client was bilingual (English/Japanese), one could set program #1 for English and program #2 for Japanese, with

program #2 having more gain for soft level inputs than program #1.

Based on a study of 102 bilingual hearing aid clients (Chasin, 2011), it was shown that people who spoke any SOV language desired 3.2 dB more gain for soft level inputs than for their English program. This was true whether the second language was Japanese, Korean, Hindi-Urdu, Iranian, or Turkish. (Somali is also a SOV language but unlike the others with this same word order, it does not have postpositions. It is possible that this same level of increase in low level input would be beneficial for speakers of Somali, but this has not yet been assessed). Specifically, hearing aid clients were asked to set the amount of gain

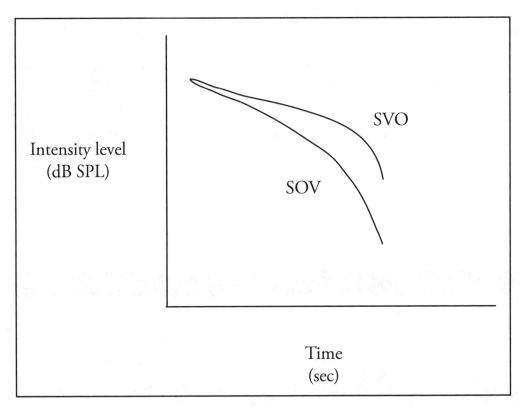

Figure 26–1. *A stylized decrease in speaking intensity as a function of time where sentence final segments and words are less intense than those in a sentence initial location. This natural decrease in vocal intensity is exacerbated in those languages that have an SOV word order with no content words (e.g., objects) near the end of the sentence.*

for soft level inputs (using a range of different commercially available hearing aids) while listing to .wav files of cold running speech in their mother tongue, after having the level set and adjusted while listening to English. The difference for each of the clients was assessed and shown in Figure 26–2. The mean difference was +3.068 dB implying that on average, a person who speaks a SOV language desires about 3 dB more gain (confidence interval 2.482–3.656) for soft level inputs than for English. There was a large variability in the data despite being statistically significant at the $\alpha = 0.01$ level. Some clients preferred no change while others, up to an 8 to 9 dB increase.

Another aspect of a dynamic non-SII related change is that some languages (again with the ubiquitous example of Japanese) have a rigid Consonant-Vowel-Consonant (CVC) morphology. It is very rare to have two vowels or two consonants that are adjacent to each other in Japanese. Even when a word is borrowed from another language with a more relaxed morphology, the rigid CVC structure is imposed. The English word "handbag" becomes "hanodobago" in Japanese. The same is true for the large hamburger chain "Mac-Donalds" but I will let the reader try to figure that pronunciation out. The intervening consonant is typically of much lower intensity than the adjacent vowel. This is especially true if the intervening consonant is a sibilant or other high frequency allophone. If the intervening consonant is a sonorant such as a nasal or a liquid, then this is less of an issue.

Although only preliminary results are in, again with the same clinical paradigm as with the SVO/SOV language issue, when bilingual English/Japanese hard of hearing clients were asked to adjust the release time of a compression circuit in a pair of experimental behind the ear hearing aids, they selected a quicker release time for Japanese than for English. This was only the case when the hearing aid was set up as a single channel device. When the hearing aids were configured as a two

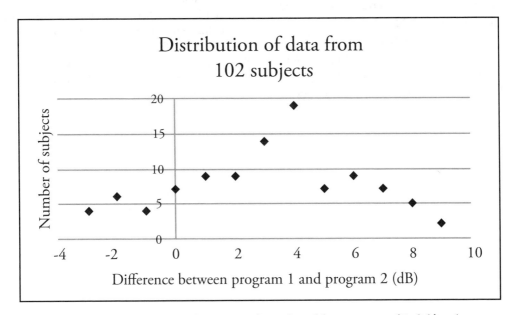

Figure 26–2. *Differences between the amount of gain desired for program #1 (English) and program #2 (SOV language) for 102 hard-of-hearing clients. The mean is 3.068 dB and is statistically significant at $\alpha = 0.01$ (confidence interval 2.482–3.656).*

channel instrument with a 2000 Hz cutoff, the differences in the selected release times did not achieve statistical significance.

These results are consistent with the need for a quicker release time for improved consonant audibility but suggest that this may no longer a clinical issue if the quieter (high frequency) consonants are treated in a different channel as the more intense (low frequency) vowels.

CONCLUSIONS

English appears to be ubiquitous, for a number of reasons: written research articles in this field are typically in English; English is prevalent on the Internet; English is a lingua-franca, meaning that it provides a common ground where the speakers have differing mother tongues; and there are a large number of countries where English is spoken either officially or as an unofficial language. Standards organizations such as the American National Standards Institute (ANSI) publish their findings and report on committee progress in English.

Yet, not everyone speaks English, and if they do, it is a second or third language. More information is required on the phonemics of a language and this can be observed in the language specific SII. It is only a matter of time before language specific SII measures are available and integrated into hearing aid fitting software. Although important for frequency response changes, the SII is limited. Syntactic issues such as sentence word order and also language specific morphological constraints may further complicate a hearing aid fitting by requiring more gain for sentence final, low level inputs, and depending on the hearing aid technology, release times should be altered in order to increase audibility.

REFERENCES

Chasin, M. (1996). *Musicians and the prevention of hearing loss.* San Diego, CA: Singular.

Chasin, M. (2008). How to set hearing aids differently for different languages. *Hearing Review*, *15*(11), 16–20.

Chasin, M. (Ed.). (2009). *Hearing loss in musicians: Prevention and management.* San Diego, CA: Plural.

Chasin, M. (2011). Setting hearing aids differently for different languages. *Seminars in Hearing*, *32*(2), 182–188.

Wong, L. A., Ho, A., Chua, E., & Soli, S. D. (2007). Development of the Cantonese speech intelligibility index. *Journal of the Acoustical Society of America*, *121*(4), 2350–2361.

Preparing Deaf Children for Regular School

Frederick S. Berg

During the last 25 years Dr. Sadanand Singh has been the foremost publisher of books for professionals who serve children with hearing disorders. His creativity, brilliance, drive, and personal touch have helped many people. This essay is dedicated to the late Dr. Singh.

INTRODUCTION

Several thousand deaf children are born annually in the United States. With the recent advent of hospital hearing screening, nearly all deaf babies are identified, the hearing losses of many of them confirmed soon afterward, and hearing aids or cochlear implants fit on them by 6 months of age. This leaves 5½ years for training these deaf children to learn spoken English and speech skills so that by age 6 , they are prepared to enter the first grade of regular school ready to learn to read, communicate orally, and progress alongside normal-hearing children. The successful implementation of these steps eliminates the need for children born deaf to receive special education and rehabilitation services (Berg, 2001, 2008, 2010).

EARLY METHODS

Before the advent of modern hearing aids and cochlear implants, a deaf child had to rely largely on lip reading to learn and use spoken English. It was integral to the success of oral deaf education in the United States, beginning in 1867 with the founding of the Clarke School for the Deaf in Northampton, Massachusetts, the first residential facility that educated deaf children without signs and finger spelling (Berg, 1970).

During 1964 a committee chaired by Homer Babbidge, president of the University of Connecticut, made a thorough investigation of the educational performance of deaf students in the United States under the auspices of the Secretary of Health, Education, and Welfare. A representative sample of residential, day school, and day class programs were visited and studied. A published report indicated that that the American people had little reason to be satisfied with the education of their deaf children (Education of the Deaf, 1965). The typical 14-year-old deaf student reads only at a third grade level (Furth, 1966).

Following the Babbidge Report, teachers of the deaf in U.S. public schools changed to using signs and finger spelling to support speech communication, whereas teachers of the deaf in U.S. private schools stepped up their use of the auditory-oral method (Berg, 2001).

By 1988 the Commission on Education of the Deaf of the U.S. Department of Education reported that the status of education for persons who were deaf in the United States was still unsatisfactory. Using signs with speech had not been successful in assisting the majority of students who were deaf to learn to read well. Only at private auditory-oral schools for the deaf, did most children with very severe hearing losses learn spoken English and become literate, and this only after years of intense auditory and speech training (Berg, 2001).

RECENT IMPROVEMENTS

During 1965 to 1966, Orin Cornett invented the Cued Speech (CS) system to enable young children who are deaf to fully recognize speech sounds and quickly learn spoken English (Moere, 2008). With CS, a speaker adds eight hand shapes and four hand positions to the shapes visible on his or her lips as he or she says speech sounds, syllables, words, and sentences (Cornett & Daisey, 1992). CS prepares a deaf child for English language comprehension and reading in a most efficient and useful way, independent of hearing aid success or failure (Berlin, 1985). However, the great majority of educators of the deaf, public and private, did not accept and use it (Berg, 2008).

During the early 1980s, researchers at Central Institute for the Deaf (CID), a private oral-aural school, sought to answer the question: Can typical deaf children achieve well above what is generally expected, even approaching the achievement of hearing children with just improved teaching? An experimental

group of CID students received concentrated, intense instruction, with a 2.3 student-teacher ratio. A control group received the typical instruction of private oral schools for the deaf, with a higher student-teacher ratio. All students wore hearing aids, and were taught through an auditory-oral approach. The findings showed that both the experimental and control subjects progressed in all areas of tested performance, but the experimental subjects made accelerated gains approaching the performance of normal hearing students (Geers, 1985).

The following decade, researchers at CID sought to answer another question: Can hearing aids, tactile speech aids, and cochlear implants facilitate the development of speech perception, speech production, and language development among deaf children at CID? A 3-year sensory aids study of 39 children was designed and implemented. At the onset of participation in the study each child (1) had a hearing loss of at least 100 dB, (2) was between 2 and 12 years of age, (3) had been born deaf or became deaf by age 3, (4) had used a hearing aid from an early age, and (5) had received early educational intervention as soon as diagnosed (Geers & Moog, 1994).

The 39 children were divided into three matched groups: 13 used Tactaid tactile aids, 13 Nucleus 22 cochlear implants, and 13 conventional hearing aids. Two years into the study another group of 13 children was added. They had hearing losses from 90 to 100 dB and used hearing aids (Geers & Moog, 1994).

These deaf children participated in an intensive auditory-oral program with daily auditory and speech instruction. At the beginning of the study, all children could detect speech through their hearing aids, but had limited speech discrimination. At the end of the study, children generally could discriminate speech better. The cochlear implant group outperformed the tactile group and the first (100+ dB) hearing aid group in speech perception, speech production, and language development, and performed similarly to the second (90–100 dB) hearing aid group. Five of 52 deaf children were able to identify words in open sets after 3 years of intense auditory and speech training. Four of the 5 were among 13 children who used cochlear implants (Geers & Moog, 1994).

A more recent study showed that a higher percentage of deaf children can identify words in open sets. Half of 181 8- to 9-year-old deaf children with cochlear implants exhibited receptive and expressive language skills similar to those of hearing 8- to 9-year-olds. Such mature language outcomes were neither typical of deaf children who used hearing aids nor of children who used sign language (Geers, Nicholas, & Sely, 2003).

During 2008 Robert Shannon, head of the Department of Auditory Implants and Perception at the House Institute, stated that the average cochlear implant recipient understood 65 percent of isolated single words in open sets. In comparison, children who use Cued Speech extensively more fully recognized isolated words in open sets (Moere, 2008; Nichols & Ling, 1982).

To ensure language development, Charles Berlin states that increasingly specialists recommend CS for the estimated 10% of deaf babies and children with Auditory Neuropathy/Dys-synchrony (AN-AD), which occurs when tests of outer hair cells suggest normal hearing but tests of the inner hair cells and auditory nerve fibers suggest deafness. Because this problem can spontaneously disappear, early cochlear implantation is only recommended where the cause is clearly hereditary and when the history of other family members justify it. Implantation can be very successful when preceded by and later supported by CS, which is always a useful tool for teaching language and syntax and clarifying the new sounds the child will hear through the implant. Berlin and staff have yet to see a child with AN-AD

show typical language development with hearing aids and Auditory-Verbal Therapy (with no visual cues) at the same rate as a deaf child with simple outer hair cell loss (Berlin, Hood, Morlet, Rose, & Blashears, 2002).

BILINGUAL APPROACHES

Notwithstanding the success of using Cued Speech or hearing aids and cochlear implants for English language development, many educators of the deaf argue that the American Sign Language (ASL) should be taught as the first language to deaf children. There is evidence that it contributes to early conceptual development for those children who have, or are provided with, access to the signing community. However, it takes an additional three to seven years for a child to develop fluency in English after learning another first language (Cummins, 2006).

Cued Speech advocates favor a proven bilingual approach to deaf education: namely, having deaf children of hearing parents learn English as a first language, and ASL as a second language. Many deaf children have become proficient in both spoken English and ASL following this approach (Cornett & Daisey, 1992).

Flexer (1999) has stated that it is unnecessary for deaf children who learn spoken English through aided listening, called the Auditory-Verbal Method, to learn CS or ASL. However, this requires that hearing aids, cochlear implants, and wireless equipment function optimally at all times, which is unrealistic. For example, young deaf children are susceptible to having speech stimulation levels that are set too high by audiologists mapping cochlear implants (Mertes & Chinnici, 2005). Also, there is a severe shortage of speech-language pathologists and auditory-oral educators to serve the needs of the thousands of deaf children who can benefit from the use of newer hearing technologies. In addition, few if any of these specialists who are available are also trained in use of CS (Berg, 2010).

SPEECH FORMATS AND HEARING TECHNOLOGIES

The vowels, diphthongs, and consonant sounds include frequencies between 125 Hz and 8000 Hz. Each of them includes one or more unique formants (maximum intensities). For example, for adults males, the /m/ has a narrow formant around 300 Hz; the /u/ has narrow formants around 300 Hz and 800 Hz; the /ɑ/ has narrow formants around 800 Hz and 1200 Hz; and the /i/ has narrow formants around 300 Hz and 2200 Hz. For male and female adults and for children, the /ʃ/ has a wide formant centered at 3000 Hz; and the /s/, a wide formant centered at 4000 Hz (Berg, 2010).

Many deaf children have enough low and mid-frequency residual hearing to fully learn spoken English by listening through a Phonak Naida BTE digital hearing aid. It includes a nonlinear frequency compression system algorithm, called Sound Recover, that compresses high frequency speech sounds such as the /s/ downward so they can be heard in the lower or mid-frequency regions (Glista, Scollie, Bagatto, Sewald, Parsa, & Jonson, 2009).

A cochlear implant, which is much more costly, has the potential of enabling most deaf children to learn to recognize all speech sounds. This potential is reached when its speech processor is accurately adjusted (mapped) to an intensity level between the child's hearing threshold and his or her comfortable listening levels for incoming electrical signals at each low-, mid-, and high-frequency electrode, followed by extensive auditory training (Berg, 2010).

A hearing aid or cochlear implant is effective for listening in quiet and preferably at close range (within 6 feet). In a noisy or reverberant environment, or beyond 6 feet, a child with a hearing aid or cochlear implant is dependent on a wireless system to more clearly understand what people are saying through hearing (Berg, 1993). A Phonak wireless transmitter will send speech via radio into a miniature receiver that links into any brand of BTE hearing aid, such as their Naida, or into a cochlear implant (Berg, 2010).

PRECISION SPEECH

The author has made extensive use of Lissajous (circular electrovisual) patterns from a Video Articulator or a Vocal Scope to supplement acoustic, lip reading, and tactile speech clues for shaping speech sounds that cannot be fully recognized otherwise. As speech is said precisely within 2 inches of its microphone, the visual display is shown as a different unique pattern for each speech sound. For a voiceless sound, for example, an /s/, each person saying it will produce the same Lissajous pattern for that sound. For a voiced sound, for example, a /z/, each person saying it will produce similar Lissajous patterns (Berg, 2008).

The author used electrovisual clues in combination with lip reading and tactile clues to shape the articulation of 36 vowels, diphthongs, and consonants of a 10-year-old boy who could not hear. At the beginning of a summer training program, his speech sounds were mainly very distorted. At the end, they were almost all precisely articulated. The author has also used Lissajous patterns to shape the speech of preschool-age deaf children (Berg. 2008).

The author has developed a Speech Shaping and Recording Target to mark the accuracies of speech responses and track progress. The target has a sector for each sound, an outer ring, an inner ring, and a bull's-eye. A substitution of another sound for the target sound, or a profound distortion of the target sound is marked off target. A moderate or severe distortion of the target sound is marked in the outer ring. A slight or mild distortion of the target sound is marked in the inner ring. A precise articulation of the target sound is marked in the bull's-eye (Berg, 2008)

A copy of the Speech Shaping Target and Recording Form may be used for each speech therapy session. Phonetic symbols for all these sounds encircle the target. They are placed just outside a sector of the target for each of these sounds. Beginning with the /ɑ/ at the top right of the target, symbols move clockwise, and end with the /r/ at the top left (Berg, 2008).

During speech shaping, go through all of these sounds with the child, beginning with the /ɑ/. Instruct the child to imitate you. Say a sound, and then look at and listen to the child as he or she imitates it. Provide the child with all helpful sensory clues: hearing, lip reading, touch, and Lissajous patterns. Reward him or her for improvements. Mark a dot in each sector of the target, based on the child's most accurate imitation. Schedule this training at least twice a week until the child can say each sound precisely. If training is begun early in the child's life, his or her speech will be highly usable in regular school (Berg, 2010).

A Speech Visualizer software program with Lissajous patterns is available free of charge from Speech Tech Ltd, A Radio Shack analog sound level meter and a paper strip are also useful visual speech indicators. Deflections of the meter needle reveal clues on intensity and duration of each speech sound. Air movement of a paper strip held in the front of the mouth reveals clues on intensities and durations of consonant sounds and the vowel /u/ (Berg, 2010)

Once a deaf child can say a vowel, diphthong, or consonant in isolation, teach him or her to sustain the sound, and say it in syllables, using correct stress patterns Teach the child to transfer this speech skill into words and sentences, including consonant blends and syllables, words, and sentences incorporating it (Berg, 2008).

The author's book entitled *Speech Development Guide for Children with Hearing Loss* includes 117 lessons. Each lesson includes: (a) the IPA symbol(s) for the speech sound or consonant blend to be taught, (b) one or more side view drawings of how the sound or blend is made, (c) one or more front view photographs of how the sound or blend is made, (d) a printed description of the sound or blend and how to teach it, (e) breath control and syllable drills or prosodic drills for the sound or blend, (f) a picture of a word that includes the sound or blend, (g) the printed form of that word, (h) a sentence to repeat and complete with the word, and (i) additional words that include the sound or blend (Berg, 2008).

A 117-item Word Test Form is used to keep track of progress in speech development. It includes IPA symbols for each speech sound and blend, printed words for each of these, and a space for recording the child's accuracy in saying each speech sound and blend (Berg, 2008).

The teaching of speech sounds and blends, as described above, refines and extends the natural development of speech sounds learned in connection with thousands of incidental situations the child experiences. Suggestions of what parents can do to utilize both natural and contrived situations with young deaf children with or without CS are specified in the book (Berg, 2008).

Once young deaf children have basic spoken English skills, train them to improve their recognition and comprehension of words, sentences, and messages in contrived tasks through auditory (A), visual (V) or lip reading, and/or AV conditions. The author has developed a course book and DVD for parents of deaf children that include tests and tasks to accomplish this (Berg, 2010).

SUMMARY

The hearing losses of most deaf children are now confirmed by audiologists soon after birth. Through intelligent and sustained utilization of newly available hearing and visual technologies, methods, and materials, these children learn spoken English and develop precise speech early in life. This prepares them to learn to read, communicate orally, and progress in regular school alongside hearing children. Such preparation of deaf children for regular school eliminates their need for later special education and rehabilitation services, resulting in a less expensive and less intrusive overall education for them.

REFERENCES

Berg, F. (1970). The locus of the education of the hard of hearing child. In F. Berg & S. Fletcher (Eds.), *The hard of hearing child: Clinical and educational management* (pp. 13–26). New York, NY: Grune & Stratton.

Berg, F. (1993). *Acoustics and sound systems in schools.* San Diego, CA: Singular.

Berg, F. (2001). Educational management of children who are hearing impaired. In R. Hull (Ed.), *Aural rehabilitation of children who are hearing impaired* (pp. 169–185). San Diego, CA: Singular.

Berg, F. (2008). *Speech development guide for children with hearing loss.* San Diego, CA: Plural.

Berg, F. (2010). *Parents of deaf children take charge. Course book, DVD, and self-instructional assignments.* Smithfield, UT: Berg.

Berlin, C. (1985). *Encouraging audiologists to recommend cued speech.* Presentation to the National Cued Speech Association, Cleveland, OH.

Berlin, C., Hood, L., Morlet, T., Rose, K., & Blashears, S. (2002). Auditory neuropathy-dyssynchrony: after diagnosis, then what? *Seminars in Hearing, 23*(3): 209–214.

Commission on Education of the Deaf, U.S. Department of Education. (1988). Toward equality education of the deaf. *Tenth annual report to Congress on the implementation of PL 94-142.* Washington, DC: Author.

Cornett, O., & Daisey, M. (1992). *The cued speech resource guidebook for parents of deaf children.* Raleigh, NC: National Cued Speech Association.

Cummins, J. (2006). The relationship between American Sign Language proficiency and English academic development: A review of research [1]. Retrieved from As/thinktank.com/files/Cummins ASL–Eng.pdf.

Education of the Deaf. (1965). *A report to the Secretary of Health, Education, and Welfare by his advisory committee on the education of the deaf.* Washington, DC: Government Printing Office.

Flexer, C. (1999). *Facilitating hearing and listening in young children.* San Diego, CA: Singular.

Furth, H. (1966). A comparison of reading test scores of deaf and hearing children. *American Annals of the Deaf, 111,* 461–462.

Geers, A. (1985). Assessment of hearing impaired children: Determining typical and optimal levels of performance. In F. Powell, T. Fietzo-Hieber, S. Fried Patti, & D. Henderson (Eds.), *Education of the hearing impaired child* (pp. 57–82). San Diego, CA: College-Hill Press.

Geers, A., & Moog, J. (1994). Spoken language results: Vocabulary, syntax, and communication. The sensory aids study at Central Institute for the Deaf. *Volta Review, 96,* 131–148.

Geers, A., Nicholas, J., & Sedy, A. (2003). Language skills of children with cochlear implantation. *Ear and Hearing, 24,* Supplement, 46S–58S.

Glista, D., Scollie, S., Bagatto, M., Sewald, R., Parsa, V., & Jonson, A. (2009). Evaluation of nonlinear compression: Clinical outcomes. *International Journal of Audiology, 48,* 632–644.

Mertes, J., & Chinnici, J. (2005, September). Cochlear implants—considerations in programming for the pediatric population. Retrieved from http://www.SpeechPathology.com

Moere, D. (2008, June 28). *Supporting auditory oral language development with cued speech.* Alexander Graham Bell Association for the Deaf and Hard of Hearing. Biennial Convention.

Nicholls, G., & Ling, D. (1982). Cued speech and the reception of spoken language. *Journal of Speech and Hearing Research, 25,* 262–269.

Speech visualizer software program. Victoria, Canada: Speech Tech, Ltd.

Educating Children ✒ with Hearing Loss in the ✒ Technology Age

Patricia M. Chute and Mary Ellen Nevins

Technology today represents the largest growing sector of the inspirational mind, transcending all aspects of daily life. Its application in social media has brought down dictators, provided outlets for those in need, and transformed the way we communicate. Technology comes in many forms, and influences the population across the age span and around the globe. Fortunately, children with hearing loss are among those affected by technology in a decidedly positive manner through innovations in listening and learning.

LISTENING TECHNOLOGIES

Not since World War II and the invention of the wearable hearing aid, has technology more drastically enhanced the auditory capacity of the individual with hearing loss (Berger, 1976). The cochlear implant represents one of the most significant developments of the late 20th and early 21st century. Like so many technologies, it has created divisive responses that both support and detract from its overall

worth. Likewise, it has created circumstances with unexpected outcomes that were never envisioned during its initial unveiling.

From the early research of Djourno and Eyries (1957) in France to the investigations several decades later in the United States (House, 1987; Michelson, 1981), the goal of bringing sound to the profoundly deaf was driven by a medical model that sought a treatment for a physical disability. The ability to apply the microsurgical techniques required to implant the device was quickly overshadowed by the material make up of the implant. The possibility of rejection of a foreign body inserted into an area close to the brain received major attention during the early clinical trials. Once the rejection issues were overcome, the promise of a decipherable acoustic signal for one who had no remaining auditory capacity became the focus of attention. It was hailed by the medical community as a cure for deafness.

The fallout from what appeared to be a technological advance was an outcry from the Deaf Community and many others who did not believe that this innovation had merit (NAD, 1991). The initial reaction of the

National Association of the Deaf (NAD) was to publish a position paper that took issue with the medical community who were perceived as individuals trying to fix the deaf to make them more like hearing people. The debate was extremely heated as members of the Deaf Community had recently captured the attention of the nation with the Deaf President Now (DPN) movement, only to find themselves struggling to maintain an ephemeral spotlight as implant technology took center stage. The conflict still exists today but has tempered considerably; for some it remains a thorny point of contention.

Regardless of the turmoil, the technology evolved from simplistic systems that could provide basic timing and intensity cues (House, 1987) to multichannel ones that offered recipients the ability to speak interactively on the telephone (Dowell et al., 1985). Clinical trials with adult populations sanctioned by the Food and Drug Administration (FDA) were expanded to include children; the capabilities and cosmetics of the device improved markedly. Once the FDA approved cochlear implants in both adults (1987) and children (1990) (Patrick et al., 2006), a new era in the treatment of hearing loss was launched. Hearing aids improved and addressed the needs of individuals with profound deafness, who had some residual hearing and did not wish to undergo surgery. Frequency transposition hearing aids (McDermott et al., 1999) evolved while digital hearing aids incorporated new sound processing schemes to reduce noise and improve perception (Engebretson et al., 1987). Simultaneously, the cochlear implant market expanded from one to three companies in the United States. Although Cochlear, an Australian based company, was the first to enter the market, the presence of Advanced Bionics, an American company and later Med El, an Austrian company, moved the technology quickly. The competition sparked rapid developments in speech processing, electrode design, programming paradigms, and device hardware. The speech processors during this period were all body-worn units that required several alkaline or specially developed lithium batteries. They were bulky and presented numerous problems, especially for small children who wore them in special harnesses under clothing. Interfacing these devices with FM systems became extremely challenging; there was a need for individually designed connecting cables, which posed problems. Early models of the body worn processors used standard dial controls or rotating wheels to set volume and sensitivity. These created issues for small children, who might purposely or inadvertently move the control dials and create a negative response.

With each generation of hardware, improvements in size and usability occurred. Device operation was supported with LEDs to display settings in a clear manner; external equipment also became more modular so that parts could be replaced more easily. Finally, in 1998, Cochlear became the first company to develop a behind-the-ear model that would be the impetus for the other companies to follow suit. In addition to the cosmetic changes that were occurring, significant alterations in speech processing were taking place. Algorithms that incorporated digitization of the signal at high speeds demonstrated better outcomes for most recipients (Briggs, 2011). The need to offer more than one type of speech processing strategy became evident as the variability in recipient performance continued to be unpredictable. All devices now had the capability of storing more than one program within the speech processor so that access to sound could be better trialed outside the confines of the clinical environment. For children, this became an important part of assessing function in the classroom. However, it added an element of complexity for teachers and speech-language pathologists managing the device at school.

In time, the implant was no longer seen as a technology that solely influenced auditory performance, but one that would enhance the academic and social development of its pediatric users (Carney & Moeller, 1998; Robbins et al., 1995). Criteria for candidacy were extended to include children with special needs, children with deaf parents, and adults born deaf. Currently, the expansion to bilateral implantation has become best practice for young children (Briggs, 2011). Today, improvements in listening technology, epitomized through the cochlear implant, have reached a temporary plateau as advances in design and efficiency can no longer match the quantum leap seen in the initial stages of development. As listening technology evolved over the years, so too did the learning technology to support its use.

LEARNING TECHNOLOGIES

During the early years of implant availability, there was a genuine gap in the knowledge base and skill set of the professionals who were asked to deliver services. It is unimaginable in today's information society that at the time of the launch of cochlear implant technology, there was no venue for systematic knowledge dissemination for front line educational personnel. Professionals were in dire need of facts regarding the device, the children for whom it was appropriate, and the strategies and techniques that would be useful in maximizing its benefit. When such information was available, it was found in professional journals for surgeons and audiologists. Early reports presented findings from hospitals and clinics where this controversial, new medical device was implanted and where therapies were provided (Berliner & Eisenberg, 1985; Tyler et al., 1986). Specialty implant meetings and national and international word of mouth

networks developed. This provided a venue for implant center habilitationists and educational consultants to hear the word and share it with teachers and speech-language pathologists in educational settings. Implant center personnel were the keepers of the information flame, recording it, analyzing it, interpreting it, ready to carry it to the next distant school, agency, or clinic where children with implants might be found. Not surprisingly, then, the responsibility for professional development of speech, hearing and educational personnel was the purview of the early implant center. A small number of visionary surgeons and implant center directors recognized that their role in the process of implantation was largely medical and clinical. They sought ways to include educational personnel as part of a team approach to implantation (Nevins et al., 1991; Parisier et al., 1994). These centers identified educational specialists who served as the conduit for exchange of ideas among the therapists and teachers with children with implants on their caseloads or in their classrooms. There were no best practices to convey in those early years, as experts were those with knowledge about the device and how it worked. Each therapist or teacher essentially served as a single case study researcher. Because educational services were not reimbursable, costs for this vital component of implant habilitation were often borne by private foundations. These supported the outreach that assisted children in achieving their fullest potential in their local schools. Over time, clarity about what the device could and could not do allowed for the identification of the nature and needs of children with implants, and the direction for training educational professionals with whom they worked (Chute & Nevins, 1996; Estabrooks, 1998; Nevins & Chute, 1996; Owens & Kessler, 1989; Tye-Murray, 1992).

As implants became readily obtainable and auditory access available to more and more children with hearing loss, greater numbers of professionals discovered that their knowledge base and skill set were out of date. They were unprepared to provide the type of intervention that would promote the development of listening and spoken language. Even recent graduates of teacher education and speech-language pathology and audiology programs were ill-equipped to meet the needs of children with implants, as the curriculum of colleges and universities had not yet been revised to reflect emerging technology and the needs of the children who received it (Chute, 2003). Furthermore, the impact of Universal Newborn Hearing Screening and its push for early intervention required a shift from an orientation that used manual communication to one that emphasized listening and spoken language. Additionally, early interventionists needed to alter the focus from the child to the parent, and learn to implement coaching strategies that would empower parents to assume the role of first teacher (Moeller, 2000). This created a desperate need for information exchange that was institutionalized, available around the clock and around the country. Most importantly, accurate information to update the knowledge base and retool the skill set of front line professionals was required. The availability of professional articles and texts aimed at school personnel working with children with implants and the willingness of seasoned professionals to travel across the country to lead in-service programming met this need for quite some time (Chute & Nevins, 2003, 2006; Cole & Flexer, 2007; Easterbrooks & Estes, 2007). Not long thereafter, local education agencies, school districts, state Departments of Education and even implant manufacturers began to assume some of the responsibility for educating the workforce. By harnessing Internet technology, learning leaders presented webinars, provided online courses, managed listserv networks and directed learning communities to enhance the delivery of information. Today, it is even possible for professionals in remote and rural areas to have access to the vital knowledge base that undergirds appropriate education for children with listening technologies.

The future of both listening and learning technology can only be speculated on at this time. From the bulky systems of 25 years ago that took hours to program, newer methods of setting the device that do not require any input from the recipient have changed the landscape of the professional working with young children. Designs for self-programming systems have been under development with promising results in the near future. Certainly the notion of the all-implantable device has reached research laboratories around the world. Simultaneously, interest in regenerating hair cells has led to new approaches, as nanotechnology and the use of human growth hormones shows progress. Regardless of where technology takes us, one thing remains clear. Children born deaf have more options than they had three decades ago. The opportunities for them to be educated alongside their hearing peers and compete intellectually and socially are now possible.

Professional learning for teachers, speech-language pathologists, and educational audiologists has matured as well. Newly created certifications for implant audiologists and professionals who specialize in working with young children with hearing loss through listening and spoken language techniques has ramped up the need for continuing education resources. These resources allow for the acquisition of the knowledge base and skill set that earns specialty certification (Goldberg et al., 2010). With a mandate to focus on the relationship of professional development to student outcomes, today's continuing education is focused and intense (Wei et al., 2009), and likely includes job-embedded mentoring. Best practices of adult learning, case-based discovery, and the creation of learning communities are the essential elements of advancing the career journey of today's sophisticated speech and hearing professional. Yet these are all additive to the ongoing need for print material, electronic or traditional, that spark conversations made possible when a common vocabulary and language are shared. The enduring power of the printed word to codify the ideas and beliefs that move generations forward in knowledge, skill, and practice cannot be overstated.

Sadanand Singh embraced that credo. His love for literature coupled with his concern for individuals with speech and hearing challenges created the impetus to develop a publishing empire. His encouragement of novice and established authors to be part of his publication family made him the ultimate teacher and mentor in his literary passion. The manuscripts he published enriched the lives of children and adults with communication disorders. Recognizing that science and education are two sides of a single coin, the vast number of books published because of Dr. Singh's visionary leadership will leave an indelible mark on the speech, hearing, and education fields.

REFERENCES

Berger, K. W. (1976). Genealogy of the words "audiology" and "audiologist." *Journal of the American Audiology Society, 2*(2), 38–44.

Berliner, K. I., & Eisenberg, L. S. (1985). Methods and issues in the cochlear implantation of children: An overview. *Ear and Hearing, 6* (Suppl.) 6S–13S

Briggs, R. J. (2011). Future technology in cochlear implants: Assessing the benefit. *Cochlear Implants International, 12,* S 22–25.

Carney, A. E., & Moeller, M. P. (1998). Treatment efficacy: Hearing loss in children. *Journal of Speech and Hearing Research, 41*(1) S61–84.

Chute, P. M. (2003). *Manpower issues affecting cochlear implantation.* Paper presented at the 8th Conference on Cochlear Implants in Children, Washington, DC.

Chute, P. M., & Nevins, M. E. (2003). Educational challenges for children with cochlear implants. In T. Schery (Ed.), *Cochlear implants in children: Ideas for intervention. Topics in Language Disorders, 23,* 57–67.

Chute, P. M., & Nevins, M. E. (2006*). School professionals working with children with cochlear implants.* San Diego, CA: Plural.

Chute, P. M., Nevins, M. E., & Parisier, S. C. (1996). Managing educational issues throughout the process of implantation. In D. Allum (Ed.), *Cochlear implant rehabilitation in children and adults* (pp. 119–130). London, UK: Whurr.

Cole, E., & Flexer, C. (2007). *Children with hearing loss: Developing listening and talking birth to six.* San Diego, CA: Plural.

Djourno, A., & Eyries, C. (1957). Auditory prosthesis by means of a distant electrical stimulation of the sensory nerve with the use of an in-dwelt coiling. *Presse Medicale, 65*(63), 1417–1423.

Dowell, R. C., Martin, L. F. A., Clark, G. M., & Brown, A. M. (1985). Results of a preliminary trial of a multiple channel cochlear prosthesis. *Annals of Otorhinology and Laryngology, 94,* 244–250.

Easterbrooks, S. R., & Estes, E. L. (2007). *Helping deaf and hard of hearing students to use spoken language.* Thousand Oaks, CA: Corwin Press.

Engebretson, A. M., Morley, R. B., & Popelka, G. R. (1987) Development of an ear-level digital hearing aid and computer-assisted fitting procedure: An interim report. *Journal of Rehabilitation Research and Development, 24*(4), 55–64.

Estabrooks, W. (1998). *Cochlear implants for kids.* Washington, DC: A. G. Bell.

Goldberg, D. M., Dickson, C. L., & Flexer, C. (2010). AG Bell academy certification program for listening and spoken language specialists: Meeting a world-wide need for qualified professionals. In K. T. Houston & C. Perigoe (Eds.) *Professional preparation for listening and spoken language practitioners. Volta Review, 110,* 129–139.

House, W. (1987). Cochlear implants: The beginning. *Laryngoscope, 97*, 996–997.

McDermott, H. J, Dorkos, V. P., Dean, M. R., & Ching, T. Y. (1999). Improvements in speech perception with use of the AVR TranSonic frequency-transposing hearing aid. *Journal of Speech, Language and Hearing Research, 42*(6), 1323–1335.

Michelson, R. P., & Schindler, R. A. (1981). Multichannel cochlear implants: Current status and future developments. *Laryngoscope, 91*(6), 886–888.

Moeller, M. P. (2000). Early intervention and language development in children who are deaf and hard of hearing. *Pediatrics, 106*, 1–9.

National Association of the Deaf (NAD). (1991). Report of the task force on childhood cochlear implants. *NAD Broadcaster, 13*, 1.

Nevins, M. E., & Chute, P. M. (1996). *Children with cochlear implants in educational settings.* San Diego, CA: Singular.

Nevins, M. E., Kretschmer, R. E., Chute, P. M., Hellman, S. A., & Parisier, S. C. (1991). The role of an educational consultant in a pediatric cochlear implant center. *Volta Review, 93*, 197–204.

Owens, E. & Kessler, D. K. (1989). *Cochlear implants in young deaf children.* Boston, MA: College-Hill Press.

Parisier, S. C., Chute, P. M., & Nevins, M. E. (1994). Pediatric cochlear implants: Surgical and rebabilitative issues. In F. E. Lucente (Ed.), *Highlights of the instructional courses* (pp. 145–154). St. Louis, MO: Mosby.

Patrick, J. F., Busby, P. A., & Gibson, P. J. (2006). The development of the Nucleus Freedom cochlear implant system. *Trend in Amplification, 10*(4), 175–200.

Robbins, A. M. Svirsky, M. A, Miyamoto, R. T., & Kessler, K. S. (1995). Language development in children with cochlear implants. *Advances in Otorhinolaryngology, 50*, 160–166.

Tye-Murray, N. (1992). *Cochlear implants in children: A handbook for parents, teachers and speech and hearing professionals.* Washington, DC: A. G. Bell.

Tyler, R. S., Berliner, K., Demorest, M., Hirshorn, M., Luxford, W., & Mangham, C. (1986). Clinical objectives and research design issues for cochlear implants in children. *Seminars in Hearing, 7*, 433–440.

Wei, R. C., Darling-Hammond, L., Andree, A., Richardson, N., & Orphanos, S. (2009). *Professional learning in the learning profession: A status report on teacher development in the United States and abroad.* Dallas, TX: National Staff Development Council.

ESSAY 29

ꙮ Listening to Words ꙮ

Event-Related Potentials Reveal Cognitive Complexity— Implications for Speech Audiometry

James Jerger and Mary Reagor

Sadanand and I were colleagues and friends for more than 40 years. He never failed to amaze me. He was an unusual combination of scholar and businessman. His research in speech production and perception was always on the cutting edge: and as a book publisher in speech and hearing he was without parallel. In a field of enterprise not renowned for its lofty ethical standards he was a faultless beacon of probity. I think that he would have liked this essay. He once told me that he thought audiology could be doing much more with speech recognition but that innovative research was sadly lacking. There is seldom a day that I do not miss him.

— James Jerger

Speech audiometry is central to the evaluation of hearing handicap, the diagnosis of auditory disorders, the evaluation of hearing aids and other amplification devices, and the assessment of cochlear-implant performance. The paradigm has changed little over the past half century. A word is presented, either in isolation, at the end of a carrier phrase, or embedded in a sentence. The listener's task is to repeat back the word or sentence heard. Each word, or key word if embedded in a sentence, is scored as either correct or incorrect. The task is essentially speech recognition. It is not cognitively demanding. Indeed, certain birds may display the behavioral response if properly motivated (from which we derive the word "parroting"). The process may be modeled as in Figure 29–1. The presentation of the word initiates a process of input phonological analysis, which immediately evokes a corresponding output phonological process leading to a verbal response. Subsequent lexical and semantic analysis and conceptualization may take place but are not necessary to the behavioral response. For example, we can repeat back words spoken in a foreign language whether or not we know the meaning of the words.

Suppose, however, that we ask the listener to do more than repeat the word back; rather, to engage in a meaningful listening task leading to a decision about what was heard. This process can be modeled as in Figure 29–2.

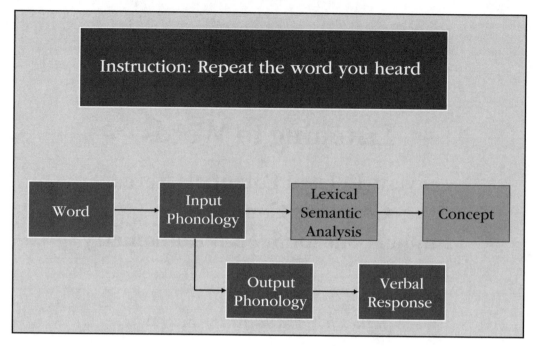

Figure 29–1. *Processing model of a speech audiometric procedure in which a word is presented and the listener repeats it back to the examiner.*

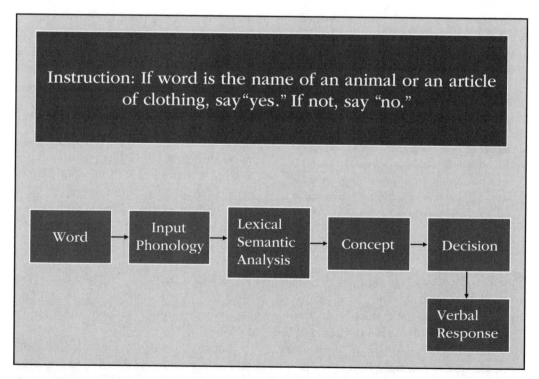

Figure 29–2. *Processing model of a speech audiometric procedure in which a word is presented and the listener is instructed to respond "yes" or "no" depending on whether the word belongs to a predefined semantic category or categories.*

If, for example we ask the listener to decide whether the word is the name of an animal, then a more complex sequence of cognitive events takes place. Now the input phonological analysis is followed by processes of lexical/semantic analysis and concept formation leading to a decision followed by a simple button push or verbal response (e.g., "yes" or "no"). It is, of course, an oversimplification to suggest a simple serial progression of these events: to be sure these cognitive events are processed in partial parallel fashion, with substantial temporal overlap of activities (Marslen-Wilson & Tyler, 1980; Van Petten, Coulson, Rubin, et al., 1999), but a serial visualization helps us to understand the totality of events involved in the process.

In the present essay we ask whether electrophysiologic responses from the brain reveal a difference between: (1) a simple repetition response to a heard word and (2) a decision based on a more complex listening task. To what extent are the additional cognitive processes invoked by the more complex task revealed in the auditory evoked potentials evoked by the heard word? Additionally, to what extent does the presence of sensorineural hearing loss affect the comparison?

AUDITORY EVOKED POTENTIALS EVOKED BY WORDS

When an isolated single-syllable word (e.g., PB word) is presented in the context of a listening task requiring recognition of a specific linguistic feature of the word, the auditory event-related potential (AERP) evoked by the word is characterized by a series of positive and negative peaks associated with various aspects of auditory processing (Figure 29–3 shows examples). Initial negative (N1) and positive (P2) peaks, at about 100 and 200 ms latencies respectively, reflect the initial detection and evaluation of the auditory event (Näätanen, Sams, Alho, et al., 1988). They are followed by a prolonged negativity, peaking at a latency of about 500 ms, thought to include more than one temporally overlapping process depending on the nature of the experimental procedure. In studies of mismatch negativity it has been termed "attentional negativity"; in studies of semantic incongruity it is simply identified by its peak latency as the "N400" response (Kutas & Hilyard, 1980). Cognitive processes implicated include attention (Näätänen, 1990), memory (D'Arcy, Connolly, Service, et al., 2004; Kutas & Federmeier, 2000), phonological processing (D'Arcy, Connolly, & Crocker, 2000; Connolly & Phillips, 1994), and semantic processing (Kutas & Iragui, 1998; Halgren, Dhond, Christensen, et al., 2002; West, O'Rourke, & Holcomb, 2008). In the present chapter we refer to all of these processes collectively under the rubric "processing negativity" (PN). In the case of target words, for example in an oddball paradigm, this negativity is partially overlapped by a later broad positivity, the late-positive component (LPC) peaking at approximately 800 ms and extending to a latency of approximately 1500 ms after word onset. The LPC response (Polich, 2007) is thought to represent processes concerned with the updating of working memory (Donchin & Coles, 1988) and the process of decision-making associated with a task involving the heard word (Kok, 1997; Nieuwenhuis, Aston-Jones, & Cohen, 2005). The extent to which this late positivity interferes with the accurate assessment of processing negativity can be minimized by considering only responses to non-target words.

We have measured such auditory evoked potentials in various tasks involving semantic category judgments. The listener hears a series of words. Some are chosen at random, others belong to a specified semantic category (e.g., names of animals, articles of clothing, body parts, etc.). It is customary to refer to the words in the specified semantic category as "targets" and the randomly chosen words as "nontargets." The a priori probability of a target word may vary from 50% to as low as 15% or 10%, depending on the cognitive component of chief interest. When the decision process is of paramount interest, the probability of a target word is purposely chosen to be small (10–20%/the "oddball" paradigm) in order to maximize the LPC component of the auditory event-related potential. If the region of chief interest is processing negativity, it is useful to increase the probability of a target in order to better engage the interest of the listener in the task so that responses to non-target words may be analyzed. In the present experiment we analyzed only responses to non-target words.

Figure 29–3 illustrates these various peaks and valleys of the waveform to a non-target word, measured at one electrode, in this case C3 in the International 10-20 System. Figure 29–4 illustrates the scalp topography across the entire array of electrodes (in this case 30 electrodes) in the 100-ms latency interval from 500 to 600-ms, encompassing the peak of the processing negativity. Maximal negativity is broadly distributed across the left hemisphere from parietal to frontal regions.

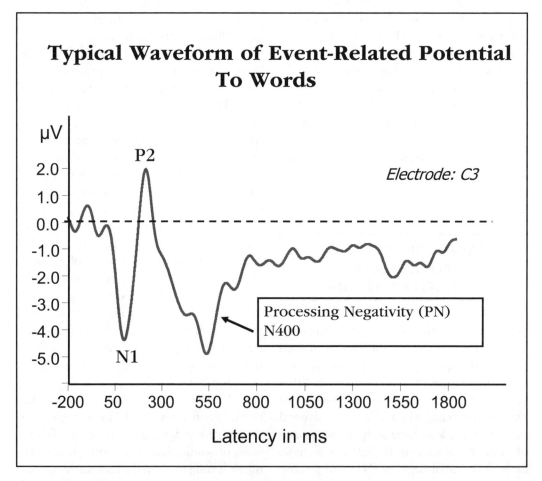

Figure 29–3. *Typical waveform to a nontarget word in a semantic category paradigm.*

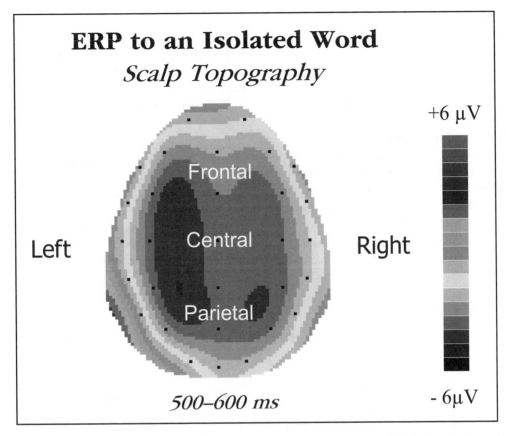

Figure 29–4. *Scalp topography in the 500 to 600-ms latency range associated with the waveform of Figure 29–3.*

A SIMPLE EXPERIMENT

In order to study the effect of the semantic category judgment task on the AERPs to words, we conducted a simple experiment. We presented a large series of words to listeners sequentially under two conditions. In one condition the listener was instructed to simply repeat each word back. In the second condition the listener was instructed to say "yes" if the word was either the name of an animal or an article of clothing: otherwise to say "no." Initial pilot study indicated that confining targets to a single semantic category was not sufficiently challenging. Hence targets from one of two predefined categories (animals and articles of clothing) were employed.

Of the total words, 26% were targets, that is, words that were either the names of animals or articles of clothing. The remaining 74% were randomly chosen nontargets. All words were common, single-syllable CVC words. The two conditions were presented in counterbalanced fashion to each participant. Electroencephalograhic (EEG) activity was recorded from 30 active electrodes affixed to the scalp according to a modification of the International 10-20 system. Data were acquired and analyzed via the Neuroscan Electrophysiological Data Acquisition System (SCAN 4.4, Neurosoft, Inc.). Data analysis was confined to the nontarget waveforms.

These two tasks were purposely constructed to provide challenge to the listener, but were not so difficult that a significant number of items were incorrectly identified: performance was uniformly above the 90% correct level.

Results

We tested two groups of participants, 7 adults with normal hearing and 7 adults with mild to moderate sensorineural hearing loss in one or both ears. Normal hearers ranged in age from 21 to 41 yr. Four were male. Hearing-impaired participants ranged in age from 21 to 67 years. All were male. Average losses (PTA, average of the HTLs at 1000, 2000, and 4000

Hz) and averaged across ears, ranged from 3 to 11 dB HTL in the normal-hearing group and from 12 to 48 dB HTL in the hearing-impaired group. Mean loss, thus defined, was 6.9 dB in the normal-hearing group and 26.7 dB in the hearing-loss group.

ADULTS WITH NORMAL HEARING

Figure 29–5 shows typical waveforms at electrode C3 for both conditions in a 31-year-old male with normal hearing. The waveform for

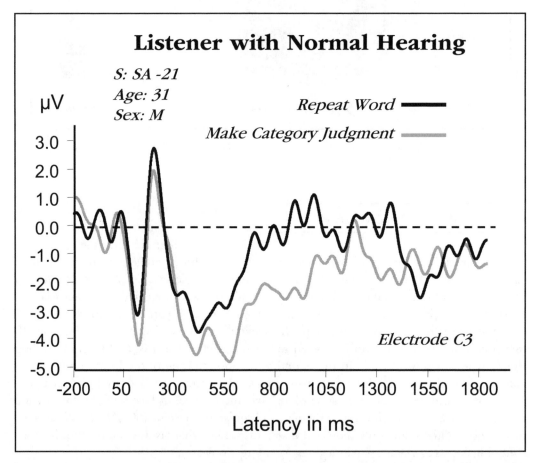

Figure 29–5. Waveforms for the two experimental conditions at electrode C3 in a 31-year-old man with normal hearing.

the *repeat-word* condition (black) shows the expected N1 and P2 peaks, indicating initial detection of an auditory event, followed by a prolonged negativity, peaking in the 400- to 600-ms latency range, then slowly returning to baseline by about 900 ms. The waveform for the *category-decision* condition (gray), shows similar N1 and P2 peaks. The subsequent negativity, however, peaks deeper and somewhat later, and remains substantially deeper until it finally returns to baseline at about 1200 ms. At first glance it would appear that the N1 peak is more negative in the second condition: this results from the fact that the N1 and P2 peaks are superimposed on a much slower negativity that begins virtually

at the onset of the word (Luck, 2005). Figure 29–6 shows grand averaged waveforms of 7 young adults with normal hearing. Again the gray waveform shows deeper negativity over the latency range from 300 to 1200 ms.

Figure 29–7 compares scalp topographies of grand-averaged activity over the 500 to 600 ms latency range in the two conditions in the normal-hearing group. In the *repeat-word* condition negativity is maximal in the left centroparietal region, but extends forward on the left side and laterally into the right centroparietal region. This result is consistent with the observation of Bentin (1987) that N400 scalp topography is maximal in frontal and central electrodes when the paradigm involves words

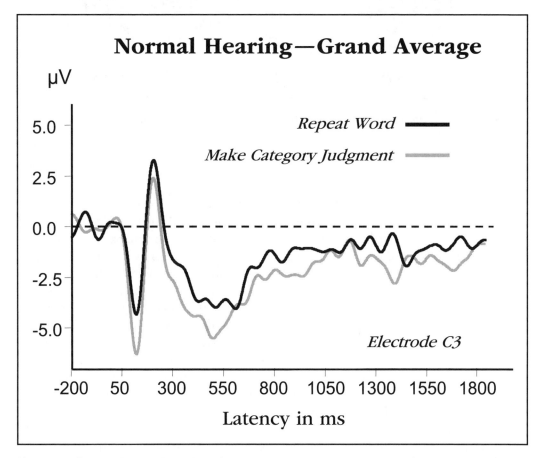

Figure 29–6. Grand averaged waveforms for the two experimental conditions in 7 adults with normal hearing.

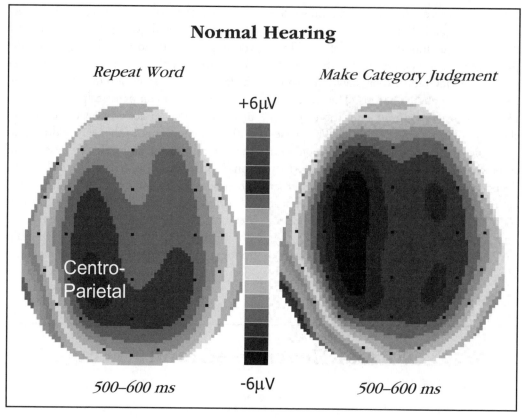

Figure 29–7. *Scalp topographies in the 500- to 600-ms latency range associated with the waveforms of Figure 29–6.*

or word pairs. In the case of the *category-decision* condition, deeper negativity extends over a greater region of the left hemisphere, and shows greater activity in the right hemisphere as well.

ADULTS WITH HEARING LOSS

Figure 29–8 shows the air-conduction audiograms and the waveforms for the two conditions at electrode C3 in a 41-year-old man with mild noise-induced sensorineural loss. The difference in processing negativity between the two conditions is striking. In the *repeat-word* condition the negativity is less than 2.5 microvolts and returns to baseline by 800 ms. In the *category-decision* condition, however, the negativity peaks at more than 8 microvolts and does not return to baseline until 1300 ms. Figure 29–9 shows grand-averaged waveforms at electrode C3 for the 7 adults with sensorineural losses. Again, the processing negativity is considerably deeper in the *make-category-judgment* condition. Figure 29–10 compares scalp topographies in the two conditions for the hearing loss group. Again, the difference between the two conditions, plotted on the same voltage scale, is substantial.

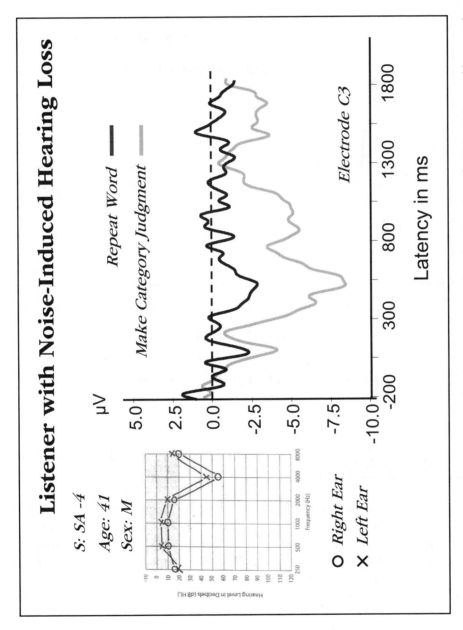

Figure 29–8. Audiograms and waveforms for the two experimental conditions at electrode C3 in a 41-year-old man with noise-induced sensorineural hearing loss.

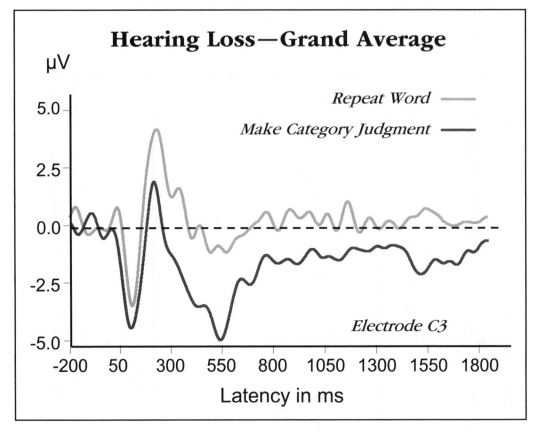

Figure 29–9. *Grand averaged waveforms for the two experimental conditions in 7 adults with sensorineural hearing loss.*

DISCUSSION

These results suggest two conclusions. First, the auditory event-related potential reflects the greater cognitive processing required to make a semantic category judgment about a word than to simply repeat the word back. The difference is apparent in the processing negativity component of the waveform, peaking in the 500- to 600-ms range and extending over 800 to 1000 ms, and in the surface topography, especially over the temporal and parietal regions of the left hemisphere. This result clearly implies that by analyzing the brain's response to a word presented in the context of a task more complex than simply repeating back, we have the opportunity to learn not only whether the word was heard correctly but to assess the cognitive effort involved in processing the word correctly, and the extra cognitive effort demanded by hearing impairment The paradigm can be extended to other speech dimensions, for example, phonemic features (Diaz & Swaab, 2006), syntactic anomalies (Friederici, Pfeifer, & Hahne, 1993), and so forth. It is, moreover, possible to obtain useful information at the level of the individual participant. In short, auditory event-related potentials can widely broaden the information derived from even the simplest speech audiometric procedure.

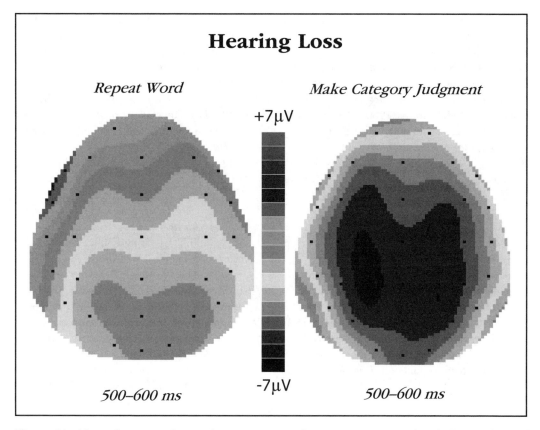

Figure 29–10. *Scalp topographies in the 500 to 600-ms latency range associated with the waveforms of Figure 29–9.*

REFERENCES

Bentin, S. (1987). Event-related potentials, semantic processes, and expectancy factors in word recognition. *Brain and Language, 31*, 308–327.

Connoly, J., & Phillips, N. (1994). Event-related potential components reflect phonological and semantic processing of the terminal word of spoken sentences. *Journal of Cognitive Neuroscience, 6*, 256–266.

D'Arcy, R., Connolly, J., & Crocker, S. (2000). Latency shifts in the N2b component track phonological deviations in spoken words. *Clinical Neurophysiology, 111*, 40–44.

D'Arcy, R., Connolly, J., Service, E., Hawco, C. S., & Houlihan, M. E. (2004). Separating phonological and semantic processing in auditory sentence processing: A high-resolution event-related brain potential study. *Human Brain Mapping, 22*, 40–51.

Diaz, M., & Swaab, T. (2006). Electrophysiological differentiation of phonological and semantic integration in word and sentence contexts. *Brain Research, 1146*, 85–100.

Donchin, E., & Coles, M. (1988). Is the P300 component a manifestation of context updating? *Behavioral and Brain Sciences, 11*, 357–374.

Friederici, A., Pfeifer, E., & Hahne, A. (1993). Event-related brain potentials during natural speech processing: Effects of semantic, morphological and syntactic violations. *Cognitive Brain Research, 1*, 183–192.

Halgren, E., Dhond, R., Christensen, N., Van Petten, C., Marinkovik, K., Lweine, J., & Dale, A. (2002). N400-like magnetoencephalography responses modulated by semantic context, word frequency, and lexical class in sentences. *NeuroImage, 17,* 1101–1116.

Kok, A. (1997). Event-related potential (ERP) reflections of mental resources: A review and synthesis. *Biological Psychology, 45,* 19–56.

Kutas, M., & Hillyard, S. (1980). Reading senseless sentences: Brain potentials reflect semantic incongruity. *Science, 207,* 203–205.

Kutas, M., & Iragui, V. (1998). The N400 in a semantic categorization task across 6 decades. *EEG and Clinical Neurophysiology, 108,* 456–471.

Luck, S. (2005). Ten simple rules for designing ERP experiments. In T. Handy (Ed.), *Event related potentials: A methods handbook* (pp. 17–32). Cambridge, MA: MIT Press.

Marslen-Wilson, W., & Tyler, L. (1980). The temporal structure of spoken language understanding. *Cognition, 8,* 1–71.

Näätänen, R. (1990). The role of attention in auditory information processing as revealed by event-related potentials and other brain measures of cognitive function. *Behavior and Brain Science, 13,* 201–288.

Näätänen, R., Sams, M., Alho, K., Paavilainen, P., & Sokolov, E., (1988). Frequency and location specificity of the human vertex N1 wave. *EEG and Clinical Neurophysiology, 69,* 523–531.

Nieuwenhuis, S., Aston-Jones, G., & Cohen, J. (2005). Decision making, the P3, and the locus coeruleus-norepinephrine system. *Psychological Bulletin, 131,* 510–532.

Petten, C. V., Coulson, S., Rubin, S., Plante, E., & Parks, M. (1999). Time course of word identification and semantic integration in spoken language. *Journal of Experimental Psychology: Learning, Memory and Cognition, 25,* 394–417.

Polich, J. (2007). Updating P300: An integrative theory of P3a and P3b. *Clinical Neurophysiology, 118,* 2128–2148.

West, W., O'Rourke, T., & Holcomb, P. (1998) Event-related brain potentials and language comprehension: A cognitive neuroscience approach to the study of intellectual functioning. In S. S. W. McIlvane (Ed.), *Perspectives on fundamental processes in intellectual functioning* (Vol. 1, pp. 131–168). Stamford, CT: Ablex.

ESSAY 30

Evidence-Based Practice in Audiology

Examples from Prevention and Treatment

Jeffrey L. Danhauer and Carole E. Johnson

Dr. Sadanand Singh, from here on affectionately referred to as Singh, was a progressive thinker and innovator who always found the positives in all individuals and pushed them to be the best they could be. Through his own research and publications, and even more so, through his support of authors (both seasoned and neophyte) by publishing their works, he propelled the communication sciences and disorders (CSD) discipline to greater heights. A perusal of the titles of the textbooks published by his companies reveals the impact that Singh has had on this and related health care fields. Most of these works underpin or set the stage for evidence-based practice (EBP) in our field. Singh always had an EBP approach to the professions, promoting science, fostering the development of clinical expertise, and creating an extended international professional and personal global family. His entire career in the academic, research, and publishing sides of the CSD discipline and related fields embodied the quest for ensuring that educators, researchers, clinicians, students, and patients all had the best sources of information available to help them make health care decisions.

His publishing companies were the first in CSD to insist that their text books were peer reviewed and his creation of ContentScan, the first search engine dedicated to evidence for our discipline, still serves as the platform for algorithms used to search the literature and scholars in the field. He saw connections and possibilities across health care professions where others perceived boundaries and obstacles; where some saw colleagues and students, he saw family.

Singh always taught the importance of research teams and the "lineage" within the profession. He was keen to point out the germinal work done by his mentor, John W. Black, and others to his students. Singh was passionate about students knowing their roots, and understanding and respecting their academic "mothers and fathers," and "brothers, sisters, and cousins." He believed that the entire profession is related with only a few degrees of separation and that the quest for knowledge is a continuum of effort initiated by our academic forefathers that will be expanded and further developed by innovations from those that follow in their footsteps.

In that light, we developed the University of California Santa Barbara/Auburn University Intercampus Audiology Research Team composed of undergraduates, Doctor of Audiology students, and colleagues to conduct research and mentor young scholars at the beginnings of their careers. This essay focuses on some of our team's lines of research, particularly involving EBP, that have been inspired by and will honor the legacy of Singh. Singh's influence is so powerful that it touches people all over the world—even those who never met nor now ever will meet the man himself. Indeed, through his publishing and promoting of the words and wisdom of others with books as the vehicle, Sadanand Singh will touch generations of people all over the world. Whether books are in their first, second, or fifth editions, they will be read, and as new scholars write the texts of the future, they will always have to refer to and cite the works that Singh helped create from his soul. Being Singh's academic son and granddaughter, it is indeed our honor to provide this essay for him.

Over the past decade, audiology has gradually moved toward EBP, which involves combining the best scientific evidence, clinical expertise, and patient and family values and preferences for clinical decision making. One particularly effective methodology used in EBP involves conducting systematic reviews (SRs) with meta-analysis on specialized topics. Indeed, SRs assess evidence about targeted interventions from a foundation of clearly formulated questions; systematically use explicit methods to identify, select, critically appraise, and narrow down a vast body of literature to focus in on only the most relevant research pertaining to the topic; and collect, analyze, aggregate, and interpret data from pertinent studies to answer the question. Some SRs use meta-analyses to aggregate the results of several studies to determine the magnitude of treatment effect. Our team has used SRs to promote EBP in audiology for the prevention,

diagnosis, and treatment of hearing disorders, as demonstrated by some examples from some of our work in these areas.

PREVENTION

Our team has used EBP and the SR methodology to evaluate a complementary and alternative medicine, xylitol, as a prophylaxis for acute otitis media (AOM) in children. AOM is prevalent in infants and young children and can lead to hearing loss that can negatively impact their speech, language, social, and academic development, and overall quality of life (QoL). Ear infections cost the United States health care system between $3 to 5 billion annually, and are especially problematic for children in underdeveloped areas having limited access to medical services. Traditional treatments for AOM involve the use of antibacterial medicines and/or surgical placement of tympanostomy tubes, which have been shown to have limited success and high costs to families and health care systems. Xylitol is a natural sugar-alcohol, that has been found to prevent AOM in children, but its use for AOM is relatively unknown to audiologists and physicians in the United States. We recently conducted two SRs on this topic which were published in the *International Journal of Audiology* (Danhauer et al., 2010a, 2011a). A few high-quality, randomized controlled trials (RCTs) provided evidence that xylitol used mainly in chewing gum chewed five times a day could serve as a prophylaxis for AOM in children. The results of that study suggested that audiologists could use this over-the-counter substance with families to help prevent ear infections in their children. Additionally, we conducted two surveys of pediatricians in the United States (Danhauer et al., 2010b; Stockwell et al., 2010), and another on all kindergarten through third grade (K–3) teachers in a school district in California (Danhauer et al, 2011b). These surveys revealed that physicians were generally not knowledgeable about and did not use xylitol with their patients and those K–3 teachers and their schools would not permit children to chew gum on campus. These limitations and the fact that children less than five years of age (i.e., those most susceptible to AOM) cannot usually chew gum made it unlikely that xylitol in chewing gum could be used successfully in AOM prevention programs. Thus, we and others have begun the search for alternative vehicles for administering xylitol to infants and young children.

The second SR we conducted on the use of xylitol as a prophylaxis for AOM involved an interdisciplinary translational mother-child transmission model borrowing evidence from the field of dentistry which has demonstrated that children of mothers who chewed gum containing xylitol had significantly fewer bacterial colonizations and dental caries than controls whose mothers did not chew the gum. Because our SRs of the hearing and dental literature revealed that xylitol in chewing gum could be a prophylaxis for AOM and dental caries in children, and as the mother-child transmission model was effective at preventing transmission of bacteria that lead to dental caries, even when the children themselves had no direct contact with the substance, we proposed that this model might also work for preventing AOM. This SR used a similar protocol to the previous one (Danhauer et al., 2010a) and found that the mother-child transmission model may also be appropriate for preventing AOM in children too young to chew gum (Danhauer et al., 2011a). In addition to rigorous SRs, other levels of evidence are also appropriate for determining whether a particular treatment or form of prevention might be warranted for a disorder. We invited critiques of the model from experts in the field. As a result, we questioned the model based on input from Dr. Alonzo Jones, a fam-

ily practitioner and pioneer in the use of xylitol in children. He suggested that while the mother-child transmission model might work, it still only places the xylitol near the source of the problem (i.e., the oral-pharyngeal cavity) which was fine for preventing dental caries, whereas a xylitol nasal spray that he developed could actually put the xylitol closer to the eustachian tube and middle ear structures where bacteria that cause AOM first enter the middle ear space. We are in the process of preparing clinical trials to evaluate its effects on preventing AOM in children. This type of interdisciplinary research involves the team spirit encouraged by Singh, which may allow audiologists to work with families and recommend non-medical preventions for this disorder.

TREATMENT

Singh always focused his energy on the most important issues in CSD affecting patients and their families. Taking his lead, our team has conducted SRs to assess the evidence pertaining to treatments for hearing loss, including traditional hearing aids and bone-anchored hearing aids (BAHAs). Untreated hearing loss often results in social isolation, problems in relationships, loss of self-esteem, and reduction in QoL, among other problems. Unfortunately, most people with hearing loss wait about 10 years after noticing a problem before getting help through hearing aids (Davis et al., 2007) due to possible stigma, cost, and feelings that hearing aids probably would not help, among other reasons (Donahue et al., 2010). Thus, a fundamental question that needed to be answered was, is there evidence that hearing aids enhance the health-related QoL for persons with sensorineural hearing loss? Members of our team collaborated with colleagues on the American Academy of Audiology Task Force on the Quality of Life Benefits of Amplification in Adults (Chisolm et al., 2007) which conducted a SR and concluded that hearing aids do indeed improve users' health-related QoL. From that SR and meta-analysis, which produced effect sizes that were in the medium range, we concluded that: (1) hearing aid use is a noninvasive, low-risk option, and the only viable treatment for sensorineural hearing loss, which can improve individuals' QoL; (2) the SR is a powerful method for assessing QoL benefits from amplification, but conclusions drawn from SRs are only as robust as the evidence that is available in the literature, and SRs must be updated periodically to reflect the timely nature of the evidence; (3) audiology has several disease-specific outcome measures focused on hearing loss and its treatment available, but needs more generic instruments that can be used across health care conditions and that can also show potential benefits of amplification; (4) investigators must exercise care in reducing sources of bias in conducting their research in order to maximize their contributions to EBP; (5) future research should be conducted with methods that will produce higher levels of evidence; and (6) all stakeholders should be encouraged that hearing aids can provide considerable QoL benefits for those with hearing loss. Our work in this area also involved conducting a SR on the nonacoustic benefits of bone-anchored hearing aids (Johnson et al., 2006), and completing an invited chapter on hearing aids and QoL in the *Handbook of Disease Burden and Quality of Life Measures* (Johnson & Danhauer, 2010).

Not all SRs produce a level of evidence from high-level studies that would suggest that clinicians should make recommendations about a particular treatment. That does not mean, however, that EBP has no role or that the treatment has no merit. It may simply mean that there were not enough studies reported in the literature to allow investigators

to make recommendations with confidence. It is important to remember that EBP is a three-legged stool and that scientific evidence is to be integrated with clinical expertise and patient preferences. For example, in a SR (Danhauer et al., 2010c) that we conducted on BAHAs and patients having congenital unilateral aural atresia (CUAA), few studies were found in the literature that provided separate results for subjects having congenital unilateral hearing losses from those with bilateral acquired losses who also used BAHAs. Furthermore, our inclusion criteria may have been too restrictive in that we were looking for studies that only employed outcome measures that would provide information about how BAHAs affected audibility, localization, and speech recognition in noise for users having CUAA. Most of the studies that were retrieved combined the results for different types of losses which made it almost impossible to answer our research question with empirical confidence. Even when looking at individual data, it was difficult to determine what patient characteristics would predict positive outcomes with BAHAs for patients with CUAA. Because these patients were born with CUAA, and surgery to correct the condition could not be done until they reached a certain age, it is likely that they had already developed strategies for directional hearing with their normal ears, which kept investigators from measuring consistent effects of the BAHAs. Although BAHAs are successful for other types of hearing losses, in this case, clinical expertise is critical in guiding patients with CUAA in determining if BAHAs are a viable treatment option. Thus, SRs are not just about finding scientific evidence, but can also be helpful in uncovering situations where clinical expertise and experience are needed to assist patients in making decisions, particularly those involving surgery, and where clinicians should exercise caution in making recommendations.

OUTCOME MEASURES

Being able to make recommendations confidently rests on outcome measures, and researchers must use standard metrics and publish their findings so that others can assess the merits of treatments. Earlier, Singh invited us to write a text book (Johnson & Danhauer, 2002) on outcomes measurement in audiology that was published by his company, Singular. In it, we described numerous measures clinicians can use to help them determine if the preventions, diagnoses, and treatments for hearing loss that they provide have positive impacts on patients' lives. Use of these measures is a vital part of EBP. Clinicians have the luxury of using standardized, normed measures from the literature or making assessments on their own patients. The point is for clinicians to do *something* to help them determine if the services they provide to their patients reduce their activity limitations and participation restrictions and enhance their health related QoL.

Other lines of research that our team is currently pursuing involve outcome measures for: (1) finding evidence for the benefit that persons with mild and moderate degrees of hearing impairment may expect from hearing aids, (2) assessing young adults' satisfaction with hearing aids and why they do and do not elect to use amplification, and (3) evaluating junior and senior high school and college students' knowledge about hearing health and use of personal listening devices such as iPods. Results of these investigations will help us counsel participants in the studies and others to seek appropriate preventions and treatments for hearing problems in order to avoid the negative consequences of hearing loss.

We hope that Singh would be proud of the contributions that his "academic offspring" are making to our profession. Each of us that he touched either directly or indirectly is so much better for having known him. The evidence is in and we can state with utmost confidence that the outcome of Singh's existence was to improve the QoL for everyone.

REFERENCES

Chisolm, T. H., Johnson, C. E., Danhauer, J. L., Portz, L. P., Abrams, H. B., Lesner, S., . . . Newman, C. W. (2007). A systematic review of health-related quality of life and hearing aids: Final report of the American Academy of Audiology Task Force on the Health-Related Quality of Life Benefits of Amplification in Adults. *Journal of the American Academy of Audiology*, *18*, 151–183.

Danhauer, J. L., Johnson, C. E., & Caudle, A. T. (2011b). Survey of K–3 teachers' knowledge of ear infections and willingness to participate in prevention programs. *Language Speech and Hearing Services in Schools*, *42*, 207–222.

Danhauer, J. L., Johnson, C. E., Corbin, N. E., & Bruccheri, K. G. (2010a). Xylitol as a prophylaxis for acute otitis media: Systematic review. *International Journal of Audiology*, *49*, 754–761.

Danhauer, J. L., Johnson, C. E., Rotan, S. N., Snelson, T. A., & Stockwell, J. S. (2010b). National survey of pediatricians' opinions about and practices for acute otitis media and xylitol use. *Journal of the American Academy of Audiology*, *21*, 329–346.

Danhauer, J. L., Johnson, C. E., & Mixon, M. (2010c). Does the evidence support use of the Baha implant system (Baha) in patients with congenital unilateral aural atresia? *Journal of the American Academy of Audiology*, *21*, 274–286.

Danhauer, J. L., Kelly, A., & Johnson, C. E. (2011a). Is mother-child transmission a possible vehicle for xylitol prophylaxis in acute otitis media? *International Journal of Audiology*, *50*, 1–12.

Davis, A., Smith, P., Ferguson, M., Stephens, D., & Gianopoulos, I. (2007). Acceptability, benefit and costs of early screening for hearing disability: A study of potential screening tests and models. *Health Technology Assessment, 11(42)*, 1–294.

Donahue, A. M., Dubno, J. R., & Beck, L. (2010). Guest editorial: Accessible and affordable hearing health care for adults with mild to moderate loss hearing loss. *Ear and Hearing, 31*, 2–6.

Johnson, C. E., & Danhauer, J. L. (2002). *Handbook of outcomes measurement in audiology.* Clifton Park, NY: Thomson Delmar Learning Singular.

Johnson, C. E., & Danhauer, J. L. (2010). Hearing aids and quality of life. In V. R. Preedy &

R. R. Watson (Eds.), *Handbook of disease burdens and quality of life measures* (Part 3, 3.9; pp. 3871–3885). Heidelberg, Germany: Springer.

Johnson, C. E., Danhauer, J. L., Reith, A. C., & Latiolais, L. N. (2006). A systematic review of the nonacoustic benefits of bone-anchored hearing aids. *Ear and Hearing, 27*, 703–713.

Stockwell, J. S., Johnson, C. E., & Danhauer, J. L. (2010). Additional data from physicians having previous experience with xylitol as a prophylaxis for acute otitis media in children. *Journal of the American Academy of Audiology, 21*, 558.

PART VI

Speech-Language Science and Speech-Language Pathology

ESSAY 31

Observations on Speech and Swallowing

William Culbertson and Dennis C. Tanner

Dr. Sadanand Singh was our favorite book publisher, and there is little doubt that he was a favorite of many other authors and readers in the field. From College-Hill Press, through Singular Publishing, and finally as leader of today's Plural Publishing he inspired us with his savvy business acumen, expressed graciously with a kind approach to all. Like us, Dr. Singh was a devotee of speech and its variations. With articulatory phonetics as a launching pad, we dedicate this essay to him as we explore the apparent relationships between speech and swallowing.

SPEECH AND SWALLOWING

The high incidence of patients having both dysarthria and dysphagia is hardly surprising. Both speaking and swallowing involve finely coordinated actions of the bulbar and respiratory musculature to perform their distinct systemic functions. Notwithstanding differences in movement patterns and behavioral origins, speech and deglutition share certain neurologic pathways and anatomical structures. It is an interesting exercise in anatomic and physiologic analysis to contemplate similarities and differences in the two functions.

PHYSIOLOGIC DIFFERENCES BETWEEN SWALLOWING AND SPEECH ARTICULATION

In this essay, we regard deglutition as that stage of swallowing during which a bolus of solid or liquid material is moved from the oral cavity to the esophagus (Culberson & Tanner, 2011), and speech as a modality of language expression in which the symbols are variations in sounds emanating from the mouth and nose. The most obvious physiologic difference between swallowing and speech is obviously systemic. The two behaviors are functions of different systems with differing ends to their movements. Speech employs the oral, nasal, and pharyngeal cavities as respiratory structures while swallowing employs them as alimentary structures, the two systems diverging at the laryngeal additus.

Neuromuscular differences between speech and swallowing involve their behavioral origins and variations in movement patterns. Speaking and swallowing movement patterns are distinct in their overall directionality and rhythm. Swallowing patterns are stereotyped and sequential, varying relatively little in action (Kennedy & Kent, 1985), and always ingressive. Speech movements are usually egressive, with air flowing out of the body even as movement patterns in syllabic articulation are constantly varying anteriorly and posteriorly in their direction. Speech movement patterns vary with the language of the speaker, but include movements that vary widely in range, direction, and velocity. Speaking and the initial stages of deglutition can be concurrent, and momentary interruptions of speech are common while a speaker clears saliva from the mouth by deglutition.

Behavioral origins of speech and deglutition arise from their diverse physiological foundations. The behavioral origins of most speech are those of widely diverse central affective motivations and neurolinguistic substrates with sensorimotor functions. Whatever the origin, once speech is underway, the speaker consciously maintains speech neuromuscular subsystem coordination and modifies ongoing patterns and intensities of contraction through afferent system feedback (Darley et al., 1975; Mysak, 1976). It is apparent, then, that most speech movements originate voluntarily and continue at least partly through conscious self-monitoring. Swallowing origins are less well understood (Logemann, 1995), but appear to involve an interplay of conscious and unconscious motivations and movements. Voluntary intake and preparation of the food bolus begin a chain of swallowing events. Once underway, deglutition becomes successively more reflexive and ultimately autonomic (Culbertson & Tanner, 2011; Tanner & Culbertson, 1999; Zemlin, 1988).

PHYSIOLOGIC SIMILARITIES BETWEEN SWALLOWING AND SPEECH ARTICULATION

It is hard to overlook the fact that, differences aside, both speech and deglutition involve coordinated contraction of comparable muscle groups supporting the same anatomical structures in the upper airway or rostral digestive tract. For both purposes, oropharyngeal muscle groups seal the upper respiratory and alimentary tracts at several sites and change its dimensions (Edwards, 1992; Logemann, 1995). For example, anterior-to-posterior lingual movements can be observed during articulation of syllables beginning with palatal approximant (sometimes referred to as palato-alveolar glides) to back vowel targets during speech, such as in the articulation of the syllable /jʌŋ/ ("young"), and rearward tongue movements can also push the bolus toward the oropharynx during deglutition. Intrinsic laryngeal muscle groups that adduct the vocal folds during vowel, approximant, glottal, and voiced obstruent consonant articulation also function sequentially to secure airway closure as a bolus passes through the pharynx. The velopharyngeal valving action that couples or uncouples the nasal cavity to the vocal tract and changes vocal tract resonance also prevents penetration of food and liquid into the nasopharynx and allows reduction of relative intraoral air pressure for sucking. Further, speakers may contract extrinsic laryngeal muscles to elevate their larynges to varying extents during pitch increases (Zemlin, 1998). These extrinsic laryngeal muscle groups also engage during transfer of a bolus from the oral cavity to the oropharynx.

NEUROPATHOLOGY OF SPEECH AND DEGLUTITION

Speech and deglutition disorders may occur simultaneously in several neurological diseases, since muscle groups associated with speech also function in the oral and pharyngeal stages of deglutition (Kennedy, Pring, & Fawcus, 1993). It is logical to expect dysarthria and neurogenic dysphagia to occur concurrently. Duffy (1995) found dysarthria to be the most frequently presented acquired neurogenic communication disorder in over three thousand patients. Miller and Langmore (1994) identified neurological disorders as the cause of most dysphagia. Almost all of Darley, Aronson, and Brown's (1975) subjects presented dysphagia as well as dysarthria, no matter what their neuropathologic classifications. Logemann (1983) observed diminished lateral and vertical lingual range of motion, reduced buccal tension, and limited rotary mandibular movement in oral stage neurogenic dysphagia. Dobie (1978) noted reduced, uncoordinated lingual movements and decreased oral sensation that affected bolus formation in the oral preparatory phase. Among a group of individuals with neurogenic dysphagia, Miller (1982) observed reduced lingual elevation, lingual range of motion, disorganized anterior to posterior lingual patterns, and limited mandibular movement in mastication during the oral phase of the swallow.

Deglutition problems in the oral stage may include difficulty with mastication, with managing and initiating bolus transfer, and with poor retention of intraoral material. These deglutition functions depend on lingual and mandibular mobility, and so does speech articulation. The vertical lingual movement required to maneuver a bolus along the palatal (maxillary) vault is also essential to palatal, postalveolar or velar consonant production as well as for close vowel articulation. Mandibular elevation is necessary for mastication and also for linguapalatal and labial juxtaposition. Such juxtaposition is required as well for close vowel formation and for palatal and labial consonant production.

Culbertson, Lambrelli, and Tanner (2010) reported a study in which they observed patterns of articulation in individuals having neurologic impairment with and without concurrent dysphagia (Table 31–1). Their findings supported the contention that some movements important in deglutition are also important in speech articulation whereas other

movements are not. In particular, there was a high incidence among the group of subjects having dysphagia of nonstandard articulation involving lingual blade elevation to palatal and prepalatal (or postalveolar) positions. This was most apparent in fricative articulation, suggested a pattern involving degradation of fine coordination in the anterior tongue musculature of these subjects. In the group of subjects having no dysphagia, articulatory problems were rare. Nishio and Niimi (2004) found a high correlation between swallowing function and all levels of speech intelligibility.

Static consonant postures during speech occur about as rarely as any single static posture occurs in deglutition. Instead, closed juncture or "Consonant-Vowel-Consonant-Vowel . . . " flow of syllables in running speech is a series of gliding movements from postures of relative vocal tract constriction associated with consonants to the more open postures associated with vowels and then back to the closed postures. Such movements require the interplay of timing and intensity with intrinsic and extrinsic oral, pharyngeal, and labial muscle groups combined with various degrees of mandibular elevation. Fricative, affricate, and plosive articulation also require increased source energy, narrow or complete vocal tract constriction and controlled breath support. Articulation of these obstruent consonants requires mandibular, lingual and labial mobility coordinated with velopharyngeal and respiratory muscle function. Depending on the phoneme, there are several configurations of intrinsic and extrinsic lingual muscle groups that accomplish these particular articulatory postures (Edwards, 1992).

Just as the sites of production for blade-alveolar and blade-prepalatal consonants involve elevation of the mandible, tongue blade or body to contact the palate or upper teeth, similar juxtapositions are seen in the transfer of material from oral cavity to pharynx in deglutition. Hamilton and McMinn (1977) and Logemann (1995) reported that the lateral

Table 31–1. Summary of Speech Articulation Patterns in Neurologically Impaired Nursing Home Residents With and Without Dysphagia

Place of Articulation	Dysphagia Group Number (%)	Nondysphagia Group Number (%)
Bilabial	18 (8%)	-0-
Labio-Dental	24 (11%)	2 (22%)
Tip-Dental	25 (12%)	2 (22%)
Tip-Alveolar	26 (12%)	3 (34%)
Blade-Alveolar	37 (17%)	-0-
Blade-Prepalatal	48 (22%)	-0-
Front-Palatal	-0-	-0-
Central-Palatal	17 (8%)	-0-
Back-Velar	20 (9%)	2 (22%)
Total	**215**	**10**
Manner of Articulation	*Number (%)*	*Number (%)*
Stop	40 (19%)	1 (10%)
Fricative	94 (45%)	5 (50%)
Affricate	32 (15%)	-0-
Glide	17 (8%)	-0-
Lateral	8 (4%)	1 (10%)
Nasal	18 (9%)	3 (30%)
Total	**209**	**10**

Source: Culbertson, Lambrelli, and Tanner (2010).

and anterior lingual dorsum is normally sealed against the palate in the initial stages of bolus transfer. If the Culbertson, Lambrelli, and Tanner (2010) results are typical, clinicians might often expect to encounter distortions of anterior fricatives in patients with dyaphagia. Furthermore, if the low incidence of articulatory problems among the nondysphagic group is typical, clinicians might also expect that, as fricative production improved, initial stages of bolus transfer might also improve. However,

the effectiveness of restorative treatment for dysphagia by speech-language pathologists has yet to be firmly established (Speyer, Baijens, Heijnen, & Zwijnenberg, 2010).

The low incidence of approximant involvement in Culbertson, Lambrelli, and Tanner (2010) suggested that the lingual excursions required for /r/ and /j/ production in running speech may be dissimilar to those required for bolus transfer. The effects of phonetic context may be such that the direction and extent of such "gliding" movements were not great enough to have an effect on speech articulation. These results bolster the position that bolus transfer may require more strength and range of movement than palatal approximant gliding.

The co-occurrence of speech articulation patterns and deglutition disorders by no means implies a relationship between phonological language functions and solid food or liquid intake. Although it is reasonable to assume that most animals swallow, the range of their phonological abilities is not presumed. It was neither within the purpose of this article to establish a relationship between phonology and motor speech disorders. We are simply observing that speech and deglutition disorders are often observed in the same patients, and describing such patterns. Future research might explore the use of concomitant articulation and dysphagia therapies in patients with dysarthria and neurogenic dysphagia.

REFERENCES

Buchholz, D. (1994). Dysphagia associated with neurological disorders. *Acta Oto-Rhino-Laryngologica Belgica, 48*, 143–155.

Culbertson, W. R., & Tanner, D. C. (2011). *The anatomy and physiology of speech and swallowing.* Dubuque, IA: Kendall Hunt.

Culbertson, W., Lambrelli, C., & Tanner, D. (2010). Patterns of Speech Articulation in Subjects with Neurogenic Dysphagia and Dysarthria. *Rehabilitation, 1*(10). WMC001042

Darley, F., Aronson, A., & Brown, J. (1975). *Motor speech disorders.* Philadelphia, PA: W. B. Saunders.

Dobie, R. (1978). Rehabilitation of swallowing disorders. *American Family Physician, 17*, 84–95.

Duffy, J. (1995). *Motor speech disorders.* St. Louis, MO: Mosby-Year Book.

Edwards, H. (1992). *Applied phonetics: The sounds of American English.* San Diego, CA: Singular.

Hamilton, W., & McMinn, R. (1977). Digestive system. In W. Hamilton (Ed.), (1976). *Textbook of human anatomy* (2nd ed., pp. 357–358). St. Louis, MO: C. V. Mosby.

International Phonetic Association. (1996). *Reproduction of the international phonetic alphabet* (Revised to 1993, Updated, 1996). Retrieved from http://www.arts.gla.ac.uk/IPA

Jinks, A. (1983). *Interactive effects of concurrent dysarthria and dysphagia treatment.* Poster presentation. Dysphagia Conference, Braintree, MA.

Kennedy, G., Pring, T., & Fawcus, R. (1993). No place for motor speech acts in assessment of dysphagia? Intelligibility and swallowing difficulties in stroke and Parkinson's disease patients. *European Journal of Disorders of Communication, 28*, 213–226.

Kennedy, J., & Kent, R. (1985). Anatomy and physiology of deglutition and related functions. *Seminars in Speech and Language, 6*, 257–272.

Kilman, W., & Goyal, R. (1976). Disorders of pharyngeal and upper esophageal sphincter motor function. *Archives of Internal Medicine, 126*, 592–601.

Logemann, J. (1983). *Evaluation and treatment of swallowing disorders.* San Diego, CA: College-Hill Press.

Logemann, J. (1995). Dysphagia: Evaluation and treatment. *Folia Phoniatrica Logopedia, 47*, 140–164.

Miller, A. J. (1982). Deglutition. *Physiological Reviews, 62*, 129–184.

Miller, R., & Langmore, S. (1994). Treatment efficacy for adults with oropharyngeal dysphagia. *Archives of Physical Medicine and Rehabilitation, 75*, 1256–1262.

Mysak, E. (1976). *Pathologies of speech systems.* Baltimore, MD: Williams & Wilkins.

Nishio, M., & Niimi, S. (2004). Relationship between speech and swallowing disorders in patients with neuromuscular disease. *Folia Phoniatrica Et Logopaedica, 56*(5), 291–304. Retrieved from http://libproxy.nau.edu/docview/85619240?accountid=12706

Speyer, R. R., Baijens, L. L., Heijnen, M. M., & Zwijnenberg, I. I. (2010). Effects of therapy in oropharyngeal dysphagia by speech and language therapists: A systematic review. *Dys-*

phagia, *25*(1), 40–65. Retrieved from http://libproxy.nau.edu/docview/733821992?accountid=12706

Zemlin, W. (1998). *Speech and hearing science: Anatomy and physiology* (3rd. ed.). Englewood Cliffs, NJ: Prentice-Hall.

ESSAY 32

✒ Oral Motor Exercises ✒

The Debate

Mary Pannbacker and Norman J. Lass

We have known Sadanand Singh as a very professional, very knowledgeable, and very dedicated academic who was highly respected by the academic community. He served as a true role model to be emulated. In addition, he was a very successful entrepreneur in the publishing industry where he administered the operations of different publishing companies that he initiated. His productivity, creativity, and initiative will influence speech-language pathology, audiology, and speech, language, and hearing sciences as well as current and future professionals in those disciplines for many years to come.

Oral motor exercises (OME) focus on the use of non-speech activities for the treatment of communication disorders. They are popular but controversial for the treatment of children and adults with speech disorders related to dysarthria, apraxia, cleft palate, and functional articulation problems (McCauley, Strand, Lof, Schooling, & Frymark, 2009; Ruscello, 2010a, 2010b). The literature on OME and its effect on nonspeech and speech activities is variable and contradictory.

One extreme point of view enthusiastically supports OME for a wide variety of speech disorders, whereas at the other extreme is the total rejection of the use of OME for the treatment of speech disorders. The former is often characterized by acceptance based on belief whereas the latter rejects OME categorically, frequently because of a lack of credible evidence based on evidence-based principles. Between these two extreme views are those that use a combination of OME and speech production activities for the treatment of speech disorders. The purpose of this essay is to answer two questions:

1. What are the different opinions about OME?
2. What are the ethical issues related to OME?

DIFFERENCES OF OPINION ABOUT OME

From a review of the literature, it appears that support for OME is primarily based on opinion (Bahr, 2008; Beckman, 2003; Beckman et al., 2005; Boshart, 1998; Marshalla, 2008; Rosenfeld-Johnson, 2001, 2005), whereas considerable experimental research does not support the use of OME (Abrahamsen & Flack, 2002; Bush, Steger, Mann-Kahn, & Insalaco, 2004; Christensen & Hanson, 1981; Colone & Forest, 2000; Guisti-Braislin & Cascella, 2005; Hayes, Savinelli, Roberts, & Caldito, 2007; Lof, 2009; Occhino & McCann, 2001; Roehrig, Suiter, & Pierce, 2004). Table 32–1 summarizes the major factors for different views about OME, which serve to differentiate supporters and nonsupporters.

Generally, clinicians and researchers have different views about OME (Muttdiah, Georges, & Brackenbury, 2011). The former usually support OME but the latter usually do not. Clinicians typically use clinical experience and opinions of colleagues more frequently

Table 32–1. Summary of Factors and Views About Oral Motor Exercises

Factor	For OME	Against OME	
Continuing education	Numerous	Lack of evidence	Watson and Lof (2009)
Certification	Required	Not required	Beckman and associates (2005)
			Brown (1993)
			Lass and Pannbacker (2008)
			Watson and Lof (2009)
Websites	Numerous	Commercial	Beckman and associates (2005)
			Boshart (1998)
			Rosenfeld-Johnson (2005)
Product promotion	Yes	No	Lass and Pannbacker (2008)
Data	Opinion	Experimental study	Lass and Panbacker (2008)
Level of Evidence	Low	Moderate	McCauley et al. (2009)
Relationship to scientific methodology	Disconnected	Connected	Lof and Watson (2008)
Outcome	Vague	Specific	Finn, Bothe, and Bramlett (2005)
			Marshalla (2008)
			Powell (2008)
			Ruscello (2010a)
Knowledge	Confirmatory	Contradictory	Ruscello (2010a, 2010b)
Methodology	Unspecified	Specified	McCauley et al. (2009)
Professional activity	Clinician	Researcher	Mackenzie, Muir, and Allen (2010)
			Muttdiah, Georges, and Brackenbury (2011)
Cost-benefit	Low-high	High-low	Lass and Pannbacker (2008)

than clinical practice guidelines or published research studies (Zipoli & Kennedy, 2005).

Clinical practice guidelines about OME are available and they are based on traditional-narrative, systematic, or evidence-based reviews (Hargrove, Griffer, & Luna, 2008). Two of these reviews were published in peer-reviewed journals (Lass & Pannbacker, 2008; McCauley et al., 2009). Lof (2009), in a traditional-narrative review, stated that OME "have not been shown to be effective and their use must be considered experimental" (p. 6). McCauley and associates' (2009) systematic review indicated "insufficient evidence exists to support or refute the use of OMEs to produce effects on speech" (p. 343). In an evidence-based review, Lass and Pannbacker (2008) reported that most support for OME was based on opinion and not on experimental studies.

Opinions and studies supporting OME frequently: (1) do not consider contradictory information; (2) provide a limited review of relevant literature; and (3) ignore new/evolving changes in our knowledge base from current literature. Speech-language pathologists and other professionals should be aware of the validity, reliability, and limitations of

OME reports, because these issues warrant consideration in clinical decision-making and treatment. Furthermore, failure to consider contradictory information and new evidence limits credibility and consequently negatively impacts client care (Finn, Bothe, & Bramlett, 2005; Lum, 2007). These issues must be considered if clinical decision making is to be credible. At best, OME should be considered experimental and should require informed consent (Table 32–2).

ETHICAL ISSUES RELATED TO OME

Speech-language pathologists have an ethical responsibility to protect the welfare of the client, to be competent, to provide accurate information, to employ credible evidence-based information, and to avoid conflicts of interest (ASHA, 2010). There are ethical issues related to using and recommending OME that are embedded in the questions presented in Table 32–3. Speech-language pathologists should seek to resolve these issues.

Table 32–2. Steps in Finding the Evidence for OME

Step	*Outcome*
1. Ask a clear, focused question.	Is OME an effective treatment?
2. Find the available evidence.	MEDLINE, CINAHL, and other databases
3. Critically appraise the evidence.	Identify levels of evidence
4. Integrate the evidence.	Conflicting and nonsupportive
5. Apply the evidence to clinical decisions.	Insufficient evidence exists to support OME
	Exclude from mainstream treatment
	Experimental treatment: informed consent
	Inform client, family, and other professionals

Table 32–3. Ethical Issues Related to OME

- Should speech-language pathologists use OME as a standard method of treatment?
- Should professional organizations be accountable for providing guidelines for experimental treatments such as OME?
- Should professional organizations be accountable for promoting products and advertisement in print and at conventions?
- Should professional organizations have evidence-based criteria for assigning continuing education credits?
- Should professional organizations develop guidelines or a position statement about OME?
- Do speech-language pathologists have a duty to reveal to consumers and other professionals about the experimental status of OME?
- Should university training programs be accountable for providing information about the pros and cons of OME?
- Do university training programs have an obligation to dispel the myths and misconceptions about OME?
- Should clients, families, and other professionals be provided with information about the risks and benefits of OME?
- Should professionals and students question the use of OME?

CONCLUSIONS AND IMPLICATIONS

Opinions about OME vary widely, from enthusiastic acceptance to complete rejection. The former tend to be based on belief and the latter are more likely to be evidence-based. Nevertheless, decisions about using and recommending OME should be based on the best experimental evidence, and not on the basis of opinion. Speech-language pathologists should be aware of the validity and reliability of reports about OME for the treatment of speech disorders. In addition, speech-language pathologists have an ethical responsibility to protect the welfare of the client by providing evidence-based information and treatments, and to avoid any potential conflicts of interest. These issues must be considered if clinical decisions are to be credible; if not, the welfare of the client will be jeopardized. OME should be considered an experimental approach rather than a standard treatment, and therefore should require informed consent. There is also a need for speech-language pathologists and related professional organizations to develop and implement guidelines for using and recommending OME.

REFERENCES

Abrahamsen, E. P., & Flack, L. (2002, November). *Do sensory and motor techniques improve accurate phoneme production?* Paper presented at the annual meeting of the American Speech-Language-Hearing Association, Atlanta, GA.

American Speech-Language-Hearing Association. (2010). *Code of ethics*. Rockville, MD: Author.

Bahr, D. (2008, November). *The oral motor debate: Where do we go from here?* Poster session presented at the annual meeting of the American Speech-Language-Hearing Association, Chicago, IL.

Beckman, D. (2003, September 4). Oral motor therapy: A protocol for speech and hearing. *Advance for Speech-Language Pathologists and Audiologists, 13*, 6–8.

Beckman, D. A., Neal, C. D., Phirsichbaum, J. L., Stratton, L. J., Taylor, V. D., & Ratusnik, D. (2005). Range of motion and strength in oral motor therapy: A retrospective study. *Florida Journal of Communication Disorders, 21*, 2–14.

Boshart, C. A. (1998). *Oral motor therapy*. Temecala, CA: Speech Dynamics.

Brown, J. (1993, June 24). Certifications and competence. *ASHA Leader, 8*, 14–15.

Bush, C., Steger, M., Mann-Kahn, S., & Insalaco, D. (2004, November). *Equivocal results of oral motor treatment on a child's articulation*. Poster session presented at the annual meeting of the American Speech-Language-Hearing Association, Philadelphia, PA.

Christensen, M., & Hanson, M. (1981). An investigation of the effects of oral myofunctional therapy as a precursor to articulation. *Journal of Speech and Hearing Disorders, 40*, 160–167.

Colone, E., & Forest, K. (2000, November). *Comparison of treatment efficacy for persistent speech disorders*. Paper presented at the annual meeting of the American Speech-Language-Hearing Association, Washington, DC.

Finn, P., Bothe, A. K., & Bramlett, R. E. (2005). Science and pseudoscience in communication disorders: Criteria and application. *American Journal of Speech-Language Pathology, 14*(3), 172–186.

Guisti-Braislin, M., & Cascella, P. W. (2005). A preliminary investigation of the efficacy of oral motor exercises for children with mild articulation disorders. *International Journal of Rehabilitation Research, 28*, 263–266.

Hargrove, P., Griffer, M. & Luna, B. (2008). Procedure for using clinical practice guidelines. *Language, Speech, and Hearing Services in Schools, 39*, 389–402.

Hayes, S., Savinelli, S., Roberts, E., & Caldito, G. (2007). Use of nonspeech oral motor treatment for functional articulation disorders. *Early Childhood Services: An Interdisciplinary Journal of Effectiveness, 1*(4), 261–281.

Lass, N. J., & Pannbacker, M. (2008). The application of evidence-based practice to nonspeech oral motor treatment. *Language, Speech, and Hearing Services in Schools, 39*(3), 408–421.

Lof, G. L. (2009, November 20). *Nonspeech oral motor exercises: An update on the controversy*. Paper presented at the annual meeting of the American Speech-Language-Hearing Association, New Orleans, LA.

Lof, G. L., & Watson, M. M. (2008). A nationwide survey of nonspeech oral motor exercise use: Implications for evidence based practice. *Language, Speech, and Hearing Services in Schools, 39*, 392–402.

Lum, C. (2007). *Scientific thinking in speech and language therapy*. Mahwah, NJ: Lawrence Erlbaum Associates.

Mackenzie, C., Muir, M., & Allen, C. (2010). Non-speech oral-motor exercise use in acquired dysarthria: Management regimes and rationales. *International Journal of Language and Communication Disorders, 45*, 617–629.

Marshalla, P. (2008, April). Oral motor treatment vs. non-speech oral motor exercises. *Oral Motor Institute Monograph, 2*.

McCauley, R. J., Strand, E., Lof, G. L., Schooling, S. T., & Frymark, T. (2009). Evidence based systematic review: Effect of nonspeech oral motor exercises on speech. *American Journal of Speech-Language Pathology, 18*, 343–360.

Muttdiah, N., Georges, K., & Brackenbury, T. (2011). Clinical and research perspectives on non-speech oral motor treatment and evidence-based practice. *American Journal of Speech-Language Pathology, 20*(1), 47–59.

Occhino, C., & McCann, J. (2001, November). *Do oral motor exercises affect articulation?* Paper presented at the annual meeting of the American Speech-Language-Hearing Association, New Orleans, LA.

Powell, T. W. (2008). The use of nonspeech oral motor treatments for developmental speech sound production disorders: Intervention and interaction. *Language, Speech, and Hearing Services in Schools, 39,* 273–279.

Roehrig, S., Suiter, D., & Pierce, T. (2004, November). *An examination of the effectiveness of passive oral-motor exercises.* Poster presented at the annual meeting of the American Speech-Language-Hearing Association, Philadelphia, PA.

Rosenfeld-Johnson, S. (2001). *Oral motor exercises for speech clarity.* Tucson, AZ: Innovative Therapists International.

Rosenfeld-Johnson, S. (2005). *Oral motor certification training.* Talk tools. Retrieved July 1, 2005, from http://www.talktools.net/egibin/talktools.storefront

Ruscello, D. M. (2010a). Collective findings neither support nor refute the use of oral motor exercises as a treatment for speech sound disorders. *Evidence-Based Communication Assessment and Intervention, 4,* 37–41.

Ruscello, D. M. (2010b). An abiding issue in the treatment of children with speech sound disorders: A comparison of oral motor and production training for children with speech sound disorders. *Evidence-Based Communication Assessment and Intervention, 4,* 65–72.

Watson, M., & Lof, G. L. (2009). A survey of university professors teaching speech sound disorders: Nonspeech motor exercises and other topics. *Language, Speech, and Hearing Services in Schools, 40,* 256–270.

Zipoli, P., & Kennedy, M. (2005). Evidence-based practice among speech-language pathologists: Attitudes, utilization, and barriers. *American Journal of Speech-Language Pathology, 14,* 208–220.

ESSAY 33

The Impact of Seeing Speech

Sharynne McLeod

Dr. Sadanand Singh was a visionary in the fields of speech-language pathology and audiology. Although his writing and research primarily addressed phonetics, phonology, measurement, and clinical procedures, his vision for dissemination of new ideas enabled authors and researchers to extend the boundaries of these fields. This chapter embraces Dr. Singh's interest in phonetics, instrumentation, and translational research. Dr. Singh coauthored two books with me: Speech Sounds: A Pictorial Guide to Typical and Atypical Speech *(McLeod & Singh, 2009a) and the companion book* Seeing Speech: A Quick Guide to Speech Sounds *(McLeod & Singh, 2009b). These books were a synthesis of our work to enable speech-language pathologists (SLPs) and others to see speech. The books combined Dr. Singh's images of speech created by acoustic (spectrographic) and cinematographic technologies with images created by electropalatography and ultrasound (Figure 33–1). Static and dynamic images were presented and described for 24 consonants, 10 vowels, and 5 diphthongs. The aim of this chapter is to discuss the importance of seeing speech, the technological advances that have enabled SLPs to see speech, and the impact that this can have when working with children and adults who have difficulties producing speech sounds.*

THE IMPORTANCE OF SEEING SPEECH

The production of consonants and vowels to generate speech is both an acoustic and articulatory event, mediated by cognitive decision making around the input and output of speech. In most clinical contexts, SLPs make auditory-impressionistic transcriptions of their clients' speech using the International Phonetic Alphabet (IPA) and the extensions to the International Phonetic Alphabet (extIPA). Transcription of speech is an efficient method to document acoustic perception of speech sounds; however, as Kent (1996, p. 7) indicates, auditory-impressionistic transcription is "susceptible to a variety of sources of error and bias." Sources of error and bias include variability due to listener characteristics, speaker characteristics, context, auditory salience, and measurement procedures. During auditory-impressionistic transcription important information can be missed, particularly when speakers have atypical or unintelligible speech:

[H]ighly unintelligible speech requires an exact description of the client's speech patterns in order to plan appropriate remediation. Some kind of direct or indirect imaging technique is indicated where impressionistic transcription leaves too wide a margin of uncertainty. (Ball, Manuel, & Müller, 2004, p. 161)

In addition to the transcription of speech, SLPs use their knowledge of tongue placement during assessment to categorize speech sound errors, and during intervention to describe changes in tongue placement to facilitate accurate productions. For example, the term "fronting" is often used to describe when children attempt to produce velar consonants (e.g., /k/) but produce alveolar consonants instead (e.g., [t]). For children who are fronting, intervention involves encouragement to put their tongue at the back of their mouth to achieve correct productions of /k/. In a recent survey, McLeod (2011) described 175 SLPs' knowledge of tongue placement for speech sound production. It was found that SLPs demonstrated good knowledge of tongue/palate contact along the midline (i.e., along the sagittal plane), but poor knowledge of contact along lateral margins of the palate (i.e., along the coronal plane). These SLPs were most accurate in their knowledge of tongue/palate contact for consonants with no contact /h, p, f/; then velar consonants /g, k, ŋ/. The remaining consonants were rarely accurate, particularly those most frequently targeted in SLP intervention for children with speech sound disorders. These SLPs did not show awareness of the central groove for the fricatives /s, z, ʃ, ʒ/, lateral bracing (side contact, or "horseshoe" contact) for alveolar consonants /t, d, n, s, z/, or posterior lateral contact for most other consonants. A recommendation from this research was for SLP education to target awareness of tongue placement for consonant production (i.e., for SLPs to *see* speech).

TECHNOLOGIC ADVANCES FOR SEEING SPEECH

Over the past 80 years, there have been numerous technologic advances that have enabled speech-language pathologists (as well as others) to see speech (Ball & Code, 1997; Ball, Gracco, & Stone, 2001). Early efforts to see speech relied on painting chalk and oil on the tongue and palate (e.g., Moses, 1939; Shohara & Hanson, 1941). Using these technologies tongue/palate contact for speech was identified along the coronal plane, indicating that alveolar consonants were produced with contact along the margins of the palate (more recently described as a horseshoe-shape contact with lateral bracing; Gibbon & Wood, 2010). Velar consonants were identified as being produced with contact across the juncture between the hard and soft palate that extended to the lateral margins of the palate. These early findings have been replicated using high-speed electropalatographic (EPG) techniques (Hardcastle & Gibbon, 1997; see McLeod & Singh, 2009a for a review of EPG images produced by speakers varying in age, language, and disorder type).

Next, acoustic technologies, using waveforms and spectrograms, were made available to see speech (e.g., Harris, Hoffman, Liberman, Delattre, & Cooper, 1958; Liberman, Cooper, Shankweiler, & Studdert-Kennedy, 1967). Dr. Singh was among the pioneers in the use of speech science technology for seeing and understanding speech production and perception (Singh & Singh, 2006). Initially, acoustic technologies were only available to those with access to speech science laboratories; however, with current technologic advancement, these analyses techniques now are available free of charge to be downloaded onto personal computers. One of the most widely used programs for this purpose is Praat (Boersma & Weenink, 2009). With accessibility of seeing speech via waveforms and spectrograms, researchers and SLPs can use this technology to check auditory-impressionistic transcriptions, as well as to measure speech. More recently, general imaging technologies such as ultrasound, medical resonance imaging (MRI), and electromyography (EMG) have been employed to see speech. Additional specialized instrumental techniques such as electromagnetic articulography (EMA) also have been developed (for a review, see Ball & Code, 1997).

Each of these instrumental measures enables SLPs to visualize speech by providing real time, objective, and detailed images of speech production (Ball et al., 2001; Ball & Code, 1997). In order to elucidate the hidden articulatory aspect of speech production, instrumental measures are often combined. For example, acoustic analyses and EPG were combined in order to understand differences in segment duration in the speech of people with Parkinson's disease compared with young and aged controls (McAuliffe, Ward, & Murdoch, 2006). Moen and Simonsen (2007) combined EPG and EMA to describe differences between the Norwegian coronal stops /t, d/ as EPG provided coronal images and EMA provided two-dimensional midsagittal images of tongue movement.

Within *Speech Sounds: A Pictorial Guide to Typical and Atypical Speech* (McLeod & Singh, 2009a) four instrumental techniques were used to provide images of speech: spectrography, cinematography, electropalatography, and ultrasound. Each of the images of /t/ in Figure 33–1 were created during the production of the word *tat*. Dr. Singh's descriptions of the spectrographic and cinematographic images have been included below, followed by an explanation of the electropalatograph and ultrasound images. Figure 33–2 provides an image of the Articulate Assistant computer screen to demonstrate the synthesis of information from acoustic, electropalatographic,

and ultrasound technologies. The EPG and ultrasound images in Figure 33–1 were created by taking the exact midpoint of the /t/ in the word-initial position of *tat*.

In the spectrogram (see Figure 33–1A), /t/ is presented in both the initial and final positions of the word *tat*. To use the words of Dr. Singh:

[T]he plosive burst for the voiceless-front stop /t/ in both the initial and final positions is above 2,000 Hz . . . there exists a presence of aspiration noise (over 100 msec), mostly concentrated above 2,000 Hz, for the voiceless stop /t/ in the initial position. At the final position, the aspiration noise is absent and a 200-msec silence is followed by a plosive burst. The speaker has the option of releasing or not releasing the final stop. (McLeod & Singh, 2009, p. 49)

In the cinematographic filmstrip,

the phoneme /t/ is at the initial and final positions of the word *tat* /tæt/. The wide lip opening starts at the first frame of the filmstrip (see Figure 33–1B). In the third frame the tongue is seen touching the alveolar ridge. The following vowel /æ/ shows a front-low tongue position with wide and open lips, accompanied by considerable excursion of the mandible. The vowel is used in the stressed position and hence can be seen sustained from frames 7 through 13. Starting with frame 14, the tip of the tongue begins to rise and continues to do so until complete contact is made with the alveolar ridge in frame 16. The remaining eight frames show the process of complete closure to accomplish the necessary durational cue for the final-voiceless-stop consonant /t/. (McLeod & Singh, 2009a, pp. 47–49)

The Reading EPG image in Figure 33–1C uses black squares to indicate tongue contact against the electrodes, and white squares to indicate no contact. The shape of the EPG

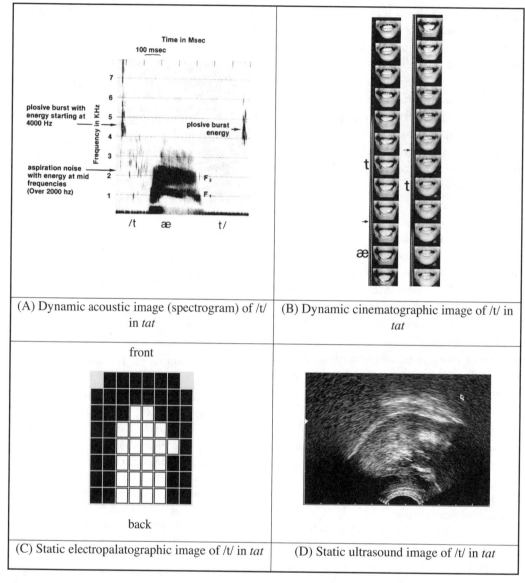

(A) Dynamic acoustic image (spectrogram) of /t/ in *tat*

(B) Dynamic cinematographic image of /t/ in *tat*

(C) Static electropalatographic image of /t/ in *tat*

(D) Static ultrasound image of /t/ in *tat*

Figure 33–1. *Seeing speech by comparing acoustic, cinematographic, electropalatographic, and ultrasound images of /t/ (McLeod & Singh, 2009a, pp. 46, 48).*

image replicates the coronal image of the hard palate, with the boundaries of the image representing the edge of the teeth along the top and sides, and the lower margin indicating the juncture between the hard and soft palate. The static EPG image (Figure 33–1C) is reminiscent of a horseshoe, with the tongue contacting the palate along the teeth. The tongue contacted the palate across the alveolar ridge (first two rows) with lateral bracing along the sides of the teeth (first and last columns).

The static ultrasound image (see Figure 33–1D), contains a bright white line showing the tongue surface during production of /t/. On the right of the image is the front of the tongue, although the tip is obscured because of the acoustic shadow of the jaw. The body of the tongue is raised in the oral cavity. Above

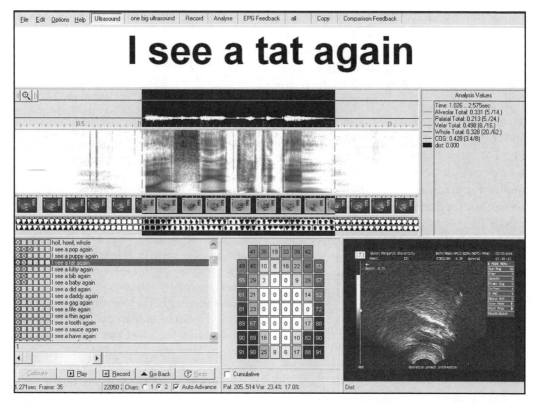

Figure 33–2. *The computer screen printout of Articulate Assistant Advanced (AAA) for combining acoustic, ultrasound, and electropalatography technologies in order to see speech in the sentence, "I see a tat again" (McLeod & Singh, 2009a, p. 354).*

the tongue is an air shadow and diagonal muscle fibres can be seen below the tongue's surface. By combining these four images, a greater understanding of the production of /t/ is gained compared with relying on acoustic impressionistic transcription.

THE IMPACT OF SEEING SPEECH IN SPEECH-LANGUAGE PATHOLOGY PRACTICE

The ability to see speech enhances SLPs' accuracy in diagnostic assessment and enables biofeedback during intervention for children and adults who have difficulties producing speech sounds. First, seeing speech has had an impact on SLPs' diagnostic accuracy. For example, Gibbon (1999) reviewed EPG studies of consonants perceived as substitutions, distortions, and even correct productions. She showed that 12 (71%) of 17 school-age children with speech sound disorders were using their tongue to cover the whole palate (undifferentiated lingual gestures). Gibbon (1999, p. 382) concluded: "Standard transcriptions do not reliably detect undifferentiated gestures, which are transcribed as speech errors . . . in some contexts, but are transcribed as correct productions in other contexts. Undifferentiated gestures are interpreted as reflecting a speech motor constraint involving either delayed or deviant control of functionally independent regions of the tongue."

Seeing speech has also had an impact on SLPs' intervention practices, particularly in the use of instrumentation as a biofeedback device (Gibbon & Wood, 2010). Instrumentation has enabled children and adults to see their own speech, compare their speech with a target that is typical of the ambient language, and change their speech production. For example, Bacsfalvi, Bernhardt, and Gick (2007) used electropalatography and ultrasound techniques for training three adolescents with severe hearing impairment to change their production of vowels. Improvements were documented using vowel formant values, EPG tongue-palate contact patterns and phonetic transcription. McAuliffe and Cornwell (2008) used EPG to enable an 11-year-old girl with a persistent lateral lisp to make consistent changes in her production of fricatives as judged by naïve listeners and documented by acoustic analysis of /s/ spectra. On a national scale, Lee et al. (2007) described how children with cleft lip and palate across Scotland benefitted from intervention using portable EPG devices to practice correct productions.

Instrumentation for seeing speech is used in research contexts, and is increasingly used in clinical contexts. Continual advancement of technologies is likely to result in less invasive, less expensive, and more informative technologies for seeing speech (Wrench, 2007), which in turn will further impact SLP assessment and intervention practices.

Acknowledgment. This chapter was written with support from Australian Research Council Future Fellowship (FT0990588).

REFERENCES

Bacsfalvi, P., Bernhardt, B. M., & Gick, B. (2007). Electropalatography and ultrasound in vowel remediation for adolescents with hearing impairment. *International Journal of Speech-Language Pathology*, 9(1), 36–45.

Ball, M. J., & Code, C. (Eds.). (1997). *Instrumental clinical phonetics*. London, UK: Whurr.

Ball, M. J., Gracco, V., & Stone, M. (2001). A comparison of imaging techniques for the investigation of normal and disordered speech production. *International Journal of Speech-Language Pathology*, 3, 13–24.

Ball, M. J., Manuel, R., & Müller, N. (2004). Deapicalization and velodorsal articulation as learned behaviors: A videofluorographic study. *Child Language Teaching and Therapy*, 20, 153–162.

Boersma, P., & Weenink, D. (2009). *Praat: Doing phonetics by computer (Version 5.1.05)* [Computer program]. Retrieved September 6, 2011, from http://www.praat.org/

Gibbon, F. E. (1999). Undifferentiated lingual gestures in children with articulation/phonological disorders. *Journal of Speech, Language, and Hearing Research*, 42, 382–397.

Gibbon, F. E., & Wood, S. (2010). Visual feedback therapy with electropalatography. In A. L. Williams, S. McLeod, & R. J. McCauley (Eds.), *Interventions for speech sound disorders in children* (pp. 509–536). Baltimore, MD: Paul H. Brookes.

Hardcastle, W. J., & Gibbon, F. (1997). Electropalatography and its clinical applications. In M. J. Ball & C. Code (Eds.), *Instrumental clinical phonetics* (pp. 149–193). London, UK: Croom Helm.

Harris, K. S., Hoffman, H. S., Liberman, A. M., Delattre, P. C., & Cooper, F. S. (1958). Effect of third-formant transitions on the perception of the voiced stop consonants. *Journal of the Acoustical Society of America*, 30, 122–126.

Kent, R. D. (1996). Hearing and believing: Some limits to the auditory-perceptual assessment of speech and voice disorders. *American Journal of Speech-Language Pathology*, 5, 7–23.

Lee, A., Gibbon, F. E., Crampin, L., Yuen, I., & McLennan, G. (2007). The national CLEFT-NET project for individuals with speech disorders associated with cleft palate. *International Journal of Speech-Language Pathology*, 9(1), 57–64.

Liberman, A. M., Cooper, F. S., Shankweiler, D. P., & Studdert-Kennedy, M. (1967). Perception of the speech code. *Psychological Review*, 74(6), 431–461.

McAuliffe, M. J., & Cornwell, P. L. (2008). Intervention for lateral /s/ using electropalatography (EPG) biofeedback and an intensive motor learning approach: A case report. *International Journal of Language and Communication Disorders*, 43(2), 219–229.

McAuliffe, M. J., Ward, E. C., & Murdoch, B. E. (2006). Speech production in Parkinson's disease II: Acoustic and electropalatographic investigation of sentence, word and segment durations. *Clinical Linguistics & Phonetics*, 20(1), 19–33.

McLeod, S. (2011). Speech-language pathologists' knowledge of tongue/palate contact for consonant production. *Clinical Linguistics & Phonetics*, 25(11–12), 1004–1013.

McLeod, S., & Singh, S. (2009a). *Speech sounds: A pictorial guide to typical and atypical speech.* San Diego, CA: Plural.

McLeod, S., & Singh, S. (2009b). *Seeing speech: A quick guide to speech sounds.* San Diego, CA: Plural.

Moen, I., & Simonsen, H. G. (2007). The combined use of EPG and EMA in articulatory descriptions. *International Journal of Speech-Language Pathology*, 9(1), 120–127.

Moses, E. R., Jr. (1939). Palatography and speech improvement. *Journal of Speech Disorders*, 4(2), 103–114.

Shohara, H. H., & Hanson, C. (1941). Palatography as an aid to the improvement of articulatory movements. *Journal of Speech Disorders*, 6, 115–124.

Singh, S., & Singh, K. (2006). *Phonetics: Principles and practices* (3rd ed.). San Diego, CA: Plural.

Wrench, A. A. (2007). Advances in EPG palate design. *International Journal of Speech-Language Pathology*, 9(1), 3–12.

ESSAY 34

Phonological Processes ☙ and Traditional Phoneme ❧ Acquisition Norms

William Culbertson

Dr. Singh was a noted figure in the field of communications sciences and disorders long before I met him in person. When I finally did meet him, it was at an annual meeting of the Council of Academic Programs in Communication Sciences and Disorders, where he threw one of his famous picnic lunches for the members. Personable, friendly, and with that intelligent twinkle in his eye that told you he knew his business, Dr. Singh had the qualities that marked him as a true leader in our field. That was back in the Singular days.

Years after that brief, "How-do-you-do?" meeting, Dr. Singh and I worked together telephonically on a Plural anatomy and physiology textbook project. I found him every bit as forthcoming and gracious as he was the first time we met. Because of this, I am pleased to present these articles in honor of a unique individual in the field of publishing.

TRADITIONAL APPROACH

Back in the 1970s, when I was a budding young speech pathologist ("language" had not yet been included in the title) we had slightly different ways of approaching placement and treatment goals. Then as now, it was crucial that criteria for treatment placement and termination be proper and backed by research. The placement paradigm was based on several studies that chronicled the acquisition of phonemes as customary parts of children's speech. The approach has solid face validity, as anyone who has observed children for any length of time can attest. Superficially, it is obvious that 3-year-olds often have more difficulty with velar plosives and with alveolar fricatives, for example, than do 7-year-olds.

Wellman (1931), Poole (1934), and Davis (1939) were the most venerable of these studies, and it wasn't until I had been using those results for several years that I discovered that Poole and Davis was the same person. Using Davis's norms, I routinely placed children who failed to differentiate /t/ from /k/ by age five, assured that by that age, they needed help to perceive and produce the velar plosives. Mildred Templin, a true pioneer in our field, published her tables in 1957, using a more reasonable 75% rate, as did Sander (1972) and Prather, Hedrick, and Kern (1975). The apparent trend among all these tables, regardless of the acquisition rate, is that mastery of adoption of phonemes into a normal child's speech seems to develop first with articulations that are easier to produce and more visible, such as the bilabial nasal, then later with more complex articulations, such as affricates. Edwards (2002) provided a neat compendium of acquisition tables. Using the phoneme acquisition tables, the primary goal of treatment is to teach the sensorimotor oral skills necessary to produce the delayed phonemes, and then to help the child assimilate the target phonemes into the phonology. Speech-language pathologists continue to rely on these tables as clinical tools to help them decide whether the children they examine are simply recapitulating the normal developmental sequence or might suffer educationally, cognitively, or socially without needed treatment.

The traditional approach to speech development is most useful for recommendations concerning treatment of children who demonstrate nonstandard articulation, targeting a few phonemes and which part or parts of the syllable structure they form. For these children, diagnostic statements that describe nonstandard productions as "substitutions, distortions, or omissions inconsistent with chronological age or local dialect," are adequate. This "five-way" structure for classifying speech sound production is widely used. For the purposes of this discussion, it is noteworthy that the classification of *distortion* implies a degree of imprecision in manner of consonant formation, brought on, perhaps, by missing dentition or immature lingual coordination, and might be described as a phonetic, rather than a phonemic error. It is important to note that, although this approach may emphasize sensorimotor development of speech articulation, it does not consider a child to have mastered a speech sound until he or she uses it phonemically. Thus, mastery of a phoneme implies inclusion into the child's phonological code as well as phonetic ability. Likewise, the traditional approach addresses the syntactic sequence of phoneme use as syllable releasers or syllable arrestors, and, in closed juncture, the so-called medial or intervocalic position in an approach similar to that of a phonotactic plan.

As the use of acquisition tables substantially predates the use of phonological development tables, it may be called the "Traditional Approach" to speech articulation treatment. Clinicians' choices of references for treatment placement support depend on their views regarding *percent of mastery*. This percentage is important information for making treatment decisions and reflects the professional standards of a clinician or a facility. For example, if a clinician finds a child's production of a phoneme is in error (not standard) and the available norms show that the child is delayed in acquisition by 6 months, it is extremely important to know if the norms listed mastery of the phoneme at the particular age by 51%, 60%, 75%, 90%, or 100% of the children sampled. Clinicians who consider placement according to extreme upper limits, such as 90 or 100%, might do so because of the likelihood that a child who is out of step with those data is late in speech development. However, the cogent question then arises about how the 5% to 10% of the children who would be expected to be developmentally delayed in phoneme acquisition were systematically eliminated from the authors' samples. On the other hand, using a 51% mastery level might appear to lack precision, as those data suggest possible placement of 49% of the population in therapy.

PHONOLOGICAL SYSTEMS APPROACH

The emphasis remained mostly on the sensorimotor aspect of the articulation processes until 1976 when David Ingram published a thin paperback entitled *Phonological Disability in Children*. In that work, Ingram presented the concept of phonological systems, a fundament of spoken language comprising all the allowable phonemes in a child's idiolect and the rules for combining them. The emphasis was shifted to the rules for articulation of the entire syllable, rather than the simpler idea of perception and production of phonemes.

Applying the works of linguistic notables such as Roman Jakobson (1942), Ingram proposed several innate *phonological processes* involved in the construction of syllables that affect classes of sounds rather than the individual sounds themselves. Others followed suit (Hodson & Paden, 1991; Grunwell, 1981; Stoel-Gammon, 1987), proposing that children naturally try various strategies at syllable building (phonotactics), and allow those that don't apply to adult phonology to become extinct.

The phonological systems approach to speech therapy regards children who persist with immature phonological processes as candidates for direct intervention. Addressing the developing child's speech-sound inventory and code system, clinicians implementing phonological treatment address a child's rule-governed or codified phonological structure in the context of the syllable. The goal of phonological therapy is to teach the child standard usage rules through phonemic contrasts.

Like phoneme mastery, phonological process development appears to follow a predictable sequence for most children. Thus, there are some trends in the disappearances or *extinction* of immature phonological processes that occur as the normal child's expanding sensory and motor abilities lead to adoption of more mature phonotactic options.

We use the term *extinction* to refer to the child's discovery that the linguistic environment no longer supports a given phonological process. With maturity of perception and refinement of production, children at later developmental stages recognize their early attempts at phonological codification are unsatisfactory. The role of the clinician in the phonological approach is to help the child discover adult phonology. In so doing, the individual "masters" phonemes in the more traditional sense.

The phonological systems approach is most useful for assessment of the speech of children who present with great differences in their individual spoken language code, or idiolect, and the standard dialect. To all but their family members, these children are unintelligible or nearly so. This unintelligibility results from a phonology that is radically different than the standard. Clinicians using the phonological approach examine speech samples in several contexts to derive rule-governed or codified phonological structures in the individual's speech, and then endeavor to teach the child the standard rules. The process of determining this phonology is often made more difficult, at least initially, by the fact that the clinician may not know the child's linguistic referent. Phonological analysis, in this regard, may be a process of discovery for both clinician and child.

Phonological diagnosis and treatment emphasizes the ontogeny of the linguistic code inherent in a child's speech, but acknowledges that a substrate of this development is sensorimotor maturation. The phonological aspect of the linguistic code evolves as a child senses the effects of coarticulation when phonemes are juxtaposed, and encodes effects that are linguistically useful. Sensorimotor maturation is required for articulation of the more complicated releasers, nuclei, and arresters of syllables.

Both the "Phoneme Acquisition" approach to speech development and the "Phonological Systems" approach have been mainstays of speech therapy practice for decades, and neither has shown any signs of supplanting the other. The fact that they are based in the simple notion that children's speech becomes more adultlike with time may be supported by both sensorimotor and neurolinguistic maturation.

Dennis Tanner, Wayne Secord, and I (1997) were among those who saw similarities in the two approaches. Notwithstanding the theoretical approach to treatment, we set out to compare the ages at which several literary sources reported the extinction of immature phonological processes in English-speaking children and the ages at which others reported a 51% and 75% rate of phoneme acquisition.

Table 34–1 contains the results of our literature review. It shows the consistency, if not a sort of qualitative concurrent validity, with which both systems compare, each supporting the other.

The authors omitted some processes described in the literature for this study. These processes include nasal assimilation, metathesis, epenthesis, and reduplication. They were omitted because of lack of data concerning the ages of extinction or, in the case of reduplication, the fact that the process is extinguished at such an early age as to be rarely encountered by school clinicians. Table 34–1 indicates the phonological processes and their mean age of extinction.

Normative data presented herein are simplified. Contextual variations such as syllabic position, phonetic environment and consonant type are left to the clinician to note. For example, the replacement of the approximant /w/ for the approximant /r/ is frequently described as *gliding of liquids*. In individual cases, this substitution may involve idiolectic alteration in the place of glide articulation, if /r/ is articulated as a glide, or replacement of the palatal approximant /r/ with a central vowel, /ɜ/, if the lips are not rounded. Such a replacement is referred to as *vocalization*. The clinician has the flexibility to apply the appropriate intervention strategies after careful observation of individual behavior.

Table 34–1. Comparison of Phonological Process Extinction and Traditional Acquisition Norms

Age (Years;Months)	Process	51% Level	75% Level
1;6		/m; w; h; n; p; b/	
1;9			
2;0		/ʃ; k; g; t; d/	
2;3			
2;6	Initial Consonant Deletion	/f; j/	
2;9			
3;0	Velar Fronting; Prevocalic Voicing	/r; s; l/	/m; w; h; n; f; ŋ/
3;3	Velar Assimilation		
3;6		/ʃ; z; tʃ/	/p; b/
3;9			/j/
4;0	Postvocalic Devoicing; Alveolar Assimilation	/v; dʒ/	/k; g/
4;3	Final Consonant Deletion		
4;6	Labial Assimilation	/θ; ð/	/d; ʃ; r/
4;9			/tʃ; s/
5;0	Cluster Reduction; Glottal Replacement		/l/
5;3	Weak Syllable Deletion; Stopping		
5;6			/t; v/
5;9			
6;0	Gliding; Vocalization	/ʒ/	/z; θ/
6;3			
6;6			/dʒ/
6;9			
7;0			/ʒ; ð/

Source: Culberson and Tanner (2001).

REFERENCES

The following authors and their studies are acknowledged for their assistance in deciding the final profile. Clinicians are encouraged to refer to these sources for detailed information about phonological development.

Culbertson, W. R., & Tanner, D. C. *Dependency of neuromotor oral maturation on phonological development.* 9th Manchester Phonology Meeting, University of Manchester, Manchester, England, May 25, 2001.

Davis, D. M. (1939). The relation of repetitions in the speech of young children to certain measures of language maturity and situational factors: Part I. *Journal of Speech Disorders, 4,* 303–318.

Edwards, H. (1992). *Applied phonetics: The sounds of American English.* San Diego, CA: Singular.

Faircloth, S. R., & Faircloth, M. A., (1973). *Phonetic science: A program of instruction.* Englewood Cliffs, NJ: Prentice-Hall.

Grunwell, P. (1981). The development of phonology: A descriptive profile. In *A first language.* Chalfont, UK: Alpha Academics.

Haelsig, P. C., & Madison, C. L. (1986). A study of phonological processes exhibited by 3-, 4-, and 5-year old children. *Language, Speech, and Hearing Services in the Schools, 17,* 110.

Hodson, B. W., & Paden, E. P. (1991). *Targeting intelligible speech* (2nd ed). Austin, TX: Pro-Ed.

Ingram, D. (1976). *Phonological disability in children.* New York, NY: Elsevier.

Jakobson, R. (1972). *Child Language, Aphasia and Phonological Universals.* The Hague & Paris: Mouton; originally published in German in 1940-1942.

Kent, R. D. (1994). *Reference Manual for Communication Sciences and Disorders.* Austin, TX: Pro-Ed.

Pool, I. (1934). Genetic development of articulation of consonant sounds in speech. *Elementary English Review, 11,* 159–161.

Prather, E., Hedrick, D., & Kern, C. (1975). Articulation development in children aged two to four years. *Journal of Speech Hearing Disorders, 40,* 179–191.

Preisser, D. A., Hodson, B. W., & Paden, E. P. (1988). Developmental phonology: 18–29 months. *Journal of Speech and Hearing Disorders, 53,* 127.

Sander, E. (1972). When are speech sounds learned? *Journal of Speech and Hearing Disorders, 37,* 55–63.

Smit, A. B., Hand, L., Freilinger, J. F., Bernthal, J. E., & Bird, A. (1990). The Iowa-Nebraska norms project and its Nebraska replication. *Journal of Speech and Hearing Disorders, 55,* 779–798.

Stoel-Gammon, C. (1987) Phonological skills of 2-year-olds. *Language, Speech and Hearing Services in the Schools, 18,* 327.

Tanner, D. C., Culbertson, W. R., & Secord, W. A. (1997). *Developmental Articulation and Phonology Profile.* Oceanside, CA: Academic Communication Associates.

Templin, M. C. (1957). *Certain Language Skills in Children.* Minneapolis, MN: University of Minnesota Press.

Wallace, W. (1971, November-December). The wabbit wost his tock. In *Mother's Manual* (pp. 28–38).

Wellman, B. L., Case, I., Mengert, I., & Bradbury, D. (1931). Speech sounds in young children. *University of Iowa Studies in Child Welfare, 5,* 42–45.

ESSAY 35

❧ Voice Research in Hong Kong ❧

Past, Present, and Future

Estella P.-M. Ma and Edwin M.-L. Yiu

The second author (EY) first came across the name of Dr. Singh as early as the 1980s, when College-Hill Press published an extensive range of speech-language pathology books that caught the eyes of the then undergraduate student (EY). The first personal encounter with Dr. Singh was related to the speech-language pathology program in Hong Kong in the late 1980s/early 1990s, during which textbooks were badly needed for the new program. With the economical climate at that time, undergraduate students in Hong Kong simply could not afford the book prices that are sold to their U.S. counterparts. Dr. Singh was very supportive of the program and arranged the first shipment of speech-language pathology textbooks to be sold at greatly reduced prices to the students. Since then, colleagues in Hong Kong have undertaken much research in the field of speech-language pathology and have become more involved in publishing. Dr. Singh provided opportunities through his publishing avenue for many researchers, writers, and academics in Hong Kong. We are grateful to have had the support of Dr. Singh to publish the Handbook of Voice Assessments *(Ma & Yiu, 2011).*

INTRODUCTION

Hong Kong had its first speech therapist in early 1960s and this speech therapist worked in an ear, nose and throat (ENT) setting (Stokes & Yiu, 1997). For 20 years (until the mid-1980s), the whole of Hong Kong, with a population of 5 to 6 million at that time, was served by only three speech therapists in the hospital setting. All of them worked in the ENT setting. Therefore, it is not surprising to find that there has been a strong influence of laryngology on the speech therapy/pathology service. With the recognition of the importance of speech therapy/pathology service in the mid-1980s, the Hong Kong Government has sent a large number of individuals to Australia for speech therapy/pathology training and funded the first and only speech therapy program in Hong Kong. This program is still the only program in China that trains the speech therapy/pathology profession.

Before 1980, there was no speech therapy/pathology training course in Hong Kong.

All the qualified speech therapists in Hong Kong received their professional training overseas, from the United Kingdom, North America, or Australia. Assessment materials and therapeutic models were undoubtedly adopted from these countries with western cultures. Obviously, adoption of these materials and management models from the western culture to a Chinese population is not always appropriate, due to the linguistic differences between Hong Kong and western countries. In Hong Kong, Cantonese is the major spoken Chinese dialect. Linguistically, Cantonese is a tone language and English is a non-tone language. They have very different phonetic and grammatical systems. The linguistic differences between English and Cantonese prompt the need for more speech and language assessment and management protocols relevant to the Cantonese population, which has led to more local research development in this area. This essay uses the Voice Research Laboratory at The University of Hong Kong as an exemplar to illustrate the development of voice research in Hong Kong over the past two decades. It first presents a historical review of the research development, followed by a review of its current research. The way our research has been translated to clinical practice is highlighted. The research roadmap of the Laboratory is also discussed.

VOICE RESEARCH IN HONG KONG: ITS PAST

The Voice Research Laboratory was first established in 1997 and has operated under the Division of Speech and Hearing Sciences at The University of Hong Kong. The Voice Research Laboratory is devoted to research related to voice science and disorders. Its mission is to improve the quality of life in individuals with voice problems by translating its research to guide best clinical practice. Research at the Voice Research Laboratory covers assessments from auditory-perceptual evaluation and instrumentation to quality of life measures, clinical trials of different voice therapy models, and also basic science. Over the years, our research has been supported from various funding bodies (Hong Kong Research Grant Council, Hong Kong Government Health and Health Services Research Fund, Hong Kong Quality Education Fund, The University of Hong Kong Endowment Fund, and The United States National Institutes of Health). Four areas of research carried out at the Voice Research Laboratory, which have contributed to clinical practice, are reviewed in the following sections.

Auditory-Perceptual Voice Evaluation

Auditory-perceptual voice evaluation is a common clinical tool used for assessing voice quality and severity. However, perceptual voice evaluation is a subjective process and it is prone to inter- and intrarater variability. A perceptual voice evaluation training program (Chan & Yiu, 2002) was developed based on the conceptual framework proposed by Kreiman and her colleagues (1993). The training program has a set of voice anchors covering normal, mild, moderate and severe severity levels of roughness and breathiness as external references for rating. The underlying principle is that the internal standards of voice quality and severity vary among listeners. Therefore, the external voice anchors serve as a common and stable reference for listeners when doing perceptual rating. This will lead to a higher reliability in auditory-perceptual evaluation. Our data revealed that the provision of external voice anchors and perceptual training are useful in improving reliability among listeners (Chan & Yiu, 2002, 2006; Yiu, Chan, & Mok, 2007).

Instrumental Voice Assessment

Apart from auditory-perceptual voice evaluation, instrumental voice analysis is frequently used for assessing vocal (dys-)function. The Voice Research Laboratory has a wide range of equipment for voice assessment and treatment, including imaging systems (videostroboscopy, color high-speed imaging systems), acoustic measurement (Computerized Speech Lab, Voice Range Profile), aerodynamic measurement (Aerophone, Phonatory Aerodynamic System), and physiologic measurement (electroglottograph, electromyography). Our research projects have generated a database of normal and disordered voice in the Cantonese population. Clinically, these data contribute to recommendations of procedural aspects and selection of instrumentation. For example, our data suggest that acoustic perturbation measures may not be sensitive enough for analyzing dysphonic voice signals (Ma & Yiu, 2005). Alternatively, voice range profile seems to be a sensitive and reliable acoustic tool for differentiating between normal and dysphonic individuals (Ma, Robertson, Radford, Vagne, El-Halabi, & Yiu, 2007). Reliability and validity of voice measurements are enhanced with more recording trials (Yiu, Yuen, Whitehill, & Winkworth, 2004) and the use of connected speech as testing stimuli (Ma & Love, 2010). The use of a high-speed imaging technique provides a more detailed and accurate analysis of vocal fold structures and functions, particularly at the voice onsets and offsets (Yiu, Kong, Fong, & Chan, 2010). Our research data using vocal attack time has also highlighted some differences between a non-tone language (e.g., English) and a tone language (e.g., Cantonese) (see Ma, Baken, Roark & Li, in press).

Voice-Related Quality of Life

Voice problems lead not only to deviant vocal structures and qualities, but also to functional and emotional impacts on the individuals. The World Health Organization has proposed a health classification scheme to classify health components of human functioning and disability. This health classification scheme was first proposed in 1980 as the International Classification of Impairments, Disabilities and Handicaps (ICIDH; WHO, 1980). The scheme then underwent several modifications before it was finalized in 2001 as the current form the International Classification of Functioning, Disability and Health (ICF; WHO, 2001). Based on this health framework, the Voice Activity and Participation Profile (VAPP; Ma & Yiu, 2001) was developed. The profile is a 28-item self-assessing questionnaire that ascertains an individual's voice activity limitation and participation restriction in carrying out various voice activities. Since its development, the VAPP has been translated into Brazilian-Portuguese (Ricarte, Gasparini, & Behlau, 2006), Finnish (Sukanen et al., 2007), and Croatian (Bonetti, Simunjak, & Bonetti, 2009). The applicability of the ICF in voice disorders has also been evaluated. Our research findings reveal that how the laryngeal system is affected or impaired (that is, voice impairment) does not necessary indicate how one perceives the impact (that is, voice activity limitation and participation restriction). Therefore, these three dimensions need to be assessed separately (Ma, 2003). This line of research has highlighted the importance of including the client's perspective in clinical decision making. The VAPP is now incorporated in a daily voice assessment protocol for evaluating the extent of impact due to the voice problems, evaluating treatment outcomes, and predicting treatment efficacy. The Voice Research Laboratory has also helped to validate the Chinese version of the Voice Handicap Index (Lam et al., 2006).

Voice Motor Learning

Hyperfunctional voice disorder is the most common type. Conservative voice therapy is considered as the first choice of treatment, which usually includes a combination of vocal hygiene and voice production training. Motor learning is involved as the individual (re) learns how to control and coordinate laryngeal muscles to produce voice more effectively. The general, nonspeech motor learning literature has documented how learning of a motor skill can be affected if learning variables are manipulated differently. A series of studies were carried out at the Voice Research Laboratory to evaluate the applicability of general motor learning principles in voice motor learning. The effects of different learning variables (timing of feedback, relative frequency of feedback, practice variability, self-controlled feedback) on learning of voice therapy tasks have been evaluated. Readers are referred to the papers for details (see Ma, Yiu, & Yiu, 2010; Wong, Ma, & Yiu, 2011; Yiu, Verdolini, & Chow, 2005). Interestingly, some of the findings seem to contradict some procedures in conventional clinical practice. For example, our data revealed that less direct feedback promotes better learning than more feedback in adults (Wong, Ma, & Yiu, 2009). The research findings contribute to refining the procedural aspect of voice production tasks. We believe this line of research would enhance voice training models and ultimately, voice therapy efficacy itself.

VOICE RESEARCH IN HONG KONG: THE PRESENT

Currently, research projects carried out at the Voice Research Laboratory are classified under three themes: (1) risk assessment and prevention, (2) alternative treatment for voice problems, and (3) pediatric voice disorders.

Risk Assessment and Prevention

As with other health problems, voice disorders are multifactorial in nature (Deary, Wilson, Carding, & Mackenzie, 2003). Preventive measures that involve the elimination of predisposed risk factors associated with the disorder and early identification of at-risk individuals have recently become important in voice research. It is critical to identify and understand risk factors that are associated with voice disorders, as it will allow health care professionals to design cost-effective preventive voice care programs by targeting those critical predisposing risk factors. Early identification of the more susceptible subpopulation is also important, as it helps to prioritize appropriate health care for them. The Voice Research Laboratory has carried out a series of studies to address this issue, by identifying and validating voice-related risk factors using the health risk assessment approach. The first study is called the *Green Voice Project*. This project is based on the risk assessment approach and a voice risk calculator is currently under development for evaluating the level of risk for voice problems. The electronic version of the voice risk calculator can be found at the Web site (http://www3.hku.hk/speech/green voice/index.htm). Another ongoing project is funded by the National Institutes of Health in the United States, to evaluate the effectiveness of resonant voice therapy in preventing voice problems in teacher trainees. The importance of voice prevention has led to the development of Apps ("YourVoice" and "YourVoice Lite") based on the Apple iOS platform. These Apps contain information on voice production and vocal hygiene, self-assessment of knowledge on vocal hygiene, video demonstration on how to practice proper voicing techniques, and self-evaluation of voicing techniques.

Alternative Treatment for Voice Problems

Hong Kong is located on the southern part of mainland China, and has a long history in development of western medicine and also embracing traditional Chinese medicine. Since 2001, the Voice Research Laboratory has begun investigating the application of traditional Chinese medicine in preventing or treating voice problems. Among a number of unsuccessful attempts, including the use of Chinese herbal supplements or extracts like ginseng, and some classical decoctions, we have found acupuncture to be promising. We published the first randomized controlled trial that demonstrated acupuncture is effective in treating vocal pathologies related to phonotrauma (Yiu et al., 2006). Results cannot be attributed to a placebo effect (Kwong & Yiu, 2010). A larger scale randomized controlled trial funded by the National Institutes of Health is currently in progress to further evaluate the long-term effectiveness of acupuncture on treating phonotrauma. Preliminary findings show that stimulating the acupoints on the skin surface is producing similar effectiveness as the real acupuncture which involves needle penetration beneath the skin at the acupoints.

Pediatric Voice Disorders

Voice problems are common in children. However, the majority of voice research data are based on the adult population. Due to the substantial structural and functional differences between adult and pediatric larynx, the normative data established from the adult population cannot be applied in the pediatric population. Our research studies have provided empirical data to guide assessment procedures in children. For example, clinician-provided coaching with verbal encouragements and a visual cue (hand-sweeping) can help children achieve their maximum phonational frequency range in fewer trials (Ma & Li, 2011). The use of connected speech stimuli at passage level leads to higher reliability for measurement of speaking fundamental frequency (Lee, Ma, & Lam, 2012). In terms of treatment, our previous work on voice motor learning in adults has been extended to the child population. Preliminary data reveal that, contrary to adults, children need more frequent feedback on their voice performance during voice training for better voice skills learning (Wong, 2012).

VOICE RESEARCH IN HONG KONG: CONCLUSIONS AND THOUGHTS FOR A FUTURE AGENDA

This essay has provided an overview of the voice research development in Hong Kong. The roadmap of voice research would continue to focus on assessment and treatment of voice disorders. One direction is to explore the applicability of a telehealth service delivery model in voice assessment and treatment. Further developments in basic science are also warranted. One example is the field of tissue engineering and regenerative medicine. This has great potential in managing vocal pathologies. In summary, there is a need for more translational research in voice for better voice assessment and treatment protocols.

REFERENCES

Bonetti, A., Simunjak, B., & Bonetti, L. (2009). Samoprocjena I objekivna procjena voka-lnih teskoca u osoba s disfonijom. *6. kongres Hrvatskog drustva za otorinolaringologiju I kirur-giju glave i vrata s medunarodnim* [in Croatian].

Chan, K. M.-K., & Yiu, E. M.-L. (2002). The effect of anchors and training on the reliabil-ity of perceptual voice evaluation. *Journal of Speech, Language and Hearing Research, 45*(1), 111–126.

Chan, K. M. K., & Yiu, E. M. L. (2006). A com-parison of two perceptual voice evaluation training programs for naive listeners. *Journal of Voice, 20,* 229–241.

Deary, I. J., Wilson, J. A., Carding, P. N., & Mack-enzie, K. (2003). The dysphonic voice heard by me, you and it: differential associations with personality and psychological distress. *Clinical Otolaryngology, 28*(4), 374–378.

Kreiman, J., Gerratt, B. R., Kempster, G. B., Erma, A., & Berke, G. S. (1993). Perceptual evaluation of voice quality: Review, tutorial, and a framework for future research. *Journal of Speech and Hearing Research, 36,* 21–40.

Kwong, E. Y.-L., & Yiu, E. M.-L. (2010). A pre-liminary study of the effect of acupuncture on salivary cortisol level in female dysphonic speakers. *Journal of Voice, 24*(6), 719–723.

Lam, P. K.-Y., Chan, K. M., Ho. W.-K., Kwong, E., Yiu, E. M., & Wei, W. I. (2006). Cross-cul-tural adaptation and validation of the Chinese Voice Handicap Index-10. *Laryngoscope, 116,* 1192–1198.

Lee, T. K.-Y., Ma, E. P.-M., & Lam, N. (2012). *The effects of speech tasks on fundamental fre-quency in Cantonese children.* Poster presented at The Voice Foundation's 41st Annual Sym-posium: Care of the Professional Voice, Phila-delphia, PA.

Ma, E. P.-M. (2003). *Impairment, activity limita-tion and participation restriction issues in assessing dysphonia.* Unpublished doctoral thesis, Univer-sity of Hong Kong, Hong Kong.

Ma, E. P.-M., Baken, R. J., Roark, R. M., & Li, P.-M. (in press). Effect of tones on vocal attack time (VAT) in Cantonese speakers. *Journal of Voice.*

Ma, E. P.-M., & Li, T. (2011). *The effects of coach-ing and repeated trials on maximum phonational frequency range in children.* Paper presented at The Voice Foundation's 40th Annual Sympo-sium: Care of the Professional Voice, Philadel-phia, PA.

Ma, E. P.-M., & Love, A. L. (2010). Electroglot-tographic evaluation of age and gender effects during sustained phonation and connected speech. *Journal of Voice, 24*(2), 146–152.

Ma, E., Robertson, J., Radford, C., Vagne, S., El-Halabi, R., & Yiu, E. (2007). Reliability of speaking and maximum voice range measures in screening for dysphonia. *Journal of Voice, 21*(4), 397–406.

Ma, E., & Yiu, E. (2005). Suitability of acoustic perturbation measures in analyzing periodic and nearly periodic voice signals. *Folia Phoni-atrica et Logopaedica, 57*(1), 38–47.

Ma, E. P.-M., & Yiu, E. M.-L. (2001). Voice activity and participation profile: Assessing the impact of voice disorders on daily activi-ties. *Journal of Speech, Language and Hearing Research, 44*(3), 511–524.

Ma, E. P.-M., & Yiu, E. M.-L. (Eds.). (2011). *Hand-book of voice assessments.* San Diego, CA: Plural.

Ma, E. P.-M., Yiu, G. K.-Y., & Yiu, E. M.-L. (2010). *Self-controlled feedback paradigm in learning of a relaxed phonation.* Poster presented at The 28th World Congress of the Interna-tional Association of Logopedics and Phoniat-rics (IALP), Athens, Greece.

Ricarte, A., Gasparini, G., & Behlau, M. (2006). *Validação do Protocolo Perfil de Participação e Atividades Vocais (PPAV) no Brasil.* Anais do XIV Congresso Brasileiro de Fonoaudiologia.

Stokes, S. F., & Yiu, E. (1997). Speech therapy and general practice in Hong Kong. *Hong Kong Practitioner, 19*(7), 374–379.

Sukanen, O., Sihvo, M., Rorarius, E., Lehtihalmes, M., Autio, V., & Kleemola, L. (2007). Voice Activity and Participation Profile (VAPP) in assessing the effects of voice disorders on patients' quality of life: Validity and reliability of the Finnish version of VAPP. *Logopedics Pho-niatrics Vocology, 32,* 3–8.

Wong, Y.-H. (2012). *The effects of relative frequency of augmented feedback on resonant voice training in adults and children with normal voice.* M.Phil. thesis. University of Hong Kong, Hong Kong.

Wong, A., Ma, E., & Yiu, E. (2009). *Effects of electromyographic terminal feedback on motor learning of the relaxed phonation task.* Paper presented at The Voice Foundation's 38th Annual Symposium: Care of the Professional Voice, Philadelphia, PA.

Wong, A. Y.-H., Ma, E. P.-M., & Yiu, E. M.-L. (2011). Effects of practice variability on learning of relaxed phonation in vocally hyperfunctional speakers. *Journal of Voice, 25*(3), 348–353.

World Health Organization. (1980). *International Classification of Impairments, Disabilities, and Handicaps (ICIDH).* Geneva, Switzerland: Author.

World Health Organization. (2001). *International Classification of Functioning, Disability and Health (ICF).* Geneva, Switzerland: Author.

Yiu, E. M.-L., Chan, K. M. K., & Mok, R. S.-M. (2007). Reliability and confidence in using a paired comparison paradigm in perceptual voice quality evaluation. *Clinical Linguistics and Phonetics, 21*(2), 129–145.

Yiu, E. M.-L., Kong, J.-P., Fong, R., & Chan, K. M.-K. (2010). A preliminary study of a quantitative analysis method for high speed laryngoscopic images. *International Journal of Speech-Language Pathology, 12*(6), 520–528.

Yiu, E. M.-L., Verdolini, K., & Chow, L. P.-Y. (2005). Electromyographic study of motor learning for a voice production task. *Journal of Speech, Language and Hearing Research, 48,* 1254–1268.

Yiu, E. M.-L., Xu, J. J., Murry, T., Wei, W., Yu, M., Ma, E., . . . Kwong, E. (2006). A randomized treatment-placebo study of the effectiveness of acupuncture for benign vocal pathologies. *Journal of Voice, 20,* 144–156.

Yiu, E. M.-L., Yuen, Y. M., Whitehill, T., & Winkworth, A. (2004). Reliability and applicability of aerodynamic measures in dysphonia assessment. *Clinical Linguistics & Phonetics, 18,* 463–478.

ESSAY 36

Translational Display of Neurophysiologic Investigations in Communication Sciences and Disorders

Reem Khamis-Dakwar

As a new scholar in the field of communication sciences and disorders, it is unimaginable not to be touched and influenced by the prolific academic work of Dr. Singh. Even though I did not have the honor to meet him in person, I feel like his work has left remarkable contribution to our field. I am honored to be part of a project to commemorate and celebrate his rich fruitful life.

INTRODUCTION

Neurophysiologic investigation in Communication Sciences and Disorders (CSD) refers to studies on the nature of a specific communication disorder, language acquisition given a specific communication disorder, as well as the assessment and intervention effects for a specific communication disorder.

In this essay, event-related potential (ERP) methodology will be introduced. Furthermore, the benefit and need for clinically driven neurophysiologic investigations in

CSD to elucidate brain processes underpinning speech-language disorders and language learning in specific communication disorders is exemplified by describing several clinically driven studies conducted at the Neurophysiology of Speech and Language Pathology Lab (NSLP Lab).

NEUROPHYSIOLOGIC INVESTIGATIONS IN CSD

Cognitive Neuroscience, CSD, and EEG: Introduction

Cognitive neuroscience refers to the scientific disciplines concerned with the study of higher cognitive functions in humans, such as memory and language, and their underlying neural bases. It "aims to understand how cognitive functions, and their manifestations in behavior and subjective experience, arise from the activity of the brain" (Rugg, 1997, p.1). The field of CSD encompasses several scientific disciplines concerned with typical human communication, speech, and language development, communication disorders, and therapy. There are relatively limited clinically driven neurophysiologic studies in CSD to date. In this essay, we maintain the fields of cognitive neuroscience and CSD can inform each other and we exemplify the incorporation of EEG/ERP methodology to relate the observed communicative behaviors to their underlying brain mechanisms in the study of CSD.

EEG and Language Correlates

Several neuroimaging techniques can be utilized to investigate brain activity. These techniques can be divided into yielding either hemodynamic or electrophysiological measures. Hemodynamic measures, such as those resulting from fMRI, identify brain activity resulting from metabolic changes, including blood flow. Electrophysiologic measures, such as those obtained in EEG and MEG, reflect cortical activity in different brain areas derived by recording electromagnetic activity across the scalp. Generally speaking, hemodynamic measures have superior spatial resolution (i.e., can more accurately measure the place of an examined brain activity), whereas measures of electromagnetic activity have better temporal resolution (i.e., can more accurately measure the timing of an examined brain activity). For example, using fMRI techniques spatial information can be obtained on a millimeter scale, but temporal resolution can only be recorded on a second scale. In contrast, EEG can provide temporal information on a millisecond range (Luck, 2005) but spatial resolution within a wider millimeter scale. Hence, studies utilizing hemodynamic brain imaging techniques are better able to more

accurately localize specific areas of the brain associated with a variety of language and/or cognitive functions, whereas studies utilizing electrophysiologic brain imaging techniques are more appropriate for identifying task-related neural activity at the millisecond level. Relative to these respective advantages, electrophysiologic measures are thought to be more effective for evaluating the subprocesses involved in language processing (Friederici, 2002). The ideal investigative approach would be to incorporate both imaging techniques, hemodynamic and electrophysiological, to obtain information with the highest temporal and spatial resolution. This essay is focused on introducing the use of EEG/ERP method in CSD (see Ward, 2010 for a review of imaging techniques).

Electroencephalography (EEG) refers to the continuous measurement of electrical activity in the brain. To acquire EEG data, in the NSLPlab, we use a HydroCel Geodesic Sensor Net (HCGSN) from Electrical Geosdesic Inc. The net enables a quick and safe way to place 32 electrodes on the scalp of participants. Nets are available in different sizes allowing for a snug but comfortable fit for each participant. In the NSLPLab we are using HCGSN nets with 32 electrodes; however, the HCGSN nets are available in densities of 32, 64, 128, and 256 channels. Figure 36–1 shows a medium 32-channel HCGSN net as viewed from the front. Each pedestal in the net contains an electrode embedded within a sponge, which decreases any potential discomfort a participant may feel. In addition, the wires connecting individual electrodes form a net enabling the whole collection of electrodes (the net) to be quickly fitted.

During the EEG recording session, participants wear the HCGSN net which is connected to an amplifier. The amplified electrical activity is recorded via EEG acquisition software. Figure 36–2 shows the data acquisition setup. On the right side of the figure, you

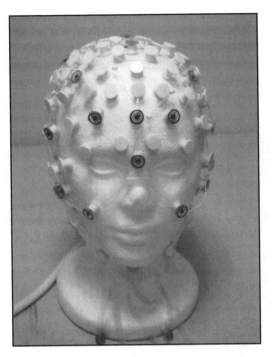

Figure 36–1. *Medium-sized HCGSN (32 channel).*

can see the participant wearing a HydroCel net (Electrical Geodesics, Inc.) with the 32 electrodes embedded in sponges. On the left side of the picture, you can see the data display of the amplified electrical activity from each of the 32 channels as it is recorded during an EEG experiment.

In EEG studies of language, we are less interested in the brain's ongoing electrical recordings (see Figure 36–2) as might be tested in a clinical setting, but more in examining the brain's responses as they are elicited with respect to a specific experimental event presentation (e.g., hearing a phonemic contrast). To do that, an offline analysis of the recorded data is performed to derive the event related potential (ERP) which is the average electrical activity correlated with the specific type of stimulus presentation. The analyses to derive the ERP responses begin with segmentation of the EEG recordings into epochs that are segments of time linked to the event

of interest, so that we get the brain responses only for the event of interest (the experimental condition). For example, if we are examining an individual's brain responses to English phonemic contrasts, and we are presenting two types of stimuli (/pa/ and /ba/), one standard step in analyzing the EEG data in this type of study is segmenting the EEG recordings that are linked to the presentation of the event of interest in the study, in this case the presentation of /pa/ and /ba/ as shown in Figure 36–3.

We also average the recorded segmented responses over all the different presentations for the same condition to derive the ERP.

There are several types of ERP components indicative of different cognitive processes. In this essay we will focus only on introducing the main correlates/ERP components associated with language.

MISMATCH NEGATIVITY (MMN)—PHONOLOGICAL REPRESENTATION AND PROCESSING CORRELATE

MMN refers to a negative preattentional frontocentral ERP component peaking around 150 to 250 milliseconds elicited by the presence of an *oddball* sound in a sequence of repetitive auditory stimuli. In the MMN task an automatic prediction of the central auditory system is violated, such as in presenting a deviant /ta/ within a train of a frequent stimulus /da, da, da, da/. Experimental studies reveal that the MMN component is associated with sensory-memory updating and change/rule violation detection (Näätänen, Kujala, & Winkler, 2010). Several studies revealed that MMN responses to deviants that constitute language-specific phonological contrasts were greater in native speakers of that language than in control participants who do not speak that particular language (for a review see

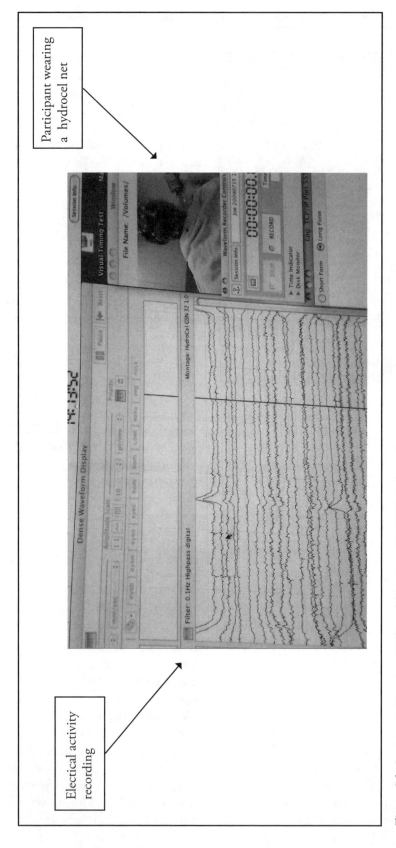

Participant wearing a hydrocel net

Electical activity recording

Figure 36–2. A participant in an EEG study wearing a HCGSN 32-channel net.

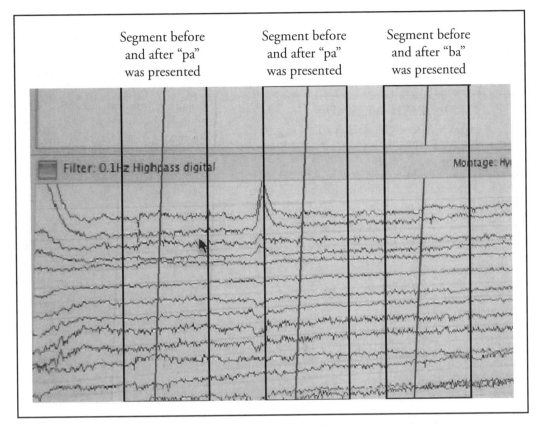

Segment before and after "pa" was presented

Segment before and after "pa" was presented

Segment before and after "ba" was presented

Filter: 0.1Hz Highpass digital

Montage: Hy

Figure 36–3. Data segmentation for /pa/ and /ba/.

Näätänen, Kujala, & Winkler, 2010). MMN is very commonly used in language studies due to its preattentional aspect, where MMN can be elicited while children are sleeping or watching a silent movie, as well as due to its robustness as a *phonological correlate.*

EARLY LEFT ANTERIOR NEGATIVITY (ELAN) AND P600: MORPHOSYNTACTIC CORRELATES

ELAN refers to an enhanced negativity over the left anterior brain regions, peaking around 100 to 200 ms after the onset of a syntactic phrase structure violation, indexing first-pass parsing processes (Hahne & Friederici, 1999). Another syntactic processing correlate is the P600, also referred to as LPC (Late Positive Complex). P600/LPC refers to a positivity detected over centroparietal regions around 500 msec after recognition of a syntactic anomaly (e.g. Friederici, Hahne, & Saddy, 2002). P600 can be elicited for several types of grammatical violations as well as for lexical codeswitching between L1 and L2 (Jackson, Swainson, Cunnington, & Jackson, 2001; Moreno, Federmeier, & Kutas, 2002), or between two language varieties in diglossic situations (e.g., Khamis-Dakwar & Froud, 2007). Hence, in addition to being considered as a correlate of grammatical processing, it is also considered to index reanalysis of syntactic and semantic information in situations carrying a high cognitive load, especially when it appears in conjunction with N400 effect (Bornkessel-Schlesewsky & Schlesewsky, 2008).

N400—LEXICAL AND SEMANTIC CORRELATE

N400 refers to a negativity detected over centroparietal regions around 400 ms after onset of a stimulus, and is considered to index lexical and semantic processing (Lau, Philips, & Poppel, 2008). It has been found to be sensitive to meaning manipulations and to the presentation of an unexpected word at both the word and sentence level in different modalities (e.g., spoken and written language), as well as with other kinds of anomalies, such as mismatches in phonology, or unexpected faces, color patches, and pictures (for a review see Kutas, Van Petten, & Kluender, 2006 or Lau et al., 2008).

CLINICALLY DRIVEN NEUROPHYSIOLOGIC STUDIES IN CSD AT THE NSLP LAB

There are only a few known clinically driven ERP investigations in CSD. Many of these studies have focused on examining the language representation and processing in a specific communication disorder such as dyslexia or stuttering (e.g., Cuadrado & Weber-Fox, 2003; Datta et al, 2010; McAnally & Stein, 1997; Weber-Fox & Hampton, 2008; Weber-Fox & Neville, 2001). Fewer studies have examined the brain changes occurring across time as language is acquired in a specific communication disorder or during the implementation of a specific treatment approach.

Building on the existing ERP research and the power of the ERP method for examining the different subprocesses of language pro-

cessing as indexed by the classic language ERP correlates, we argue that further incorporation of ERP studies in the field of CSD is beneficial. There is a need to expand ERP studies not only to enhance our understanding of the nature of specific communication disorders, but also to understand the course of language learning in specific communication disorders and the different SLP therapy effects.

Toward that end, the NSLP Lab in Adelphi University was established in 2008. As the director of the lab, part of my mission is to inform colleagues and students within the Adelphi University community about the ERP method and to encourage them to make use of the EEG system in the NSLP Lab to address their clinically based inquiries. Research at the NSLP Lab focuses on examining the neural underpinnings of language learning in specific sociolinguistic situations (such as Arabic diglossia), specific communication and language disorders (such as apraxia of speech), as well as during rehabilitation (such as in accent modification therapy) using event-related potentials (ERPs).

LEXICOSEMANTIC DEFICITS IN CHILDREN UNDERGOING INSULIN TREATMENT FOR DIABETES

Difficulties in vocabulary development have been reported in children with insulin-dependent diabetes mellitus (IDDM) (Northam, Anderson, Wether, Warne, Adler, & Andrewes, 1998). Using a word-picture semantic processing task, we examine differences in the brain responses of children with IDDM after initial and long-term exposure to insulin treatment. This study aims to clarify whether reported deficits in vocabulary development in this population reflect changes in neural organization for linguistic processing, which have potential clinical implications in terms of the need for preventive service delivery for children with diabetes, beginning at the earliest stages of insulin therapy.

LANGUAGE DEVELOPMENT IN CHILDREN WHO ARE INTERNATIONALLY ADOPTED (CWIA)

The effects of immersing an internationally adopted (IA) child in the new language of the environment (LE) whereas ceasing exposure to the language of adoption (LA, or first language), are not fully understood. A recent meta-analytic examination of language skills in CWIA revealed that IA children show poorer language performances during the school-age years (and beyond) as opposed to their nonadopted peers (Scott, Roberts, & Glennen, 2011). To evaluate whether later language difficulties might be related to differences in phonemic system organization, an investigation of auditory MMN responses from five CWIA (3–5 years old) adopted from China and exposed to LE for at least 2 years, and five matched nonadopted monolingual English-speaking children was conducted (Khamis-Dakwar & Scott, in preparation). Words were presented in a randomized order in passive listening oddball paradigms under three conditions: (1) Chinese only phonemic feature (/maai5/tone 5 (buy) & /maai6/tone 6 (sell), based on tonal differences present in Mandarin and not in English; (2) English-only phonemic feature not represented in Mandarin (/mad/ vs. /mat/); and (3) phonemic contrast evident in both languages (/mad/ and /man/). MMN was derived from 32-channel EEG recordings by averaging and montaging to frontocentral sensors and subtraction of averaged standard responses from averaged deviant responses within each condition.

Enhanced MMN responses were observed for tonal differences in CWIA children, but not for the control group. The English phonemic contrasts were associated with delayed MMN responses for the CWIA group, but not the control group. These preliminary findings reveal differences in the phonological representations in CWIA children that were not identifiable based on behavioral testing of language and phonological performance.

THERAPY EFFECTS

A growing body of anecdotal evidence reveals positive effects of using yoga in speech therapy with children and adults (see Kaley-Isley, Peterson, Fischer, & Peterson, 2010 for a review). Reported effectiveness of incorporating yoga intervention techniques in SLP treatment can be underlined by direct effect on the language processing system or indirect effect on general cognitive skills. In a pilot study, we examined the effects of yoga intervention using ERP on an 11-year-old child presenting with a language delay and ADHD. EEG data were recorded while the participating child was presented with two sets of stimuli in a picture-word paradigm while practicing a previously learned relaxation technique developed as a part of yoga-based therapy for that child. The first set of stimuli represented a congruous condition composed of 25 pairs of auditory word representations and matching picture presentations (congruous condition). The second stimuli set represented an incongruous condition in which 25 pairs of auditory words did not match the visual representation on a display (incongruous condition). The study findings reveal that the implementation of the yoga-based relaxation techniques during exposure to the lexical task was correlated with a P300 enhancement indexing attentional resource allocation, as compared with

ERP responses elicited from a child serving as a control participant (i.e., matched for typical language development for gender, age, socio-economic status, and region of residence). Viewed from a neurophysiologic perspective, these pilot results showing a P300 enhancement correlated with yoga therapy, rather than an N400 enhancement (an index of lexical processing) suggests that the reported positive effects of incorporating yoga for this child are likely due to general cognitive enhancement during linguistic processing.

CONCLUSION

Since the establishment of the NSLPlab, my mission has been to open the lab for colleagues and students to make use of ERP method to enhance their understanding of a specific clinical question of interest. My intention here has been to provide examples of studies developed and conducted in the lab in collaboration with colleagues and students that exemplify the power and range of potential benefits to be gained from incorporating the ERP method in CSD studies.

REFERENCES

Bornkessel-Schlesewsky, I., & Schlesewsky, M. (2008). An alternative perspective on "semantic P600" effects in language comprehension. *Brain Research Reviews, 59*(1), 55–73.

Cuadrado, E., & Weber-Fox, C. (2003). Atypical syntactic processing in individuals who stutter: Evidence from event-related brain potentials and behavioral measures. *Journal of Speech, Language, and Hearing Research, 46,* 960–976.

Datta H., Shafer, V. L , Morr, M. L., Kurtzberg, D., & Schwartz, R. G. (2010.) Brain discriminative responses to phonetically similar long

vowels in children with SLI. *Journal of Speech Language Hearing Sciences, 53*(3), 757–777.

Friederici, A. D. (2002).Towards a neural basis of auditory sentence processing. *Trends in Cognitive Science, 6,* 78–84.

Friederici, A. D., Hahne A., & Saddy, D. (2002). Distinct neurophysiological patterns reflecting aspects of syntactic complexity and syntactic repair. *Journal of Psycholinguistic Research, 31*(1), 45–63.

Hahne, A., & Friederici, A. D. (1999).Electrophysiological evidence for two steps in syntactic analysis:Early automatic and late controlled processes. *Journal of Cognitive Neuroscience, 11,* 194–205.

Jackson, G. M., Swainson, R., Mulin, A., Cunnington, R., & Jackson, S. R. (2004). ERP correlates of receptive language-switching tasks. *Quarterly Journal of Experimental Psychology, 57A*(2), 223–240.

Kaley-Isley, L. C., Peterson, J., Fischer, C., & Peterson, E. (2010). Yoga as a complementary therapy for children and adolescents: A guide for clinicians. *Psychiatry, 7*(8), 20–32.

Khamis-Dakwar, R., & Froud, K. (2007). Lexical processing in two language varieties: An event related brain potential study of Arabic native speakers. In Mughazy, M. (Ed.), *Perspectives on Arabic linguistics* (pp. 153–166). Amsterdam: John Benjamin.

Khamis-Dakwar, R., & Scott, K. *Neural correlates of language acquisition in internationally adopted children.* Poster presented at Cognitive Neuroscience Symposium. San Fransisco, April 2011.

Kutas, M., Van Petten, C., & Kluender, R. (2006). Psycholinguistics electrified II: 1994–2005. In M. Traxler & M. A. Gernsbacher (Eds.), *Handbook of psycholinguistics* (2nd ed., pp. 659–724). New York, NY: Elsevier.

Lau, E. F, Phillips, C., & Poeppel, D. (2008)A cortical network for semantics: (De)constructing the N400. *Nature Reviews Neuroscience, 9*(12), 920–933.

Luck, S.L. (2005). *An introduction to the event-related potential technique.* Cambridge MA: Massachusetts Institute of Technology.

McAnally, K. I., & Stein, J. F. (1997). Scalp potentials evoked by amplitude-modulated tones in dyslexia. *Journal of Speech, Language, and Hearing Research, 40,* 939–945.

Moreno, E. M., Federmeier, K. D., & Kutas, M. (2002). Switching languages, switching palabras (words): An electrophysiological study of code-switching. *Brain and Language, 80,* 188–207.

Näätänen , R., Kujala, T., & Winkler, I. (2010). Auditory processing that leads to conscious perception: A unique window to central auditory processing opened by the mismatch negativity and related responses. *Psychophysiology, 48,* 4–22.

Northam, E. A., Anderson, P. J., Wether, G. A., Warne, G. L., Adler, R. G., & Andrewes, D. (1998). Neuropsychological complications of IDDM in children 2 years after disease onset. *Diabetes Care, 21,* 379–384.

Rugg, M. D. (1997). *Cognitive neuroscience.* Hove, East Sussex, UK: Psychology Press.

Scott, K., Roberts, J. A., & Glennen, S.(2011). How well do children who are internationally adopted acquire language? A meta-analysis. *Journal of Speech, Language, and Hearing Research, 54,* 1153–1169.

Ward, J. (2010). *The student's guide to cognitive neuroscience.* Hove, East Sussex, UK: Psychology Press.

Weber-Fox, C., & Hampton, A. (2008). Stuttering and natural speech processing of semantic and syntactic constraints on verbs. *Journal of Speech, Language, and Hearing Research, 51*(5), 1058–1071.

Weber-Fox, C., & Neville, H. J. (2001). Sensitive periods differentiate processing for open and closed class words: An ERP study in bilinguals. *Journal of Speech, Language, and Hearing Research, 44,* 1338–1353.

ESSAY 37

An Acoustic Analysis of a Case of Amusia

Robert Goldfarb and Lawrence J. Raphael

Research in auditory processing at the cortical level has focused primarily on speech and language. There is a distinction between abilities to process musical information and segmental speech, such as consonants and vowels, but there is also a relationship between processing of music and intonation associated with speech prosody. Furthermore, there is a distinction between congenital amusia, also called tone deafness, and acquired amusia following brain damage. The 19th-century German anatomist, August Knoblauch, described nine disorders of perception and production of music, coining the term "amusia" (cited in Johnson & Graziano, 2003). Much of the subsequent research followed the case report format, with the purpose of localizing music in the brain. Although the etiology was occasionally musicogenic epilepsy (e.g., Bautista & Ciampetti, 2003; Sparr, 2003), most studies, including the present one, focused on cases of cerebrovascular accident, or stroke.

The question of cerebral localization, identifying which regions of the brain correspond or participate in the perception and production of music, is not resolved. Case reports of amusia following brain infarctions have implicated the following areas: anterior portion of bilateral temporal lobes (Satoh, Takeda, Murakami, Onouchi, Inoue, & Kuzuhara, 2005); right frontoparietal cortex, cerebellum, and lenticular nucleus of the right hemisphere (Nicholson, Baum, Kilgour, Koh, Munhall, & Cuddy, 2003); bilateral temporoparietal region (Tanaka, Yamadori, & Mori, 1987); and focal lesion in the left superior temporal gyrus (Piccirilli, Sciarma, & Luzzi, 2000). This last report is somewhat unusual, in that the subject was not a professional musician. Left-hemisphere damage resulting in amusia was often reported in case reports of musicians (e. g., Hofman, Klein, & Arlazoff, 1993; Mavlov, 1980); early reports proposed both language and music representation in the left hemisphere (Tzortzis, Goldblum, Dang, Forette, & Boller, 2000).

There are several oversimplifications in the literature regarding amusia, which may be summarized as follows: Presence or absence of aphasia or agnosia; site of lesion in the right or left hemisphere; and specific areas of damage in either or both hemispheres do not predict presence, type, or severity of amusia (Brust, 1980). Amusia is neither associated with musical naiveté following right-hemisphere damage (RHD), nor with musical sophistication following LHD; there is no shift from right to left hemispheres as a function of increase in musical sophistication. Language dominance does not determine receptive amusia (purportedly following damage to language-dominant temporal lobe) versus expressive amusia (purportedly following damage to nondominant frontal lobe).

Neurological examinations of amusia included CT scan (Nicholson et al., 2003; Tzortzis, et al., 2000), and fMRI (Nakada, Fujii, Suzuki, & Kwee, 1998). Another technique used to identify cognitive strategies for processing melodic and temporal musical information is Musical Instrument Digital Interface (MIDI). MIDI acts much like a player piano roll, used to specify the actions of a synthesizer, whereas the tone or effect is generated by the instrument itself. Schuppert, Munte, Wieringa, and Altenmüller (2000) used MIDI to determine melodic and temporal processing deficits in their participants with brain damage. More than two-thirds of participants showed impairments; those with LHD had significant deficits in both melodic and temporal processing, whereas those with RHD had significant deficits in the temporal conditions. Finally, brain potentials may identify auditory cortical processing. Munte, Schuppert, Johannes, Wieringa, Kohimetz, and Altenmüller (1998) used P300 event-related potentials (ERPs) to evaluate 12 poststroke patients, half of whom had amusia. The P300 is elicited when a participant detects infrequent stimuli presented in a series of frequent stimuli (P3b), but also when a participant does not detect and only listens passively to infrequent stimuli (P3a). Although the P3a has front-central scalp maximum and a short latency, the P3b has parietal scalp maximum and a long latency. The authors reported that patients with amusia had a significant decrement in amplitude for P3a, relative to controls, and patients without amusia had an impairment of early stimulus evaluation. The P3b was reduced for both patient groups, relative to controls.

The lack of agreement among brain researchers suggests a paradigm shift may be necessary for a deeper understanding of amusia. In the present essay, we report results of acoustic analysis to measure temporal aspects of the piano recordings of James P. Johnson, pre- and poststroke.

JAMES P. JOHNSON

James P. Johnson, born February 1, 1894, died November 17, 1955 (according to Queens General Hospital; date is contested), was known as the "Father of Stride Piano," a style which bridged ragtime and jazz. As a composer and accompanist in more than 400 recordings, he is best known for his era-defining song, "The Charleston," in the 1920s. Harlem Stride Piano style required the left hand to make rapid octave runs and jumps, and the right to sweep half the keyboard. Johnson's compositions and musicianship served as a link between the ragtime of Scott Joplin and the jazz of Duke Ellington and Thelonius Monk. Ellington considered his mastery of the technically challenging étude, "Carolina Shout," to be equivalent to a semester in a conservatory.

Johnson's discography runs from August 1921 in New York through September 1949 in Los Angeles. According to the only published full-length biography (Brown, 1984), Johnson suffered a mild stroke (possibly a transient ischemic attack or TIA) in 1940. The physical symptoms of a TIA tend to be reversible, and there are no reports that Johnson exhibited any hemiparesis. He resumed public appearances in the early 1940s, but his performance style was reportedly less clean and precise. Johnson began using a drummer for songs previously recorded as solo piano pieces, presumably to help him maintain rhythm. There are gaps in Johnson's discography from 6/47 through 8/49, and one may speculate that he had a second TIA or cerebrovascular accident during this time.

ACOUSTIC ANALYSIS

The selections were recorded digitally into the CSL, model 4500, at a sampling rate of 11,025 Hz. Wideband spectrograms (bandwidth: 323 Hz.) were made of equivalent portions of the pre- and poststroke recordings. Figure 37–1 is a composite of two pictures (waveform and time-linked spectrogram). The time elapsed between Johnson's left-hand beats (indicated by the distance between the vertical lines in Figure 37–1) was measured for sequences of at least 10 consecutive beats. Standard deviations of Johnson's timings were calculated for both the pre- and poststroke recordings and are displayed in Table 37–1.

Acoustic analysis of pre- and poststroke recordings of the same compositions (see Table 37–1) yielded much larger standard deviations after the strokes. In other words, Johnson was rhythmically more variable in his poststroke recordings. There were, respectively, 28, 20, 32, and 36 data points in the analyses of the *Keep Off the Grass, Carolina Shout, You've Got to Be Modernistic,* and *Jingles*. We attempted to analyze "identical" passages from the pre- and post-stroke recordings; but Johnson was an improviser, and it is doubtful that anything he played came out exactly the same way in any two versions. They are equivalent, if not identical.

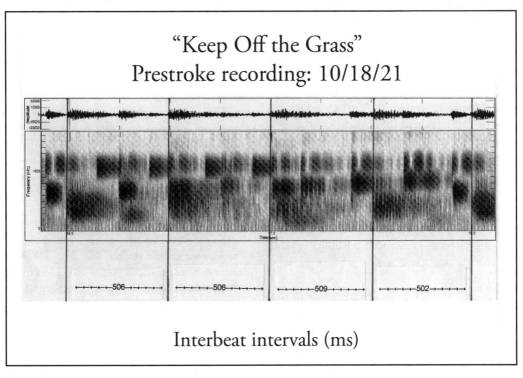

Figure 37–1. Waveform and time-linked spectrogram.

Table 37–1. Analyses of Pre- and Poststroke Recordings of the Same Compositions

Composition	Standard Deviations (ms.)	
	Prestroke Recordings	*Poststroke Recordings*
Keep Off the Grass	+/– 6.4	+/– 13.2
Carolina Shout	+/– 12.0	+/– 39.8
You've Got to Be Modernistic	+/– 18.7	+/– 35.3
Jingles	+/– 8.7	+/– 24.2

DISCUSSION

There currently is no adequate theoretical explanation for the occurrence of amusia. Proposed etiologies for the condition have ranged from frontotemporal dementia, in the case of Maurice Ravel, to brain tumor (George Gershwin), to cerebrovascular accidents (James P. Johnson). In addition, the wildly diverging points of view regarding brain centers responsible for musical ability indicates that a behavioral approach to the study of the disorder may be more fruitful than a neuropathological one. We suggest acoustic analysis of musical recordings may be a strategy for increasing our understanding of this complex and perplexing disorder.

In the present analysis, we investigated only the temporal aspects of Johnson's playing. Although it would have been possible to examine the melodic contours using narrowband spectrograms or an f-zero contour, we have not yet attempted such an analysis because of our current focus on timing and rhythm. Future studies of amusia may consider another measure, for pitch intervals, which is not subject to acoustic analysis, and also seems to fall outside the limited scope of this essay.

REFERENCES

Bautista, R., & Ciampetti, M. (2003). Expressive aprosody and amusia as a manifestation of right hemisphere seizures. *Epilepsia, 44,* 1128–1157.

Brown, S. (1984). *A case of mistaken Identity: The life and music of James P. Johnson.* Institute of Jazz Studies, Rutgers University. Lanham, MD: Scarecrow Press.

Brust, J. (1980). Music and language: Musical alexia and agraphia. *Brain, 103,* 367–392.

Hofman, S., Klein, C., & Arlazoroff, A. (1993). Common hemisphericity of language and music in a musician. A case report. *Journal of Communication Disorders, 26,* 73–82.

Johnson, J., & Graziano, A. (2003). August Knoblauch and amusia: A nineteenth-century cognitive model of music. *Brain and Cognition, 51,* 102–114.

Mavlov, L. (1980). Amusia due to rhythm agnosia in a musician with left hemisphere damage: A non-auditory supramodal defect. *Cortex, 16,* 331–338.

Munte, T., Schuppert, M., Johannes, S., Wieringa, B., Kohimetz, C., & Altenmüller, E. (1998). Brain potentials in patients with music perception deficits: Evidence for an early locus. *Neuroscience Letters, 256,* 85–88.

Nakada, T., Fujii, Y., Suzuki, K., & Kwee, I. (1998). "Musical brain" revealed by high-field (3 tesla) functional MRI. *NeuroReport, 9,* 3853–3856.

Nicholson, K., Baum, S., Kilgour, A., Koh, C., Munhall, K., & Cuddy, L. (2003). Impaired processing of prosodic and musical patterns after right hemisphere damage. *Brain and Cognition, 52,* 382–389.

Piccirilli, M., Sciarma, T., & Luzzi, S. (2000). Modularity of music: Evidence from a case of pure amusia. *Journal of Neurology, Neurosurgery, and Psychiatry, 69,* 541–545.

Satoh, M., Takeda, K., Murakami, Y., Onouchi, K., Inoue, K., & Kuzuhara, S. (2005). A case of amusia caused by the infarction of anterior portion of bilateral temporal lobes. *Cortex, 41,* 77–83.

Schuppert, M., Munte, T., Wieringa, B., & Altenmüller, E. (2000). Receptive amusia: Evidence for cross-hemispheric neural networks underlying music processing strategies. *Brain, 123,* 546–559.

Sparr, S. (2003). Amusia and musicogenic epilepsy. *Current Neurology and Neuroscience Reports, 3,* 502–507.

Tanaka, Y., Yamadori, A., & Mori, E. (1987). Pure word deafness following bilateral lesions: A psychophysical analysis. *Brain, 110,* 381–403.

Tzortzis, C., Goldblum, M-C., Dang, M., Forette, F., & Boller, F. (2000). Absence of amusia and preserved naming of musical instruments in an aphasic composer. *Cortex, 36,* 227–242.

ESSAY 38

Birdsong and Human Speech and Language

What the Zebra Finch Uses, Loses, and Regains

Leonard L. LaPointe, Frank Johnson, Malcolm R. McNeil, and Sheila Pratt

Sadanand Singh traveled a mighty journey from Bihar, India. His contributions to our field are magnanimous and continuing, and have been at the levels of academics, publishing, and philanthropy. In the spirit of the Hindu proverb, he has indeed "used his wealth, his thought, and his speech to advance the good of others." Those others have been all of us who toil in the vineyards of communication science and disorders.

I knew Sadanand Singh as a close friend and colleague. I first met him at a conference in Buenos Aires. We became fast friends and toiled together through three publishing houses and through tragedies and laughter and not a few good bottles of Bordeaux. We rode wild horses in the mountains of India, explored the Taj Mahal in bare feet, and enjoyed fish curry on the beaches of the Arabian Sea in Goa. I miss him every day.

—LLL

INTRODUCTION

How similar is birdsong learning to human speech and language acquisition? Can destabilized birdsong inform us about recovery of speech and language in humans? When birds have an impairment of learned song motifs because of brain damage, how do they recover it? Do they lose the individual notes or syllables? Do they lose the order or the syntax of notes in the song? Is their destabilized singing characterized by imprecise movements in attempts to produce notes? How long does it take for a bird to recover his song to its presurgical state? Does destabilized birdsong relate to neurologically destabilized speech and language in humans? Would birds be a viable animal model for manipulations or interventions that could alter the quantity and quality of recovery? What are the limitations of a bird-song-human language analogy?

These are questions that have piqued our curiosity about similarities and differences between the tuneful noises that birds generate and the communicative audible patterns of sound that humans produce. A group of us at Florida State University and the University of Pittsburgh have been pondering these issues for several years. Our initial findings are more than mildly interesting and cautiously encouraging. Perhaps an animal model of dissolution and recovery of birdsong would allow us to explore a variety of intrinsic (neural) and extrinsic (social and facilitative) manipulations that might inform us about correlates in human communication recovery after brain damage.

BIRDS AND HUMANS

Speech has long been thought of as a uniquely defining characteristic of humans. Yet songbirds, like humans, communicate using learned signals (song, speech) that are acquired from their parents by a process of vocal imitation. Both song and speech begin as amorphous vocalizations (subsong, babble) that are gradually transformed into an individualized version of the parent's speech, including dialects (Ziegler & Marler, 2008).

Species-specific vocal production represents one of many strategies by which organisms communicate. Only a few (including oscine passerines and humans) develop their vocal behavior through experience against the backdrop of time-sensitive sensory and motor experiences (Goldstein, King, & West, 2003). Human speech and birdsong have numerous rather striking parallels. Both humans and songbirds learn their complex vocalizations

early in life, exhibiting a powerful dependence on hearing the adults they will imitate, as well as themselves as they practice, and a fading of this dependence as they develop and become more proficient and practiced in their emissions (Kuhl, 2003). As pointed out by Berwick et al. (2011) unlike our primate relatives, many species of bird share with humans this significant capacity for vocal learning, a crucial factor in speech acquisition. Striking and perhaps unexpected behavioral, neural and genetic similarities exist between auditory-vocal learning in birds and human infants. Only relatively recently have the linguistic parallels between birdsong and spoken human language begun to be investigated. Although both birdsong and human language are hierarchically organized according to particular syntactic constraints, birdsong structure is best characterized as "phonological syntax," resembling aspects of human sound structure (Berwick et al., 2011). Crucially, birdsong for the most part, lacks semantics and words except for the "Polly wants a cracker" learned mimical repetitions of some bird species. Formal language and linguistic analysis remains an essential comparative endeavor in linguistic analyses of birdsong and a bone of contention as to the relevance of comparative investigations of human language and birdsong. Figure 38–1 presents the time line of zebra finch song acquisition. The condensed time of crystallized song acquisition, along with the compressed time of recovery of destabilized birdsong presents a unique opportunity to explore characteristics of acquisition, impairment, and recovery of learned vocalizations.

Birdsong as a model system for human speech and language may not be perfect for the study of the brain and cognitive evolution, but the model lends itself to manipulations that are ethically unavailable to investigations of dissolution and recovery of linguistic structures in humans.

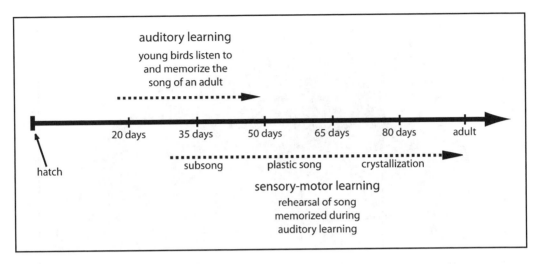

Figure 38–1. Time line of zebra finch song acquisition.

In birdsong, individual notes can be combined as particular and meaningful sequences into syllables, syllables into "motifs," and motifs into complete song "bouts." Birdsong thus can be characterized and described as a number of chains of discrete acoustic elements arranged in a specific temporal order. In the zebra finch, these songs consist of fixed sequences with only sporadic variations. In other bird species (e.g., nightingales, starlings, or Bengalese finches), more variable sequences may be generated where a song element might be followed by several alternatives, with overall song structure describable and somewhat predictable by probabilistic rules between a finite number of factors (Berwick et al., 2011).

Neural Similarities

In the past few decades, scientists have learned that the basis of much of what was previously understood about bird brains, that they were largely comprised of the most primitive and instinctual of brain structures, was not completely correct. Perhaps 75% of the brains of parrots, hummingbirds, and thousands of other species of songbirds are actually made up of a sophisticated information processing system that works in many of the same ways as does the cortex and basal ganglia networks of humans (Jarvis et al., 2005; Nixdorf-Weiberger & Bischof, 2007; Ziegler & Marler, 2008).

Different orders of birds have evolved networks of brain regions for song learning and production that have a surprisingly similar gross anatomy. These networks of song acquisition and production have invited analogies to human cortical regions and basal ganglia. Comparisons between different songbird species and humans seem to indicate both general and species-specific principles of vocal learning and have acknowledged common neural and molecular substrates, including the forkhead box P2 (*FOXP2*) gene (Bulhuis, Okanoya, & Scharff, 2010).

Figure 38–2 depicts a sagittal view of the zebra finch brain and highlights major components of the vocal-motor circuit. Song is produced by two premotor streams that convey stereotyped and variable patterns of neural activity. The two pathways converge on a common output that ultimately controls the vocal and respiratory musculature.

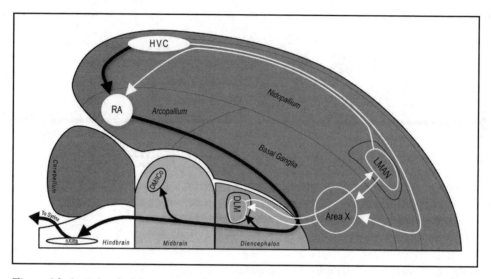

Figure 38–2. *Zebra finch brain. Sagittal view showing major components of the vocal-motor circuit. All regions and connections are bilateral and anatomically symmetric. Abbreviations: HVC, acronym is proper name; RA, robust nucleus of the arcopallium; LMAN, lateral magnocellular nucleus of the anterior nidopallium; Area X, Area X of the avian basal ganglia; DLM, medial dorsolateral nucleus of the thalamus; nXIIts, tracheosyringeal portion of the hypoglossal nucleus.*

Adult songs are therefore vocal composites that reflect the integrated activity of two contrasting premotor streams: one that drives the learned song pattern and one that can drive quite variable sequences of vocal sounds. This latter pathway plays a key role in vocal exploration during juvenile learning (Aronov et al. 2008, Thompson et al. 2011) but also enables vocal plasticity in adulthood (Tumer & Brainard, 2007; Andalman & Fee 2008). The centers in the nido- and arcopallium (HVC, LMAN, RA) are generally analogous to cortical structures in the human brain, and Area X and DLM are homologous to basal ganglia and thalamic structures, respectively. Note that both pathways originate anatomically from within HVC (a telencephalic nucleus located at the dorsal most aspect of the caudal nidopallium) and terminate in RA. The nidopallium, meaning nested pallium (no pun intended), is the region of the avian brain that is used mostly for some types of executive

functions but also other higher cognitive tasks. The region was renamed nidopallium in 2002 during the Avian Brain Nomenclature Consortium because the prior name (neostriatum) suggested that the region was used for more primitive functions as does the subcortical neostriatum in mammalian brains. Projection neurons from RA provide the primary vocal/motor output of the telencephalon, activating populations of hindbrain motor neurons that control muscle groups involved in respiration and the production of vocal sounds from the avian sound generator, the syrinx.

ZEBRA FINCH SONG ACQUISITION

One unique vocal learning birdsong exemplar is the zebra finch (*Taeniopygia guttata*, family *Estrildidae*, suborder *Oscines*, order *Pas-*

seriformes). The process of vocal learning in zebra finches demonstrates some remarkable similarities to language acquisition in human infants. Zebra finch song learning occurs during two overlapping phases: auditory learning (posthatch days 20 to 50) and sensorimotor integration (posthatch days 35 to 80). During auditory learning, the juvenile bird attends to and memorizes a tutor (male) vocal pattern, followed by a sensory-integration phase where the bird practices singing, similar to the babble stage of human speech-language acquisition, and gradually modifies output toward a stabilized pattern. Zebra finch song is composed of one to several short, introductory or call notes, followed by 4 to 7 individually distinct and more complex "syllables" or note complexes, which are typically produced without repetition and in a fixed sequence. This comprises the songbird's "motif," which can be sung one to several times in rapid succession (referred to earlier as a song "bout"). After puberty, there is very little change in the acoustic structure of individual notes, but occasional variation in note number and sequence persists (Brainard & Doupe, 2001; Glaze & Troyer, 2006; Kirn, 2010; Lombardino & Nottebohm, 2000; Nordeen & Nordeen, 1992, 1993; Williams, 2004, 2008).

Parallels to the evolution, acquisition, and characteristics of birdsong and human communication have been drawn by numerous researchers (Doupe & Kuhl, 1999; Jarvis, 2004; Kuhl, 2003; Miller et al., 2008; Pytte & Suthers, 2000; Saito & Maekawa, 1993). Furthermore, it has recently been reported that similar to human speech, adult birdsong is maintained by error correction (Sober & Brainard, 2009). These researchers perturbed the pitch (fundamental frequency) of auditory feedback in adult finches using custom-designed headphones. Birds compensated for the imposed auditory error by adjusting the pitch of song. When the perturbation was

removed, pitch returned to baseline. These results suggest that adult birds correct vocal errors by comparing auditory feedback to a sensory target and seem to indicate that life-long error correction is a general principle of learned vocal behavior. Similar adjustments to pitch-shifted auditory feedback have been documented in humans as well (Bauer & Larson, 2003; Sivasankar, Bauer, Babu, & Larson, 2005).

Also interesting is the recent research with birdsong that has manipulated the characteristics of tutor song. How well a songbird learns a song appears to depend on the formation of a robust auditory template of its tutor's song. Using functional magnetic resonance neuroimaging, Voss, Salgado-Commisariat, and Helakar (2010) examined auditory responses in two groups of zebra finches that differed in the type of songs they learned after being tutored by birds producing stuttering-like syllable repetitions in their songs. Birds that learned to produce the stuttered syntax showed attenuated blood oxygenation level-dependent (BOLD) responses to tutor's song, when compared to birds that produced normal song. The production of variant songs with stuttered syllables has important implications for the further study of dysfluency, phonetic-phonological aberrations, and perhaps linguistic disturbances in humans.

Despite increasing attention to comparative cognitive ethology, very little attention has been paid to parallels that may or may not exist in the dissolution and recovery patterns of communication in human and non-human vocal learners. A recent issue of *Brain and Language* (2010) was devoted to the consideration of comparative issues of birdsong and human language. As the editors who introduced this special issue stated, the issue was devoted to a consideration of birdsong and its potential relevance to human speech and language. Commentaries by two eminent pioneers in the field of birdsong research (Konishi, Notte-bohm) were featured. The primary aim of the special issue was to provide researchers who study human language with a current over-view of the state of research on vocal learn-ing and behavior in songbirds; to help build appropriate links; and to identify important limitations when relating birdsong research to human speech and language. The issue was well seasoned with caution and emphasized that definitive comparative conclusions were imperfect at this time, but that we appear to be on a threshold of a thoughtful consider-ation of possible links between birdsong and language, and more generally, to the potential utility of a comparative approach to the neu-robiology of communicative systems.

An animal model of dissolution and recovery of verbal learning might allow the generation of hypotheses regarding intrinsic and extrinsic factors that could affect both acquisition and recovery patterns of learned verbal patterns. As White (2009) has indicated, future work in songbirds will rely on increas-ingly sophisticated technologies for altering gene expression with temporal and anatomic precision during phases of song development. This could help clarify as well as refine our understanding of song control circuitry and consequences of destabilization. Furthermore, these advances might allow testing functional consequences on song learning and mainte-nance, and we would add, on recovery patterns after dissolution. As this technology becomes routine, it will be important to make specific hypotheses about how song might be altered, and to provide data from outside song control areas to determine whether disruption within song control regions specifically affects only song, or causes general disruption of com-mon neuronal function. Perhaps as interest-ing would be the potential to determine the interrelationships of extrinsic variables, such as practice, re-exposure to tutors, or ambi-

ent stimulus environment with these intrin-sic genetic manipulations. Another tempting investigative pathway that a viable animal model would offer would be the potential to explore and manipulate variables that influ-ence neurogenesis and neuroplasticity. These potential biologic and environmental interac-tions make an even more compelling case for the attempt to clarify patterns of dissolution and recovery of verbal learning in songbirds.

BIRDSONG DESTABILIZATION AND RECOVERY

The birdsong laboratory in the Program in Neuroscience at Florida State University has a research agenda that includes systematic ablation of discrete, interconnected telence-phalic nuclei underlying vocal learning and production of the zebra finch (Thompson & Johnson, 2007, Thompson, Wu, Bertram, & Johnson, 2007). Of particular interest to us is the trajectory of disruption and subsequent recovery of song patterns (5 to 8 days). The nature of paradigmatic (syllables, notes, or units of meaning) and syntagmatic (order or sequence) changes that characterize postsurgi-cal destabilization and recovery of zebra finch song and how these changes might compare to human language dissolution and recovery are in need of examination for their poten-tial to inform processes in human speech. We have begun a preliminary investigation of the destabilization of elements of birdsong in the zebra finch along with its postsurgical recovery patterns in an attempt to foster understanding of these patterns of birdsong use and recovery. After description of the methods and nature of birdsong destabilization and recovery we dis-cuss possible implications for human speech-language loss and recovery.

METHODS

Surgical Manipulation and Audio-Recording

Complete details of experimental manipulations can be found in Thompson & Johnson 2007, Thompson et al., 2007, and Thompson et al., 2011. Briefly, our experimental manipulations focus on HVC (see Figure 38–2). The HVC contains neural populations that sequence the rigid temporal structure of the zebra finch song pattern (Hahnloser et al., 2002; Long & Fee, 2008). In this regard, there may be a partial functional resemblance between songbird HVC and vocal premotor cortical regions in humans (e.g., Broca's area). Under deep anesthesia, an electrolytic stereotaxic surgical procedure is used to produce targeted partial ablation (~10% by volume, microlesion) within HVC bilaterally. The HVC contains three subpopulations of neurons (those that project to RA, those that project to Area X, interneurons) that are arranged in a mosaic, and microlesions therefore produce proportional damage across the three populations.

For purposes of audio recording, adult male zebra finches are housed individually for the duration of each experiment in acoustic isolation chambers where environmental conditions (ventilation, ambient temperature, photoperiod) are monitored and maintained at constant values by computer control. Housed under these conditions, adult male zebra finches produce hundreds of song bouts each day (termed "undirected" because no conspecific is present), which are captured by a microphone and a computer running sound event-triggered recording software. In this way, the totality of each bird's vocal output can be captured and measured over the course of an experiment.

Syllable Identification

A semiautomated procedure is used to isolate sound files that contain singing from sound files that captured only calls and/or other noises made by birds (e.g., wing flaps, beak wipes). Details of this procedure are available in Wu et al. (2008). Sound Analysis Pro (SA+) software (Version 1.04, Tchernichovski et al., 2000) is then used to measure the duration and spectral properties of each syllable produced prior to and following the surgical manipulation. After a thresholding step where a specific amplitude value is used to determine the start and stop of each syllable as it is produced preoperatively, all subsequent singing is measured relative to the preoperative acoustic structure of each syllable in each bird's vocal pattern. The sequence of syllables produced is preserved during this process, allowing measurement of the temporal organization of the syllable pattern.

The SA+ measurement of each syllable produced on each day of singing includes duration (in ms) and four spectral features: **pitch** (a measure of the frequency structure of sound), **FM** (a measure of frequency change in the temporal structure of sound), **entropy** (a measure of the nonharmonicity or "noisiness" of sound), and **pitch goodness** (a measure of the harmonic structure of sound). The SA+ calculates these spectral features as mean values for each syllable using an FFT window of 9.27 ms and a window advance of 1.36 ms. Pitch, FM, entropy, and pitch goodness were selected because songbirds demonstrate the ability to make behavioral discriminations in response to variation in all four of these spectral features and because these four features are sufficient to effectively individuate zebra finch syllables.

For each day of singing, the duration and spectral feature values for each syllable are used to create four scatter plots. Within these plots, each data point represents a single syllable and thus discrete clusters of data points signify repeated instances of a specific syllable type. Figure 38–3 shows an example of typical preoperative singing, where five distinct syllable clusters are generated by a bird with a five-syllable song: the clustering is most evident in the scatter plot for entropy, which was then used to identify the syllables in the three other scatter plots.

Two-Dimensional Statistical Characterization of Song Phonology

Scatter plots allow the comparison of large sets of syllables to determine the rate (rapid or gradual) and structure (degradation or cohesion) of changes to the vocal pattern over time. To track changes in the vocal pattern of each bird, feature scatter plots are treated as random samples from a two-dimensional probability distribution and compared to one another; this allows use of the Kullback-Leibler (K–L) distance, a powerful tool for comparing two probability distributions (Wu, Bertram, Thompson, & Johnson, 2008). The K–L distance is expressed in units of bits, with values near 0 indicating a high degree of similarity (as is measured when two pre-operative days of singing are compared) and values of 4 to 6 bits indicating a large difference (as is measured when a day of destabilized singing is compared to a day of preoperative singing). Together, use of these quantitative and statis-

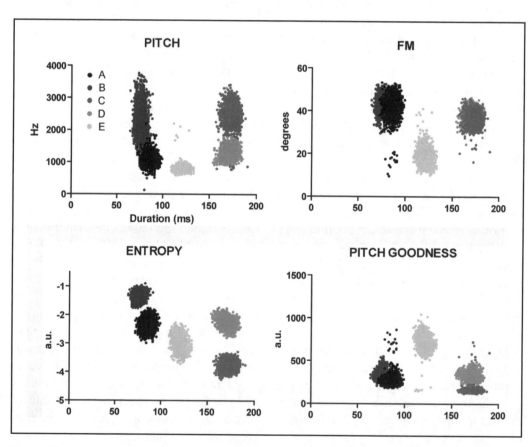

Figure 38–3. Duration x spectral feature scatter plots of normal zebra finch song.

tical approaches provides an objective means by which to measure change in the acoustic structure of birdsong.

CHARACTERISTICS OF VOCAL DESTABILIZATION AND RECOVERY

Figure 38–4 depicts acoustic spectrogram exemplars across conditions of pre- and post-

HVC microlesion surgery from an individual bird. Panels A and D of this figure represent preoperative and recovered acoustic birdsong spectrograms, whereas panel B is the first utterance postoperatively, and C represents recovering vocalization. Following HVC microlesions an obvious loss of vocal patterning is evident and the unstructured sequences of sound are in some ways reminiscent of the babbling phase (subsong) of juvenile bird. Destabilized motifs are still produced in the context of discrete bouts and bouts still begin with the

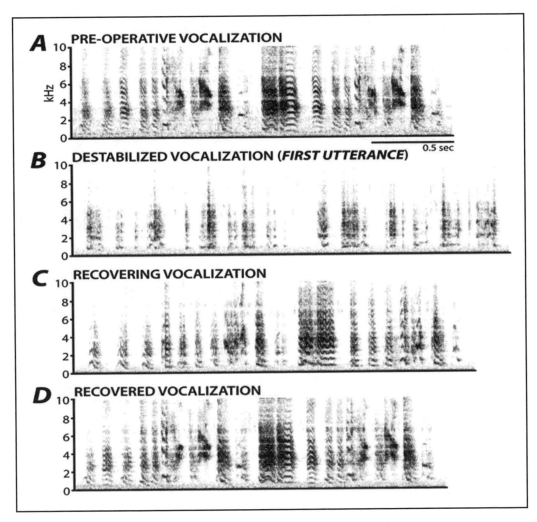

Figure 38–4. Exemplar preoperative and postoperative vocalization spectrograms for a single bird following HVC microlesions.

production of introductory notes, although introductory notes appear to be generated at a slower rate. Thus, although HVC microlesions may have had some effect on the underlying mechanisms that drive the initiation of a song bout, microlesion effects on syllable and motif structure were more pronounced. In all birds, vocal patterning recovers gradually over the course of several days despite the loss of approximately 10% of the HVC neural population. It should be noted, however, that vocal recovery is not always complete in all birds (see Figure 38–6, below).

Because birds were maintained in complete social isolation for the duration of the experiment, only "undirected" (i.e., not directed toward a female) songs were recorded and used for analysis. It is unknown if the

presence of a female and the production of female-directed song during the first few days following surgery might have prevented or lessened the severity of the destabilization, but this extrinsic manipulation falls into the category of potential future experimental manipulations that might be carried out to explore factors in birdsong recovery.

Figure 38–5 illustrates the transition from selected individual spectrograms of singing to quantitative scatter plot analysis of the spectral and sequential properties of song measured across whole days of singing. In this example, measurement of destabilization and recovery is shown by comparing duration x pitch scatter plots. Statistical comparison of any day of presinging against singing produced on Post Day 1 produces K–L distances values between

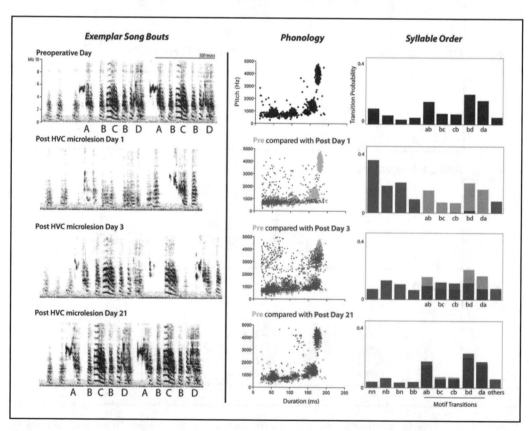

Figure 38–5. Examples of pre- and postoperative spectrograms and scatterplots for bird 611.

4 and 5 bits, whereas the same comparison on Post Day 21 produces values that are near 0 bits. Similarly, there is a near-complete loss of normal syllable ordering at Post Day 1 that has also recovered at Post Day 21.

Recovery Time

Although all birds that received HVC microlesions demonstrated a similar level of motif destabilization and recovery, an analysis of hour by hour change in several acoustic features (pitch, FM, and entropy) revealed that motif recovery could be surprisingly rapid in some birds (within 3 days). In the initial study (Thompson & Johnson, 2007) we concluded that:

a. bilateral HVC microlesions in adult male zebra finches destabilized song motifs;

b. motif impairment was surprisingly short-lived as all HVCml birds recovered most aspects of vocal stereotypy within a 2-week postoperative period; and,

c. an hourly analysis of recovery in selected birds indicated that this recovery could occur within 3 days.

Whereas the death of RA-projecting neurons in HVC can trigger a subsequent increase in their incorporation into HVC by a process of neurogenesis (Scharff et al., 2000), the available data suggest that this is a process that requires at least 2 to 3 weeks (Kirn et al., 1999). Therefore, a rapid lesion-induced remodeling of synaptic connectivity within the song control system (cf. Kittelberger & Mooney, 1999) would seem a more likely candidate for mediation of the vocal recovery that we observed. However, whatever the exact nature of the underlying processes of recovery, these processes appear to depend on auditory feedback. When birds are deafened (via bilateral cochlea removal) following HVC microlesions they are unable to recover their pre-operative motif, and persist in the production of relatively unpatterned sequences of unstructured syllables (Thompson et al., 2007).

The programmatic research ongoing at the Florida State University Birdsong Laboratory has afforded a relatively clear picture of the course of surgical destabilization and subsequent recovery of the zebra finch birdsong. Representative documentations of the results of surgical destabilization and recovery can be found in the *Journal of Neurobiology* (Thompson & Johnson, 2007) as well as in the *Journal of Neuroscience* (Thompson, Johnson, Wu, & Bertram, 2007; Thompson et al., 2011). As detailed in these publications, maintenance of stable vocal patterns (motifs) in adult male zebra finches depends on an integrated forebrain neural network that appears to include distinct pathways for stereotypy and plasticity of vocal production, including the important centers and pathways of zebra finch brain labeled the HVC and LMAN.

DESTABILIZED SONG FOLLOWING LESIONS TO MULTIPLE SONG CONTROL REGIONS

Quantitative analysis of the destabilized vocalizations of birds that received HVC microlesions revealed pervasive effects on the structure of song motifs including decreased acoustic and temporal similarity to preoperative motifs and increased variation in the acoustic and temporal structure of motifs. This suggested that the vocal effects of HVC microlesions may not be due entirely to damage to HVC, but rather a direct or indirect amplification of the highly variable stream of premotor neural activity that is normally conveyed by LMAN to RA (Olveckzy et al., 2005, see Figure 2).

If so, we hypothesized that the destabilizing effects of HVC microlesions might be mitigated or reduced in the absence of LMAN. This hypothesis appears to be confirmed by the data. When HVC microlesions were made in birds that received prior ablation of LMAN only relatively minor effects on syllable spectral quality were observed and vocal patterning remained intact on the first day of postoperative singing (Thompson & Johnson, 2007). Similarly, when HVC microlesions were followed by LMAN ablation a sudden (1 to 2 day) recovery of the vocal pattern was observed, as soon as the first postoperative utterance in some birds (Thompson et al., 2007). Even though syllable spectral quality did not completely return to preoperative levels in all birds, there was still significant improvement over a far more rapid course of recovery. As the only vocal deficit that we were able to detect in birds that received both HVC microlesions and LMAN ablation, degraded syllable spectral quality could be a product of HVC damage alone.

MOTIF SYLLABLES PRE- AND POSTOPERATIVELY

One of the questions that intrigued us at the initiation of this research related to the features of birdsong that were destabilized and recovered. Do zebra finches lose the precision, clarity, or sequencing of their note or syllable productions? Are birdsong motifs characterized by omission or addition of notes or syllables? The neurolinguistic features of paradigmatic or lexical-semantic disruption of song as opposed to syntagmatic or sequencing would appear to be an intriguing level of analysis. Our working hypotheses prior to more fine-tuned acoustic analysis centered on expectations that the disruptions would be characterized by altered precision, durations,

or sequencing of syllables (notes) within the zebra finch motifs.

Paradigmatic Disruption

One of the findings that has surprised us is the characteristic of syllable omission and commission during the postoperative destabilization and recovery phase of birdsong. Destabilized birds apparently have difficulty producing their limited repertoire of syllables or notes immediately postsurgically as well as during the recovery phase. Figure 38–6 presents percentage of total syllables produced by bird 560 plotted against a 12-day course of recovery. We include bird 560 here as one of the more dramatic examples of incomplete vocal recovery that we have observed following HVC microlesions. The syllables in this bird's repertoire (A, B, C, and D) can be seen to be relatively invariant during the two preoperative recorded sessions Pre1 and Pre2. However, during the postsurgical sessions, the large corpus of destabilized zebra finch productions are characterized by omitted syllables and the surprising introduction of new or novel syllables that were never a part of the presurgical birdsong repertoire. These new or novel syllables are also depicted in Figure 38–6.

As can be seen in this illustration, destabilization of the song was most evident on Day Post1 during which syllables B, C, and D were completely omitted from the repertoire and new syllables constituted approximately 85% of the utterances or productions. Syllables B, C, and D are then reintroduced rather rapidly and in increasing proportion during the recovery phase. By Day Post3 new syllables, never before recorded in the syllable repertoire of the bird's learned motif, still constitute approximately 50% of the syllables produced. This characteristic of the introduction of novel syllables, foreign to the usual birdsong repertoire, continues but diminishes

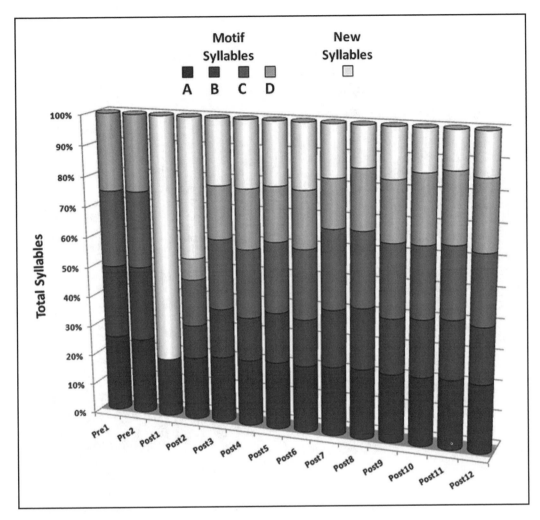

Figure 38–6. Syllables of bird 560.

throughout the Post12 days of measurement. Even at Post12, when the zebra finch motif has regained most of its presurgical syllabic character, previously omitted syllables are back, but approximately 15% of its motif productions are novel syllables. This introduction of new notes or syllables is similar in some respects to the neologistic jargon or paraphasic utterances of some persons with aphasia. Words such as "ferbis," "appleholtent," "baybeeay," "veeches," and "newbolt" are among the rich utterances reported by persons with jargon aphasia. They are nonsemantic para-

phasias that are unlikely to appear in a dictionary and have been characterized as linguistic "word salad" by some (LaPointe, Murdoch, & Stierwalt, 2010).

Figure 38–7 illustrates the characteristics of bird 560's motif syntax (order) and transitions from syllable-to-syllable for two measurement sessions preoperatively followed by 12 measurement sessions postoperatively. To quantify syllable transitions, we used a syllable cluster template to identify syllable-types in a scatter plot from a baseline day of singing (e.g., see the duration x entropy scatter plot

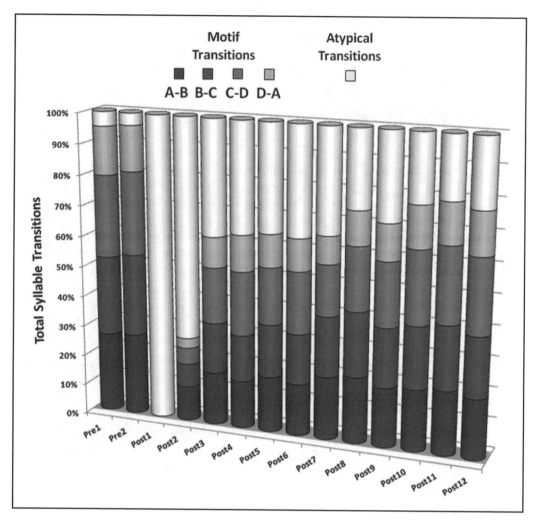

Figure 38–7. Syllable transitions of bird 560.

in Figure 38–3). Boundaries are traced around each cluster to distinguish one syllable from another. These syllable boundaries are then used to objectively identify syllable types and the order in which they were produced on each subsequent day of singing. Within Figure 38–7 the typical motif transitions for the syllables A, B, C, and D are depicted as follows: A-B; B-C; C-D; and D-A. Atypical transitions are also depicted. As can be seen only a small percentage (~3%) of transitions are atypical in the two preoperative measurement sessions. In Day 1 postoperatively, all syntax transitions (100%) are atypical. During subsequent recov-

ery, typical transitions from syllable to syllable then begin to emerge rapidly, and from Day 3 through Day 12, atypical transitions characterize the birdsong syntax from approximately 40 to 25%. It is interesting to note that, unlike syllable recovery, syntax (transition) recovery never fully recovers to preoperative levels across 12 days of measurement. This may speak to the relative robustness of syllable or note recovery postoperatively compared to the lesser strength of postoperative recovery of characteristics of syntactical transitions from one syllable to another. At any rate, the relative disruption and recovery of syllable (note) production compared to syntax (transition) can be appreciated and plotted over time and may serve as a baseline for future empirical interventions.

CAVEATS AND OPTIMISM

Birdsong is not human speech and language. Significant differences exist, particularly in the area of lexical-semantic richness. The complexity of human language is unparalleled among biological communication systems, and there are no completely suitable animal models. Recognizing these limitations is crucial and we do not want to overstate the case or the aptness of human speech and language to that of songbird learned vocalizations. However, songbirds are considered by many to be the best animal model as they are unique among nonhumans in their combination of vocal sophistication and experimental accessibility (including a sequenced genome, Warren et al., 2010). Scientists now realize that structures highly analogous to mammalian cortex also dominates the songbird's brain. The zebra finch's learning to produce songs is anything but instinctual and involves complex interactions between the cortex analogues and other brain regions. Research laboratories, such as that at Florida State University, are bringing sophisticated clarification to what is known about the birdsong brain in dissolution and recovery of its song. A consortium of leading scientists has outlined well the biological and biomedical rationales for the pursuit of research on birdsong (Clayton, 2005).

NEUROGENESIS

Among these rationales are potential applications in adult neurogenesis. In 1984 Goldman and Nottebohm showed that the adult song-

bird brain makes new neurons. This was at a time when neurogenesis in the adult mammalian brain was a topic broached with extreme caution, if not discounted entirely. Now neural plasticity, particularly based on experiential exposure, is fully one of the most promising and exciting areas of neural and rehabilitative science. Stem cell research and other intrinsic manipulations appear to have a rich promise for the empirical study of synaptogenesis and changes in neural architecture. The adult songbird telencephalon remains a promising avenue to study the functional significance and control of adult neurogenesis because of well-defined circuits linked to specific behaviors (Nottebohm, 2004). Many human disorders arise from disruptions to the brain regions involved in lexical-semantic acquisition and use as well as in the learning and producing complex of sequential behaviors. Discerning the relative neuroconnectivity that produces the rich varieties of lexical-semantic symbolic behavior has been a long-time goal of neurolinguistics and neuroscience in general. Parkinson disease (PD) arises when specialized neurons and neuroconnectivity in the basal ganglia begin to die. Among other signs and symptoms for this and a myriad of other motor speech disorders, patients lose control of learned movements and vocalizations. These are continuing targets of empirical research that are hindered by the lack of a clear animal model.

ECOLOGY

The relation of ecology to human health is a not so obvious potential area of research on songbirds and humans. Songbirds are conspicuous, diurnal species that are open to study in the wild. Songbirds hold a prominent place in studies of reproduction, behavioral and population ecology, and perturbations of the environment. Many neurologic diseases including several movement disorders such as Parkinson disease and ALS have been associated with perturbations of the environment, especially as these relate to environmental toxins. This is an area where an animal model might be useful in determination of potential effects on the nervous system. It also introduces the realm of extrinsic variables that might be introduced that have an influence on acquisition, dissolution, or recovery of learned vocalizations. Does a songbird recover faster when housed with the tutor from whom it learned? Could changing the amount, duration, or variability of exposure influence recovery? Are there other environmental extrinsic variables that could be introduced to study changes in the speed or efficiency of recovery of learned vocalizations? A rich variety of extrinsic manipulation of variables can be proposed and brainstormed and can be converted to testable hypotheses due to the experimental accessibility and short recovery period of songbird vocalizations.

EXPERIMENTAL ACCESSIBILITY

By far, the most thoroughly studied single songbird species is the zebra finch, which are small, have short generation time (4 months) for a complex vertebrate, and breed easily in captivity. Each zebra finch male sings a unique learned song as part of the courtship ritual and to maintain a monogamous bond with his mate. To develop a normal song, the young male must hear both an adult tutor (typically his father) and his own vocal performance, during a critical period in adolescence. Once the song is learned, it is sung stably throughout adult life, and new learning ceases. The relatively brief time frame of juvenile learning and the lifelong adult stability of song offer unique opportunities for understanding how the processes of vocal imitation, vocal sequencing, and vocal memory can be managed by a vertebrate brain.

Perhaps not so surprisingly, the first gene to date linked to speech disorders in humans (FoxP2) is also expressed in the neural song circuit, especially at times of vocal learning where it can be studied much more fruitfully than in humans. There are few organisms that rival the songbird for experimental study of genomic mechanisms underlying evolution and expression of vocal learning, speech communication and related cognitive processes. An array of potential intrinsic and extrinsic experimental variables exist that could be targets of empirical research on learned vocalizations.

This field may be expanded by our findings that not only movement and syntactical transitions are destabilized and subsequently recovered in the zebra finch, but notes or syllables are also omitted and replaced with novel syllabic utterances somewhat like the neologistic paraphasias seen in aphasia. Furthermore, the durational and velocity changes in destabilized birdsong might have analogs in motor speech disorders in humans. These characteristics of destabilization and recovery deserve to be studied further as do the variables that might influence impairment and restitution of the precious world of song and speech.

REFERENCES

Andalman, A. S., & Fee, M. S. (2008). A basal ganglia-forebrain circuit in the songbird biases motor output to avoid vocal errors. *Proceedings of the National Academy of Science, 106*(30), 12518–12523.

Aronov, D., Andalman, A. S., & Fee, M. S. (2008). A specialized forebrain circuit for vocal babbling in the juvenile songbird. *Science, 320*(5876), 630–634.

Bauer, J., & Larson, C. R. (2003). Audio-vocal responses to repetitive pitch-shift stimulation during a sustained vocalization: Improvements in methodology for the pitch-shifting technique. *Journal of the Acoustical Society of America, 114,* 1048–1054.

Berwick, R. C., Okanoya, K., Beckers, G. J. L., & Bolhuis, J. J. (2011) Songs to syntax: The linguistics of birdsong. *Trends in Cognitive Sciences, 15,* 113–121.

Brainard, M. S., & Doupe, A. J. (2001). Postlearning consolidation of birdsong: Stabilizing effects of age and anterior forebrain lesions. *Journal of Neuroscience, 21,* 2501–2517.

Bulhuis, J. J., Okanoya, K., & Scharff, C. (2010). Twitter evolution: Converging mechanisms in birdsong and human speech. *Nature Reviews Neuroscience, 11,* 747–759.

Clayton, D. F. (2005). Proposal to sequence the zebra finch genome. Retrieved September 23, 2011 from http://www.genome.gov/Pages/Research/Sequencing/SeqProposals/ZebraFinchSeq2.pdf

Doupe, A. J., & Kuhl, P. K. (1999). Birdsong and human speech: Common themes and mechanisms. *Annual Review of Neuroscience, 22*0, 567–631.

Glaze, C. M., & Troyer, T. W. (2006). Temporal structure in zebra finch song: Implications for motor coding. *Journal of Neuroscience, 26,* 991–1005.

Goldman S. A., & Nottebohm, F. (1983). Neuronal production, migration, and differentiation in a vocal control nucleus of the adult female canary brain. *Proceedings of the National Academy of Sciences, 80,* 2390–2394.

Goldstein, M. H., King, A. P., & West, M. J. (2003). Social interaction shapes babbling: Testing parallels between birdsong and speech. *Proceedings of the National Academy of Sciences, 100*(17), 9645–9646.

Hahnloser, R. H., Koshevinkov, A. A., & Fee, M. S. (2002). An ultra-sparse code underlies the generation of neural sequences in a songbird. *Nature, 419*(6902), 65–70.

Jarvis, E. D. (2004, June). Learned birdsong and the neurobiology of human language. *Annals of the New York Academy of Sciences, 1016,* 749–777.

Kittelberger, J. M., & Mooney, R. (2005). Acute injections of brain-derived neurotrophic factor in a vocal premotor nucleus reversibly disrupt adult birdsong stability and trigger syllable deletion. *Journal of Neurobiology, 62,* 406–424.

Kirn, J. R. (2010). The relationship of neurogenesis and growth of brain regions to song learning. *Brain and Language, 115,* 29–44.

Kirn, J. R., Fishman Y., Sasportas, K., Alvarez-Buylla, A., & Nottebohm F. (1999). Fate of new neurons in the adult canary high vocal center during the first 30 days after their formation. *Journal of Comparative Neurology, 411*(3), 487–494.

Kuhl, P. K. (2003). Human speech and birdsong: Communication and the social brain. *Proceedings of the National Academy of Sciences, 100*(17), 9645–9646.

LaPointe, L. L., Murdoch, B. E., & Stierwalt, J. A. G. (2010). *Brain-based communication disorders.* San Diego, CA: Plural.

Long, M. A., & Fee, M. S., (2008). Using temperature to analyse temporal dynamics in the songbird motor pathway. *Nature, 456* (7219), 189–194

Lombardino, A. J., & Nottebohm, F. (2000). Age at deafening affects the stability of learned song in adult male zebra finches. *Journal of Neuroscience, 20,* 5054–5064.

Miller, J. E., Spiteri, E., Condro, M. C., Dosumu-Johnson, R. T., Geschwind, D. H., & White, S. A. (2008). Birdsong decreases protein levels of FOXP2, a molecule required for human speech. *Journal of Neurophysiology, 100*(4), 2015–2025.

Nixdorf-Bergweiler, B., & Bischof, H. J. (2007). *A stereotaxic atlas of the brain of the zebra finch, taeniopygia guttata.* Bethesda, MD: National Center for Biotechnology Information.

Nordeen, K. W., & Nordeen, E. J. (1992). Auditory feedback is necessary for the maintenance of stereotyped song in adult zebra finches. *Behavioral and Neural Biology, 57,* 58–66.

Nordeen, K. W., & Nordeen, E. J. (1993). Long-term maintenance of song in adult zebra finches is not affected by lesions of a forebrain region involved in song learning. *Behavioral and Neural Biology, 59,* 79–82.

Nottebohm, F. (2004). The road we travelled: Discovery, choreography, and significance of brain replaceable neurons. *Annals of the New York Academy of Sciences, 1016,* 628–658.

Olveczky, B. P., Andalman, A. S., & Fee, M. S. (2005). Vocal experimentation in the juvenile songbird requires a basal ganglia circuit. *PLoS Biology 3,* e153.

Pytte, C. L., & Suthers, R. A. (2000). Sensitive period for sensorimotor integration during vocal motor learning. *Journal of Neurobiology, 42*(2), 172–189.

Saito, N., & Maekawa, M. (1993). Birdsong: The interface with human language. *Brain Development, 15*(1), 31–39.

Scharff, C., Kirn, J. R., Grossman, M., Macklis, J. D., & Nottebohm, F. (2000).Targeted neuronal death affects neuronal replacement and vocal behavior in adult songbirds. *Neuron, 25*(2), 481–492.

Sivasankar, M., Bauer, J. J., Babu, T., & Larson, C. R. (2005). Voice responses to changes in pitch of voice or tone auditory feedback. *Journal of the Acoustical Society of America, 117,* 850–857.

Sober, S. J., & Brainard, M. S. (2009). Adult birdsong is actively maintained by error correction. *Nature Neuroscience, 12,* 927–931.

Tchernichovski, O., Nottebohm, F., Ho, C. E., Pesaran, B., & Mitra, P. P. (2000). A procedure for an automated measurement of song similarity. *Animal Behavior, 59,* 1167–1176.

Thompson, J. A., Basista, M. J., Wu, W., Bertram, R., & Johnson F. (2011). Dual pre-motor contribution to songbird syllable variation. *Journal of Neuroscience, 31,* 322–330.

Thompson, J. A., & Johnson, F. (2007). HVC microlesions do not destabilize the vocal patterns of adult male zebra finches with prior ablation of LMAN. *Developmental Neurobiology, 67,* 205–218.

Thompson, J. A., Wu, W., Bertram, R., & Johnson, F. (2007). Auditory-dependent vocal recovery in adult male zebra finches is facilitated by lesion of a forebrain pathway that includes the basal ganglia. *Journal of Neuroscience, 27*(45), 12308–12320.

Tumer, E. C., & Brainard, M. S. (2007). Performance variability enables adaptive plasticity of "crystallized" adult birdsong. *Nature, 450*(7173), 1240–1244.

Voss, H., Salgado-Commissariat, D., & Helekar S. A. (2010). Altered auditory BOLD response to conspecific birdsong in zebra finches with stuttered syllables. *PLoS One, 5,* 14415.

Warren, W. C., Clayton, D. F., Ellegren, H., Arnold, A. P., Hillier L. W., Künstner A, . . . Wilson R. K. (2010). The genome of a songbird. *Nature, 464*(7289), 757–762.

White, S. A. (2010). Genes and vocal learning. *Brain and Language, 115,* 21–28.

Williams, H. (2004). Birdsong and singing behavior. *Annals of the New York Academy of Sciences, 1016,* 1–30.

Williams, H. (2008). Birdsong and singing behavior. In H. P. Zeigler & P. Marler (Eds.), *Neuroscience of birdsong* (pp. 32–49). London, UK: Cambridge University Press.

Wu, W., Thompson, J. A., Bertram, R., & Johnson, F. (2008). A statistical method for quantifying songbird phonology and syntax. *Journal of Neuroscience Methods, 174,* 147–154.

Ziegler, P., & Marler, P. (2008). *Neuroscience of birdsong.* Boston, MA: Cambridge University Press.

ESSAY 39

Defense Mechanisms and Coping Styles in Aphasia

Dennis C. Tanner

I was honored to have Dr. Sadanand Singh write the Foreword to one of my books. As most authors do, I sought someone with a national reputation and impeccable credentials to write it. I was understandably nervous when I approached him with the Foreword proposition. However, I was soon treated to one of the most warm and gracious individuals with whom I have been professionally associated. In my telephone conversations with him, I was struck by his absolute grasp of intent of the book. What I received from Dr. Singh was a Foreword that capsulized the spirit of the book and focused on the humanity of communication and its disorders. This statement from the Foreword expressed his commitment to the marvelous act of human communication and the impact of communication disorders on those who suffer them: "What I admire about Dr. Tanner is that he explores fully the connections among all aspects of normal human communication, and the impact on the individual, family, caregiver, and society when this connection is lost. This is what our field is all about." Dr. Sadanand Singh was truly a compassionate visionary who has left an indelible mark on the lives of all who had the great fortune to know him.

Over the years, I have seen thousands of patients with aphasia. Although I have understandably been concerned for their communication abilities, I have always been intrigued by the psychology of this devastating disability. Do persons with aphasia have the same types of psychological reactions as people with intact language, and if not, what is the nature of their adaptation to this often-times life-altering communication disorder? As a doctoral student at Michigan State University, I minored in psychiatry with a focus on how patients cope with loss of language. Several years later, I took a sabbatical with a psychiatrist and addressed sites of brain lesions and the psychological manifestations of them. In my interactions in the world of psychiatry, I was repeatedly exposed to the concepts of psychological conflicts and defenses, referred to by some as "coping styles."

There are three determinants for the psychological reactions and adjustment challenges facing many persons with aphasia (Figure 39–1). First, the brain damage which causes aphasia may affect the patient's psychological well-being and coping abilities. These

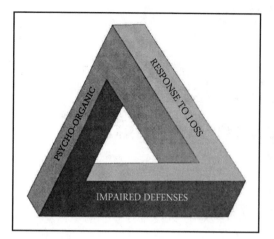

Figure 39–1. The psychological determinants of aphasia

psycho-organic factors can cause or be associated with psychological reactions ranging from euphoria to anxiety-depression. Second, most patients suffering from significant aphasia experience a deep sense of *loss*. For many patients, there is a loss of self, a detachment from valued objects, and separation from loved ones as a consequence of the communication disorder. Like all people, they grieve over the unwanted changes and pass through several predictable *stages of grief*. Third, aphasia can be a substantial psychological stressor and tax the patient's premorbid *coping styles and psychological defenses*. Verbal coping styles and psychological defenses can be impaired or eliminated because of the loss of language and leave the patient without habitual methods of adapting to the disorder. In many cases of aphasia, psycho-organic factors, impaired coping styles and defense mechanisms, and response to loss and the unwanted life changes combine to affect the patient's adjustment to the disorder (Tanner, 1980, 2003, 2010; Tanner & Gerstenberger; 1988). This essay addresses the types of external and internal stressors experienced by persons with aphasia and their typical coping styles and defense mechanisms.

DEFENSE MECHANISMS AND ADAPTABILITY TO APHASIA

Sigmund Freud introduced the concept of defense mechanisms in 1895 (Encyclopædia Britannica, 2011). According to Porcerelli and Hibbard (2004), he conceptualized them as collection of mental forces that oppose unacceptable ideas or feelings, and would cause significant distress if acknowledged. Today, although there is general agreement that defense mechanisms play an important role in mental health (Boyd, 1998), they remain controversial as do most of Freud's early groundbreaking psychological concepts. However, most authorities agree that defense mechanisms help people protect themselves from anxiety, exclude disturbing thoughts from conscious awareness, and support self-esteem. Defense mechanisms are used by people to cope with reality and the concept has stood the test of time (Porcerelli, Thomas, Hibbard, & Cogan, 1998).

Today, defense mechanisms and coping styles are recognized as patterned thoughts, feelings, reactions, and behaviors that arise in response to perceived or real internal or external threats. They can be placed on a continuum of adaptability. Some are immature, neurotic, maladaptive, and radical and they are employed when life stressors, and the individual's ability to cope with them, become overwhelming. Other defense mechanisms and coping styles are mature and adaptive, and lead to positive adjustment and mental health. However, even mature defense mechanisms and coping styles can be maladaptive when used inappropriately. Some defense mechanisms and coping styles clearly require intact language functioning to employ, whereas others can be activated without language.

Patients with aphasia, particularly those with global aphasia, are unable to employ verbal defense mechanisms and coping styles.

They have special adjustment challenges not experienced by persons with intact language functions. Even aphasic patients with partial language functioning may be impaired in the utilization of verbal defense mechanisms or find that they are less accessible. In the discussion that follows, several psychological defense mechanisms and coping styles are reviewed relative to their application to patients with global aphasia with the understanding that patients with partial language will have correspondingly reduced ability to employ them. When the threats are primarily from external sources, patients with aphasia can activate *avoidance, ego restriction, physical escape,* and *autistic fantasy* with little or no impairments as a result of the loss of language. These defense mechanisms and coping styles involve avoiding or escaping from the threats and are readily available to all patients including those with global aphasia.

COPING WITH PREDOMINANTLY EXTERNAL THREATS

Avoidance is a basic and innate defense mechanism and coping style; the person simply tries to avoid the threat. Although turning away from disturbing situations is a response to external threats, pure avoidance lies at the core of many defense mechanisms and coping styles. The *avoidant personality disorder* involves the extreme use of avoidance and many of these patients try to distance themselves from painful and negatively reinforcing experiences (Millon & Meagher, 2004). In many patients with aphasia, there is much to avoid. There are often invasive diagnostic procedures, painful physical therapies, and confrontation with disabilities. To protect themselves from unpleasantness, patients may postpone or refuse confrontation with the negativity. While encouraging patients to par-

ticipate fully in rehabilitation through support and counseling, clinicians should understand the defense of avoidance and its use in psychological protection. When used sparingly, avoidance through postponement and refusal can be adaptive ways of coping with the stressors associated with aphasia and it is available to all patients.

Ego restriction, a type of avoidance, occurs when a patient refuses or abandons an activity in response to extreme anxiety and the risk of failure. The anxiety is based on perceived threats to self-esteem. Patients with aphasia who recognize they cannot perform many day-to-day activities previously enjoyed may limit their interactions to safe ones that carry little or no possibility of failure. Consequently, some patients with aphasia may refuse or abandon family, occupational, and social activities even thought they may likely succeed at them. For some patients, the threats to self-esteem are simply too great to attempt them. Certainly, patients should be encouraged to attempt new and possibily threatening activities, but it also should be recognized that ego restriction can serve an important ego-protection function and reduce anxiety, which may be as important to the patient as the activities themselves.

Physical escape can provide psychological relief and is employed when simple avoidance is impractical. Physical escape is also an innate defense mechanism and coping style, providing immediate relief from threatening situations. For patients with aphasia, these threatening situations may occur in therapy activities. The threats may be related to confronting the disorder, or aspects of it, which may be harmful to their self-esteem. Some patients with aphasia may not be prepared to confront limitations in word recall, agraphia, alexia, or other aspects of the syndrome of aphasia. Patients with aphasia may request a break from therapy or physically show signs of the need to escape from the confines of the therapy suite. Requests to go to the bathroom or feigning illness may also be indications for the need to physically escape unpleasantness.

Eisenson (1984) noted that a catastrophic reaction, a psychobiological breakdown, may result in the patient losing consciousness. Loss of consciousness, fainting, is the ultimate escape from unpleasantness and the patient completely escapes the psychologically threatening confrontations. By allowing physical escape, and even encouraging it in some cases, clinicians can prevent catastrophic reactions. Physical escape can provide the patient who has adjustment challenges with necessary relief from the negativity and stress associated with aphasia.

Autistic fantasy is a form of escape through daydreaming. It is a symbolic way of meeting psychological needs and a substitute for more appropriate actions to deal with emotional conflicts (Burgess & Clements, 1998). During fantasy escape, the patient symbolically deals with threats to the self-concept and self-esteem.

Fantasy escapes are retreats into a fantasy world which can include gratifying occupational, athletic, sexual, financial, social, and other imaginary activities. During these escapes, the patient with aphasia is temporarily spared the emotional negativity associated with the disorder. For neurotypical persons, the retreat into a fantasy world is considered undesirable and immature, especially when used in excess or to the exclusion of realistically dealing with psychological issues. However, for patients with aphasia, the fantasy defense mechanism and coping style can be desirable, mature, and adaptive given the extreme circumstances associated with the devastating communication disorder. For patients with aphasia, fantasy escape can bridge the gap between of the reality of their disorder and what they desire. At least temporarily, it can help them obtain needed relief from the frustration associated with aphasia. Although some patients may appear to be "blanking out," detached, and not focused on therapeutic activities, they may simply be engaging in autistic fantasy as a way of coping with the disorder. Despite the fact that language may help structure elaborate fantasy escapes, most patients with aphasia can use visualization to satisfy their psychological needs.

COPING WITH PREDOMINANTLY INTERNAL THREATS

There is no clear distinction between threats of an external and internal nature because external threats are also accompanied by the thoughts and emotions associated with them. However, this distinction is appropriate when addressing defense mechanisms and coping styles in patients with aphasia because discovery and analysis of the perceived threats are hindered by the communication barrier. When the perceived threats are primarily prompted by internal thoughts or memories, the defense mechanisms and coping styles involve blocking, suppressing, or in some way, repressing them.

The following major defense mechanisms and coping styles do not require language to protect from predominantly internal threats. Consequently, they are available to most patients with aphasia, even those with global involvement.

Denial: Denial is the blocking from conscious awareness of threatening and unpleasant memories, events, and situations. Denial is integral to many defenses mechanisms and coping styles that do not result from brain injury (anosognosia, or denial of impairment). Denial protects the ego, reduces anxiety, and keeps unacceptable thoughts and emotions from conscious awareness.

Repression: Repression is excluding negative thoughts, feelings, drives, memories, and ideas from conscious awareness by inhibiting them before or after they reach consciousness. Carlat (1999) considers repression a way of forcing the emotion out of conscious awareness.

Regression: Psychological regression is the retreat to a more secure and comfortable level of adjustment. In regression, the patient returns to an immature stage of psychological adjustment to avoid anxiety and threats to self-esteem. It involves thoughts, behaviors, and emotions on the part of the patient.

Displacement and *Projection:* Both displacement and projection involve the subconscious attempt to reduce anxiety by shifting negative emotions from one person or object to another or attributing them to someone else. According to Stuart (2001), the negative emotions are displaced to a less threatening or dangerous person or object. Projection reduces anxiety and guilt by projecting negative thoughts and emotions onto others.

Sublimation and *Substitution:* Both of these defense mechanisms and coping styles enable the person to redirect negativity to personally or socially acceptable thoughts, attitudes, and behaviors.

The above defense mechanisms and coping styles are used to protect the patient with aphasia from the negativity associated with the communication disorder. Certainly, they could be more effectively activated with the use of language, but they are available, more or less, to all patients with aphasia including those with global involvement. Although in neurotypical persons, these defense mechanism and coping styles might appear immature and maladaptive, in patients with aphasia

they can be adaptive and mature ways of dealing with the disorder, primarily because the ones listed below are unavailable to them.

MAJOR DEFENSE MECHANISMS AND COPING STYLES UNAVAILABLE TO PATIENTS WITH APHASIA

Rationalization and intellectualization, suppression, undoing, and *humor* are defense mechanisms and coping styles partially compromised or largely unavailable to language-deprived individuals. Because they require language, they are unable to be used by persons with aphasia, particularly those with global aphasia.

Rationalization and intellectualization are attempts to elevate self-esteem by avoiding disturbing emotions. They disguise motivations and mask emotions.

Suppression is the voluntary exclusion of disturbing thoughts from conscious awareness. Unlike repression, which is done involuntarily, suppression is a conscious act. Suppression is more compromised in patients with perseveration due to the lack of mental flexibility and inability to shift.

Undoing is a symbolic attempt to partially or completely undo a previous act. The patient endeavors to deal with emotional conflicts by making amends. It is a subconscious attempt to take back an unacceptable action or communication.

With humor, an amusing aspect of a conflict or stressor is used to remove or minimize negativity. Carlat (1999) considers the use of humor as an overt expression of emotions without personal discomfort to be a mature psychological defense and coping style. One of the reasons it is beyond the ability of patients with aphasia is that they tend to be on a concrete level and some humor is highly abstract.

OTHER DEFENSE MECHANISMS AND COPING STYLES

Certainly, the above defense mechanisms and coping styles are not the only ones potentially available to persons with aphasia. Passive aggression, altruism, several types of dissociation, and others may or may not be available to individuals with aphasia. They may be partially available, compromised, impossible to observe accurately, or completely unavailable, and their functions in adaptability depend on the aphasia, types of stressors, and the patient's reactions to them.

SUMMARY

Aphasia can be psychologically devastating to some individuals. Psycho-organic factors and responses to loss and unwanted change can create major adjustment challenges for some patients. Although it is impossible to know how patients with severe aphasia "think," assumptions can be made about their responses to the stressors associated with the disorders. It is logical to conclude that psychological defense mechanisms and coping styles that do not require language remain available to help patients protect themselves from anxiety and threats to their self-esteem. Clinicians should appreciate these patients' unique adjustment challenges and integrate them into all clinical interaction.

REFERENCES

Boyd, M. (1998). Biopsychosocial aspects of stress and crisis. In M. Boyd & M. Nihart (Eds.), *Psychiatric nursing*. Philadelphia, PA: Lippincott.

Burgess, A., & Clements, P. (1998). Stress, coping, and defensive functioning. In A. Burgess (Ed.), *Psychiatric nursing*. Stamford, CT: Appleton & Lange.

Carlat, D. (1999). *The psychiatric interview*. Philadelphia, PA: Lippincott Williams & Wilkins.

Eisenson, J. (1984). *Adult aphasia* (2nd ed.). Englewood Cliffs, NJ: Prentice-Hall.

The Neuro-Psychosis of Defence. (2011). In *Encyclopædia Britannica*. Retrieved from http://www.britannica.com/EBchecked/topic/1522880/The-Neuro-Psychosis-of-Defence

Millon, T., & Meagher, S. (2004). The millon clinical multiaxial inventory-III (MCMI-III). In M. Hilsenroth & D. Segal (Eds.), *Comprehensive handbook of psychological assessment, Volume 2: Personality assessment*. Hoboken, NJ: John Wiley & Sons.

Porcerelli, J., Thomas, S., Hibbard, S., & Cogan, R. (1998). Defense mechanisms development in children adolescents, and late adolescents. *Journal of Personality Assessment, 71*, 411–420.

Porcerelli, J., & Hibbard, S. (2004). Projective assessment of defense mechanisms. In M. Hilsenroth & D. Segal (Eds.), *Comprehensive handbook of psychological assessment, Volume 2: Personality assessment*. Hoboken, NJ: John Wiley & Sons.

Stuart, B. (2001). Anxiety responses and anxiety disorders. In G. Stuart & M. Laraia (Eds.), *Principles and practice of psychiatric nursing* (7th ed.). St. Louis, MO: Mosby.

Tanner, D. (1980). Loss and grief: Implications for the speech-language pathologist and audiologist. *Journal of the American Speech and Hearing Association, 22*, 916–928.

Tanner, D. (2003). Eclectic perspectives on the psychology of aphasia. *Journal of Allied Health, 32*, 256–260.

Tanner, D. (2010). *Exploring the psychology, diagnosis, and treatment of neurogenic communication disorders*. New York, NY: iUniverse.

Tanner, D., & Gerstenberger, D. (1988). The grief response in neuropathologies of speech and language. *Aphasiology, 1*(6), 79–84.

ESSAY 40

The Impact of Augmentative ❧ and Alternative Communication ❧ (AAC) Technology

Cindy Geise Arroyo

Although I did not know Dr. Singh personally, I have used many of his publications as a student and as an educator through the years. As I learned more about Dr. Singh's personal and professional life in preparation for this essay, I was struck by his accomplished career, passion for education, and especially by his human spirit. I am grateful for the opportunity to participate in this deserved tribute.

It is estimated that 8 to 12 individuals per 1,000 experience severe communication impairments at some point in their lives that may require AAC intervention (ASHA, 2008). The purpose of AAC is to temporarily or permanently compensate for the impairment, activity limitations and participation restrictions of individuals with severe disabilities of speech-language production and/or comprehension. AAC involves an ongoing program of decision-making and strategies that considers individuals' needs, their methods of communication and the effectiveness of their communication with a variety of communication partners in multiple communication environments (ASHA, 2004).

A guiding principle in AAC is that communication is the essence of human life (ASHA, 1991) and that all people have the basic right to communicate regardless of the severity of their disability (National Joint Commission for the Communication Needs of Persons with Severe Disabilities, 1992). Consequently, all individuals are viewed as potential candidates for AAC, consistent with a zero exclusion policy. Access to effective methods of AAC is viewed as essential to individuals' quality of life, self-determination, and ability to participate in decision-making affecting their lives (Light & Gulens, 2000). "The silence of speechlessness is never golden. Communication is a basic human need, a basic human right, and much more than that it is a basic human power" (Williams, 2002, p. 248).

My personal introduction to AAC was in the late 1970s, as a speech-language pathologist in a cerebral palsy center, working closely with the rehabilitation engineering department. Rehabilitation science and engineering may be defined as "the field of study that encompasses basic and applied aspects of the health sciences, social sciences and engineering related to restoring functional capabilities in a person and improving their interactions with the surrounding environment" (Brandt & Pope, 1997, p. 24). In a clinical application, there is a synthesis of knowledge from several disciplines to address the needs of individuals with disabling conditions. The engineer creates an alteration in the environment (internal or external) to make it more supportive. These altered environments can replace or compensate for the compromised or lost function (e.g. communication) through engineered technologies and devices. The objective of rehabilitation is to facilitate and emphasize an *enabling* process, rather than a *disabling* circumstance. As part of the rehabilitative process, methods of "technological" support can be traced back at least 3500 years to the Egyptian civilization. Ancient drawings have depicted scenes such as an individual with a weakened leg using a long pole as a mobility aid (Childress, 2002). AAC is an area of practice that has evolved and expanded from early electromechanical communication and writing systems to communication and language boards and sophisticated computer-based options (Vanderheiden, 2002). It has emerged as an internationally acknowledged clinical and academic area of concentration addressing individuals with complex communication needs who are widely diverse in their diagnoses, age, ethnicity, and cultural backgrounds (Blackstone, Williams, & Wilkins, 2007).

In recent years, terminology has emerged to represent ways to bridge the gap between research and practice in order to improve quality of life for individuals with disabilities by developing and facilitating the use of technology and services and informing policies and practices for the disabled. *Knowledge translation* refers to the process of developing a new knowledge and applying that knowledge to society (Higginbotham et al., 2009). *Technology transfer* is the transmittal of developed ideas, products, and techniques from a research environment to one of practical application, disseminated to the greater community (Brandt & Pope, 1997). The Rehabilitation and Engineering Research Center on Communication Enhancement (AAC-RERC) is an organization that has been working to increase the number of research and development ideas that are transferred from the labs to the real world (e.g., consumers). They have implemented a Technology Transfer Plan by collaborating with manufacturers, researchers and AAC users. The collaboration of professional fields such as rehabilitation engineering and speech-language pathology presents opportunities for initiating and disseminating effective technologies, physical, and social-communicative strategies for individuals with severe communication impairments. The area of AAC evolved clinically from speech-language pathologists presenting a problem and rehabilitation engineers collaborating to solve it, with the components that were available at that time. As the problem is identified, ideas need to be generated to solve the problem. There may be numerous solutions to the problem and the challenge is to find the solution that best meets the needs of the person with a disability. Technological advances have resulted in more options for individuals with disabilities but it has also complicated the process of AAC evaluations and interventions/ recommendations.

AAC options must be available for individuals who are considered beginning communicators as well as for individuals who encounter complex communication needs towards the end of their life span. Effective AAC interventions require the identification of an appropriate system, but also the development of the individual's communicative competence and psychosocial concerns (Blackstone & Wilkins, 2009). Young children are developing their communication and language skills rapidly during the first years of life and it is crucial that AAC needs be addressed early to develop communicative competence (Branson & Demchak, 2009). The ability to express wants, needs, and emotions and exchange information with others supports the development of social closeness with others at any age, which is essential to the development of communicative competence. In turn, social closeness leads to an increase in interpersonal relationships and inclusion in a larger social and cultural community (Light, Parsons, & Drager, 2002).

Prior to the 1980s and the availability of AAC, individuals with severe communication impairments such as those associated with cerebral palsy and ALS, struggled to communicate in a functional manner. The significant advances in technology over the last three decades have resulted in a wide range of communication options, with the most recent impact of sophisticated and efficient eye-gaze systems. Many AAC devices also now have the capability of interfacing with the telephone, internet and social media allowing for a broader range of social contexts, leisure activities, and communication partners (Blackstone et al., 2007).

Recent research in the area of AAC has increasingly focused on issues of quality of life (O'Keefe, Kozak & Schuller, 2007). Quality of life is an individual's own perception of his or her well-being which may be measured by the ability to communicate in different social situations; the development of relationships through communication; employment opportunities; general life satisfaction and psychosocial well-being (Markham & Dean, 2006; O'Keefe, Kozak & Schuller, 2007).

Quality of life considerations are becoming increasingly important in the evaluation of healthcare interventions (Markham & Dean, 2006). Clinicians can enhance quality of life through the sensitive and evidence-based implementation of AAC practices. This should include education and ongoing support for AAC users and their families/caregivers and facilitating AAC users and their family members to feel competent, especially for families from diverse cultural backgrounds. Practices such as programming vocabulary from the native language spoken in the home and consideration for family members' unique communication styles and preferences should be priorities when working with culturally and linguistically diverse families. Providing information and training materials in the native language can also facilitate a partnership between professionals and families and enhance quality of life for the individual with a disability (Saito & Turnbull, 2007). Improvement in quality of life for all individuals with disabilities may be considered the optimal outcome of AAC interventions (Schlosser, 2003).

As clinicians implementing the use of AAC technology for individuals with complex communication needs, how can we support the development of communicative competence and an improved quality of life? Based on interviews with family members/caregivers of adolescents using AAC, expectations were that AAC users would experience increased independence and communicative competence; an enhanced ability to express feelings; and the opportunity for increased communication opportunities. The families also expressed their desire to be involved in AAC decision-making, to have more education and training, and to have ethnicity and cultural practices considered (Bailey, Parette, Stoner, Angell & Carroll, 2006). Barriers to effective AAC use and development of communicative competence have been identified by individuals with disabilities. These include a lack of public awareness of communication disabilities and knowledge of AAC (Datillo, Estrella, Estrella, Light, McNaughton, & Seabury, 2008). Negative attitudes toward individuals with disabilities can create barriers to the development of communicative and social competence and communication opportunities (McCarthy & Light, 2005; McDougall,

DeWit, King, Miller, & Killip, 2004). Individuals with disabilities, especially those with complex communication needs, often experience rejection, bullying, and social isolation and thereby, diminished self-esteem.

Although AAC users have reported that communication via AAC systems can be time consuming and that their communication partners often become impatient or interrupt their communication attempts, they acknowledged that their AAC devices were their biggest social support, giving them opportunities for involvement and independence (Datillo et al., 2008). AAC technology can also be perceived as difficult to learn and overwhelming (Murphy, 2004), but users have commented, "It helps me make friends" and, "It is my voice" (Clarke, McConachie, Price, & Wood, 2001).

AAC intervention should be dynamic rather than static, accommodating to the changing needs of the individual with complex communication needs. AAC systems should be continuously updated, modifying messages, adding vocabulary, and integrating family perspectives and cultural considerations (Johnson, Inglebret, Jones, & Ray, 2006).

Despite the technological advances that have occurred over the last four decades, many individuals with severe physical disabilities and/or significant cognitive disabilities still do not have access to communication technology options and services and are limited in their communication partners, opportunities, and environments (Williams, Krezman, & McNaughton, 2008). Increasingly, digital independence is necessary to participate in these environments, therefore individuals must be able to integrate and access activities such as email, cell phones, and E-books with their communication device. Practices such as knowledge translation and technology transfer may facilitate increased awareness of AAC and more opportunities for appropriate applications and services for individuals with complex communication needs. As technol-

ogy continues to expand and develop, we must ensure that the individual with disabilities and complex communication needs is not lost in the translation.

REFERENCES

American Speech-Language-Hearing Association (ASHA). (1991). *Report: Augmentative and alternative communication, 33* (Suppl. 5), 9–12.

American Speech-Language-Hearing Association (ASHA). (2004). *Roles and responsibilities of speech-language pathologists with respect to augmentative and alternative communication.* (Technical report).

American Speech-Language-Hearing Association (ASHA). (2008). *Communication facts: Special populations: Augmentative and alternative communication.*

Bailey, R., Parette, H., Stoner, J., Angell, M., & Carroll, K. (2006). Family members' perceptions of augmentative and alternative device use. *Language, Speech, and Hearing Services in the Schools, 37,* 50–60.

Blackstone, S., & Wilkins, D. (2009). Exploring emotional competence. *Perspectives in Augmentative and Alternative Communication, ASHA, Division 12, 18*(3), 73–77.

Blackstone, S., Williams, M., & Wilkins, D. (2007). Key principles underlying research and practice in augmentative and alternative communication. *Augmentative and Alternative Communication, 23*(3), 191–203.

Brandt, E., & Pope, A. (1997). *Enabling America: Assessing the role of rehabilitation science and engineering.* National Academy of Science: National Academic Press.

Branson, D., & Demchak, M. (2009). The use of AAC methods with infants and toddlers with disabilities: A research review. *Augmentative and Alternative Communication, 25,* 274–286.

Childress, D. S. (2002). Development of rehabilitation engineering over the years: As I see it. *Journal of Rehabilitation Research and Development, 39*(Suppl. 6), 1–10.

Clarke, M., McConachie, H., Price, K., & Wood, P. (2001). Views of young people using AAC systems. *International Journal of Language and Communication Disorders, 36*(1), 107–115.

Datillo, J., Estrella, G., Estrella, L., Light, J., McNaughton, D., & Seabury, M. (2008). "I have chosen to live life abundantly:" Perceptions of leisure by adults who use AAC. *Augmentative and Alternative Communication, 24*(1), 16–28.

Higgenbotham, D. J., Beukelman, D., Blackstone, S., Bryen, D., Caves, K., Deruyter, F., . . . Williams, M. B. (2009). AAC technology transfer: An AAC-RERC report. *Augmentative and Alternative Communication, 25*(1), 68–76.

Johnson, J., Inglebret, E., Jones, C., & Ray, J. (2006). Perspectives of speech-language pathologists regarding success vs. abandonment of AAC. *Augmentative and Alternative Communication, 22*(2), 85–99.

Light, J., & Gulens, M. (2000). Acceptance of AAC by adults with acquired disorders. In D. Beukelman, K. Yorkston, & J. Reichle (Eds.), *Augmentative and alternative communication for adults with acquired neurological disorders* (pp. 107–136). Baltimore, MD: Paul H. Brookes.

Light, J., Parsons, A., & Drager, K. (2002). In D. Reichle, D. Beukelman, & J. Light (Eds.), *Exemplary practices for beginning communicators: Implications for augmentative and alternative communication.* Baltimore, MD: Paul H. Brookes.

Markham, C., & Dean, T. (2006). Parents' and professionals' perceptions of quality of life in children with speech and language difficulties. *International Journal of Language and Communication Disorders, 41*(2), 189–212.

McCarthy, J., & Light, J. (2005). Attitudes towards individuals who use augmentative and alternative communication: Research review. *Augmentative and Alternative Communication, 21*, 44–55.

McDougall, J., DeWit, D., King, G., Miller, L., & Killip, S. (2004). High school-aged youth's attitudes toward their peers with disabilities: The role of school and student interpersonal factors. *International Journal of Disabilities, Development, and Education, 51*, 287–301.

Murphy, J. (2004). "I prefer contact this close:" Perceptions of AAC by people with motor neurone disease and their communication partners. *Augmentative and Alternative Communication, 20*(4), 259–271.

National Joint Committee for the Communicative Needs of Persons with Severe Disabilities. (1992). Guidelines for meeting the communication needs of persons with severe disabilities. *ASHA, 34*(Suppl. 7), 1–8.

O'Keefe, B., Kozak, N., & Schuller, R. (2007). Research priorities in AAC as identified by people who use AAC and their facilitators. *Augmentative and Alternative Communication, 23*(1), 89–96.

Saito, Y., & Turnull, A. (2007). AAC practice in the pursuit of family quality of life : A review of the literature. *Research and Practice for Persons with Severe Disabilities, 32*(1), 50–65.

Schlosser, R. W. (2003). Outcome measurement in AAC. In J. Light, D. Beukelman, & J. Reichle (Eds.), *Communicative competence for individuals who use augmentative and alternative communication* (pp. 479–513). Baltimore, MD: Paul H. Brookes.

Vanderheiden, G. C. (2002). A journey through early augmentative communication and computer access. *Journal of Rehabilitation Research and Development, 39*(6), 39–53.

Williams, B. (2002). More than an exception to the rule. In M. Fried-Oken & H.A. Bersani (Eds.), *Speaking up and Spelling it out: Personal essays on augmentative and alternative communication* (pp. 245–254). Baltimore, MD: Paul H. Brookes.

Williams, B., Krezman, C., & McNaughton, D. (2008). "Reach for the stars": Five principles for the next 25 years of AAC. *Augmentative and Alternative Communication, 24*(3), 194–206.

Using Set Theory in SLP Diagnosis and Treatment

Robert Goldfarb and Mary Jo Santo Pietro

Mathematics has informed clinical practice in speech-language pathology in many ways. For example, LaPointe (1977) recommended a base-10 model to document the effects of therapy in individuals with aphasia. More recently (Goldfarb & Davis, 2010), we used mathematical concepts from Euler and Lagrange in recommending an oceanographic model for visualizing regional cerebral blood-flow of the middle cerebral artery in aphasia. The concept of the lemma has had broad application in both mathematics and psycholinguistics. In the present essay, we examine how set theory can apply to diagnosis and treatment in communication disorders associated with Alzheimer disease, aphasia, and fluency disorders.

Georg Cantor (1845–1918) published the first of six papers in 1874 which would collectively be referred to as set theory (Enderton, 1977). His radical notion was that the word *infinite* had two meanings. The first denotes a magnitude that increases beyond any indicated limit. Cantor called this the *improper set*, because the magnitude is always finite, although variable. The second meaning of infinite refers to the idea of real numbers,

and is called the *proper* or *completed infinite*, which leads to a rigorous theory of infinite collections. Cantor concluded that real numbers could not be defined without reference to a completed infinite set. The apparent theoretical paradoxes of sets can be resolved in any of three ways: demonstrable, disprovable, or undecidable. Godel (1947) found the last alternative most likely, because the difficulties with set theory might not be purely mathematical.

A set is a collection of things where we regard the collection as a single object. Accordingly, we are all members of the set of human beings, and may also be members of subsets, such as adults and scholars, but we are not all members of the subset of females. In linguistics, the meaning of a predicate is a set. For example, the predicate, *is large*, refers to all things which are large. In addition if we consider that large is a size, then we can think of a set containing all things that have all sizes. Enderton (1977, pp. xiii–xiv) lists 168 mathematical symbols that express relationships in set theory.

Cantor's general theory of sets refers to what is known as the concept of the cardinal number, or the continuum problem (Godel, 1947), with the following question: How many points are there on a straight line in Euclidean space? The question only makes sense if the concept of "number" extends to infinite sets, and the number of objects belonging to the same set is constant. That is, even if properties (e.g., color, distribution in space) of the objects in some class change, their number does not. Two sets will have the same cardinal number if their elements or characteristics have or can be brought into a one-to-one correspondence. Theoretically, in sets A and B, the characteristics of A can be transformed into a set which is indistinguishable from B, and then both sets will have the same cardinal number.

This concept of the continuum problem applies to a paper by Bloodstein (1960), although he did not refer to set theory. According to Bloodstein's continuity hypothesis, which has been subsequently rejected (see for example Goldfarb, 2006a), behaviors commonly described as stuttering (let's call this set A) cannot distinguish stuttering from disfluencies in children who speak with typical fluency but may also show these same speech disruptive behaviors (set B). In terms of fluency, sets A and B will have the same cardinal number (Set A = Set B). Those who were eventually labeled as individuals who stutter were those who stuttered severely and persistently. Therefore, according to the continuity hypothesis, diagnosis is a futile and meaningless exercise.

The hypothesis of a recent study (Bakker, Myers, Raphael, & St. Louis, 2011), that "cluttering, exceptionally rapid speech, and normally fluent speech are different points on the same clinical continuum" (Bakker et al., 2011, p. 46), provides another opportunity to apply set theory in a critical analysis. The three sets of participants, people who clutter (we can call them set A), people with exceptionally rapid speech (set B), and people with typi-

cal fluency (set C), engaged in conversational speech analyzed acoustically, production of diadochochinetic trains and related real words, and comfortable versus faster oral reading of the "Rainbow Passage." As described, Sets A, B, and C are disjoint sets, having no elements in common. Measurements of speech rates, clarity, and fluency were considered preliminary, with statistical analysis refuting membership in the same set only in some instances.

The one-to-one correspondence between sets will seldom, if ever, occur in the behavioral sciences. Problems may lie in the identification of the continuum, the nature of the task, and the nature of the analysis. For example, Bloodstein's (1960) continuum of time and severity tracked disfluencies produced by children who did and did not ultimately stutter. The correspondence found in whole-word repetitions would not hold if part-word repetitions were analyzed. Similarly, the continuum of speech rate (Bakker et al., 2011) showed some discrete points of behaviors by the three populations tested, but mostly showed overlaps, based on the task.

Overlaps between two collections yields more familiar applications of set theory. We use braces to denote sets, so {0, 1} is the set containing the elements 0 and 1. Santo Pietro and Goldfarb (1995) used this language of sets to demonstrate a specific treatment strategy. A patient receiving treatment for aphasia and a clinician are each asked, independently, to list their most important five goals of language rehabilitation. The patient indicates the desire to improve the ability to:

1. Recite hymns and prayers in church.
2. State bids while playing games of bridge.
3. Retrieve names and relationships of family members.
4. Verbalize activities of daily living.
5. Speak and understand conversational speech on the telephone.

The clinician's goals for the patient are to improve the ability to:

3. Retrieve names and relationships of family members.
4. Verbalize activities of daily living.
5. Speak and understand conversational speech on the telephone.
6. Read and understand the newspaper.
7. Write legibly with the left hand.

Selecting appropriate target goals can be aided by examining the two sets of goals arithmetically. If Set A = {1,2,3,4,5} and Set B = {3,4,5,6,7}, then the intersection of these two sets of goals is {3,4,5}, or Set C. Expressed in symbols A ∩ B = C, or {1,2,3,4,5} ∩ {3,4,5,6,7} = {3,4,5}, where ∩ (read "cap") is the symbol for intersection. The three goals in Set C {3,4,5} might be expected to elicit maximal motivation and cooperation between patient and clinician.

John Venn (1834–1923) is best known for his development of diagrams, later named after him, depicting relationships between sets. We have used Venn diagrams to illustrate strategies of clinical intervention in individuals with communication disorders following Alzheimer disease (Ostuni & Santo Pietro, 1991), aphasia (Santo Pietro & Goldfarb, 1995), and stuttering (Goldfarb, 2006a).

The diagram in Figure 41–1, which incorporates a Venn diagram, portrays a person (P) with a language impairment (I) communicating (C) with a communication partner (CP) within an environment (E). None of the components should be treated independently of the others. The clinician who works only to build skills lost as a result of the neurological impairment (treating to deficit) is addressing only (I). However, (I) is contained completely within the set of the person (P), who is contained completely within an environment (E). It also intersects the communication (C)

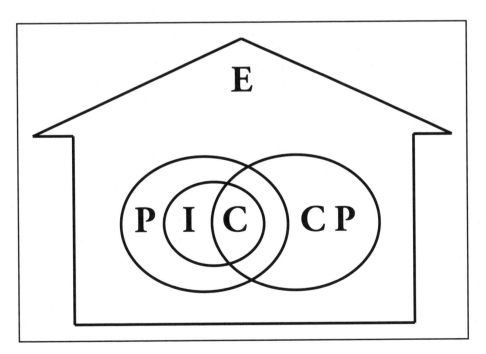

Figure 41–1. The interaction of sets.

between the person and the communication partner (CP) as well as the communication partner alone. Rebuilding skills lost or absent through impairment will have a direct effect on the total person (P), the person's communication partner (CP), the level of communication between them (C), and their shared environment (E). Conversely, (P), (CP), (C), and (E) will have a direct effect on level of impairment as the skill-(re)building proceeds.

To be effective, therapy must address all intersections to maximize the person's unimpaired communication skills (treating to strength), repair communication acts between persons and communication partners, educate and support the partners, repair the communication-impaired environment to provide opportunities for communication, and treat the whole person to reduce psychosocial handicap.

Set theory may also apply to diagnosis and evaluation. Recently (Goldfarb & Serpanos, 2009), we identified five rules for diagnosis: (1) Say what the client does, not what the client is; (2) Be an educated consumer of tests and measures; (3) Beware of "clinicese," where clients may exhibit behaviors in the clinic that they do not generalize outside of the speech and hearing center; (4) Do differential diagnosis when appropriate; and (5) Obey the limits of our scope of practice.

The third and fourth rules above, in particular, express aspects of set theory. Regarding Rule 3, a working hypothesis for carryover (or generalization of linguistic skills acquired in therapy to other communication environments) might be for the two sets of clinical communication and communication in another environment to approximate the same cardinal number. Deciding where among diagnostically related groups the observed language behavior best fits (Rule 4) offers the opportunity to examine intersections along a continuum. For example, Goldfarb (2006b,) presented the following case:

An elderly homeless man, identified as Mr. X because he cannot say his name, has been admitted with what the emergency room physician described as disorganized language. The patient has no identification, no documented medical history, and has not yet had brain imaging studies. You have been asked to determine if the disorganized language represents fluent aphasia, the language of schizophrenia, or the language of dementia. (p.106)

The patient is referred to a speech-language pathologist at University Hospital. Evaluation of Mr. X's language reveals preservation of prosody, phonology, morphology, and syntax, with disturbances in semantics and pragmatics. This still fits the pattern of the diagnostically related groups of fluent aphasia, the language of Alzheimer and frontotemporal dementia, and the language of chronic undifferentiated schizophrenia.

The Venn diagram in Figure 41–1 also illustrates two major points of applying set theory to diagnosis and evaluation of fluency disorders (Goldfarb, 2006a, p. 25): (1) Diagnosis must be comprehensive. The whole person as well as the communication partners and environment must be considered; and (2) The individual's needs and wishes must be an integral component in determining approaches to treatment.

Various approaches to communication therapy can be viewed as sets. For example, speech-language pathologists have traditionally employed an approach that Lubinski (1995) labeled a *skills model* to treat individuals with speech and language disabilities. In the skills model, the speech-language pathologist accompanies the patient to a quiet treatment room and teaches a set of discrete skills designed to improve communication abilities over time to a *normal* level. The skills model puts responsibility for change on the patient, with the goal of carryover to real-life encounters.

Lubinski pointed out that the skills model might not prove very useful for adults with communication disorders secondary to chronic disabilities, such as aphasia, Alzheimer disease, or chronic undifferentiated schizophrenia. She reasoned that patients with chronic neurologic impairments are unlikely ever to improve to normal, and, furthermore, that they are seldom in a position to choose or manage their interactions with others. Lubinski suggested that a better approach for treating adult neurologically impaired individuals would be a *communication model* where both patient and caregiver are coached to improve the quality of communicative acts between them. This is a more functional approach that, while encouraging the practice of skills, sets the primary goal as successful communication between the patient and the communication partner. If accurate communication is achieved, the therapy has been successful. The sets of skills of both patient and communication partner overlap to produce a successful outcome set called *communication*, whose Venn diagram is shown in Figure 41–2.

Lubinski went on to point out, however, that neither the skills approach nor the communication approach can be efficacious unless patients have *communication opportunities* to use their skills and communication partners with whom to achieve successful communication. By necessity, the sets of *communication skills* and *communication acts* overlap with the set of *communication opportunities*. Neither the skills nor the communication acts can be realized without an overlapping set of communication opportunities.

Building on Lubinski's observation of the need for communication opportunities, Santo Pietro and Ostuni (2003) and others

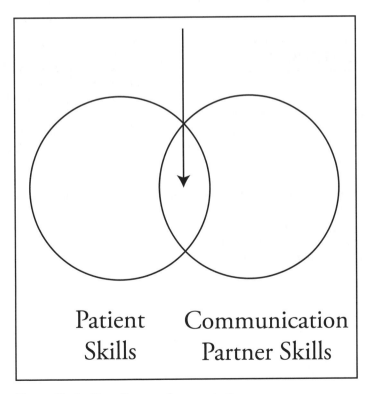

Figure 41–2. Venn diagram of communication.

have extended that paradigm and placed the above Venn diagram into a larger set labeled *environment* to form a working therapeutic model for adults with neurogenic communication disorders. In creating evidence-based treatments for persons with Alzheimer disease, Santo Pietro and Ostuni illustrated how therapeutic changes in the physical and psychosocial environment profoundly affect the ability of patients and caregivers to develop communication skills, and how the environment either enables or discourages the success of communication acts between patients and their communication partners. This is true for both institutionalized patients and for patients living in the community. Acknowledgement of the overlapping of approaches has led to in-depth examination of the specific effects of environmental factors on communication and ways to constitute communication-friendly environments and direct environmental treatments for communication disabilities.

REFERENCES

Bakker, K., Myers, F. L., Raphael, L. J., & St. Louis, K. O. (2011). A preliminary comparison of speech rate, self-evaluation, and disfluency of people who speak exceptionally fast, clutter, or speak normally. In D. Ward & K. Scaler Scott (Eds.), *Cluttering: A handbook of research, intervention and education* (pp. 45–66). East Sussex, UK: Psychology Press.

Bloodstein, O. (1960). The development of stuttering. II. Developmental phases. *Journal of Speech and Hearing Disorders, 25,* 366–376.

Enderton, H. B. (1977). *Elements of set theory.* New York, NY: Academic Press.

Godel, K. (1947). What is Cantor's continuum problem? *American Mathematical Monthly, 54,* 515–525.

Goldfarb, R. (2006a). Diagnosis. In R. Goldfarb (Ed.), *Ethics: A case study from fluency* (pp. 13–26). San Diego, CA: Plural.

Goldfarb, R. (2006b). Differential diagnosis of adults with neurogenic communication disorders. In E. M. Walsh (Ed.), *Topics in Alzheimer's disease* (pp. 89–109). New York, NY: Nova Science.

Goldfarb, R., & Davis, R. (2010). Oceans of the brain. *Journal of Experimental Stroke and Translational Medicine, 3,* 22–26.

Goldfarb, R., & Serpanos, Y. (2009). *Professional writing in speech-language pathology and audiology.* San Diego, CA: Plural.

LaPointe, L. L. (1977). Base-10 programmed stimulation: Task specification, scoring, and plotting performance in aphasia therapy. *Journal of Speech and Hearing Disorders, 42,* 90–105.

Lubinski, R. (1995). Environmental considerations for elderly potients. In R. Lubinski (Ed.), *Dementia and communicaton* (pp. 257–278). San Diego, CA: Singular

Ostuni, E., & Santo Pietro, M. J. (1991). *Getting through: Communicating when someone you care for has Alzheimer's disease.* Vero Beach, FL: Speech Bin.

Santo Pietro, M. J., & Goldfarb, R. (1995). *Techniques for aphasia rehabilitation generating effective treatment (TARGET).* Vero Beach, FL: Speech Bin.

Santo Pietro, M. J., & Ostuni, E. (2003). *Successful communication with persons with Alzheimer's disease: An in-service manual* (2nd ed.). St. Louis, MO: Butterworth-Heinemann.

ESSAY 42

❧ Verbotonal Worldwide ❧

Carl W. Asp, Madeline Kline, and Kazunari J. Koike

With warm affection, the first author acknowledges the late Dr. Sadanand Singh as an inspiration and a special friend.

BREIF HISTORY

In 1939, Petar Guberina completed his dissertation at the Sorbonne University, Paris, which established how vocal pitch change (intonation) affected the meaning of a phrase, and discussed how spoken language affected the learning of written language. His study became the theoretical foundation of a practical strategy called the Structural-Global-Audio-Visual (SGAV) method for teaching normal hearing people to speak before reading a foreign language (Renard & Van Vlasselaer, 1976). More popularly used in Europe, the methodology was later expanded to teach people with hearing impairment how to speak their native language by learning to listen first. This methodology has been coined "The Verbotonal Method."

In 1963, Guberina was appointed visiting Professor at Ohio State University, Columbus (OSU). For four years, 1963 to 1967, Carl

Asp was his clinical research assistant on a federal OSU research grant with Professor John Black (Black, 1963). Professor Guberina taught Verbotonal theory to all PhD students including Carl Asp and Sadanand Singh. Following this exposure, Dr. Singh published the 1981, *Verbotonal Method for Communication Problems* (Asp, Guberina, & Pansini, 1981, revised 2011) with College-Hill Press, and in 2006, *Verbotonal Speech Treatment* (Asp, 2006, revised 2011) with Plural Publishing. Dr. Singh established himself as a well-known academician, researcher, publisher, and philanthropist (Dr. Sadanand Singh Fund) in the field of communication disorders.

Interaction with Professors Guberina and Black along with fellow student, Dr. Singh, inspired Dr. Asp to pursue further research in Verbotonal theoretical principles, and in 1967, he acquired a federal research grant as a certified professor (CCC-A and CCC-SLP) at the University of Tennessee, Knoxville (UTK) (Asp, 1967). This research grant became a cornerstone of spreading Verbotonal. For the past 70 plus years (1939 to present), Verbotonal has developed in many countries with various languages and cultures. For example, the UTK Web site (Verbotonal.utk.edu) identifies

15 languages, two books in English, one book in Chinese, one in Arabic, and one in Russian, videotapes, pictures, Facebook, YouTube, 2000 plus research titles, 15 different Web sites, equipment, training, and certification. Numerous Croatian and French articles have been translated and published into English and also Japanese (Roberge, 1973), although terminology has been modified to increase understanding in the language of the reader. Verbotonal is used worldwide!

INTRODUCTION

What is Verbotonal? It's an auditory-based strategy that maximizes the listening skills of children and adults with hearing impairment, while simultaneously developing intelligible spoken language through binaural listening (Asp, 2006, revised 2011). The strategy implies the clinician's use of refined listening skills to analyze the client's error(s) and correct those errors with use of various tools based on theoretical and scientific evidence.

Verbotonal has five areas of applications: (1) children with hearing impairment (peripheral or central), (2) adults with hearing impairment, (3) diagnostic therapy, (4) speech-language disorders (e.g., articulation, stuttering, aphasia, autism), and (5) foreign languages (e.g., English as a Second Language, ESL). The theory and tools are adjusted to the severity of the problem. The clinical setting may be in public schools, private or residential schools, clinics, or even home schooling. Verbotonal focuses on therapy by the trained teacher/clinician. Parents are, of course, involved through individualized parent education, in order to maximize what the child has learned in the therapy session.

Five basic principles of Verbotonal are described in the following paragraphs in an attempt to explain why and how it is applied to the aforementioned areas with focus on application to the hearing-impaired: (1) neuroplasticity of the human brain, (2) vibrotactile phase of listening, (3) listening through rhythm and intonation, (4) error analysis and correction, and (5) listening through spoken language.

NEUROPLASTICITY OF THE HUMAN BRAIN

The brain of all species constantly reorganizes new neural connections throughout life. This maturational process is often referred to as *neuroplasticity*. Because of neuroplasticity, children five years old and younger are more easily adapted to learn to speak two different languages, since their neural maturational process is still evolving and, in a sense, is optimal (Piaget, 1973) to different neural stimulation (e.g., foreign spoken language). After puberty, however, the child's brain becomes an adult brain that is less plastic for learning a new language without systematic teaching approaches (e.g., SGAV, Rosetta Stone, etc.).

Verbotonal considers this concept of neuroplasticity a very important principle in the application of therapy to the hearing impaired, and looks for what is optimal stimulation to each individual brain (Asp, Guberina, & Pansini, 1981, revised 2011). Hearing impairment is primarily a peripheral disorder; however, the rewiring of the brain's neural connectivity is considered to be the ultimate Verbotonal goal. For example, it has been observed that young children or adults with high frequency hearing losses can learn to perceive low and high tonality (pitch) words (e.g., bow vs. cease) through the most sensitive frequencies below 1000 Hz. We theorize that this clinical phenomenon is possible because auditory perception within the brain has been rehabilitated (rewired).

Table 19–1 in Essay 19 illustrates body movements and speech modification based on the seven perceptual parameters for error analysis and correction of binaural listening through spoken language.

VIBROTACTILE PHASE OF LISTENING

Figure 42–1 shows the human brain receiving neural information from the vestibular, auditory and speech channels. With the adding of proprioception, the human brain goes through developmental neuroplasticity as the developing infant matures to childhood and then adolescence. As an infant, the vibrotactile channel (vestibular) is a more dominant sense than hearing (cochlear), whereas hearing becomes more dominant in the older child. Verbotonal considers that the utilization of this early dominant sense (vibrotactile phase) is a foundation toward the development of good sound awareness, which is the critical step for later development of good spoken language through listening.

Figure 42–2 shows the Verbotonal Listen Control Panel. It has five channels: wideband, low-pass, low-peaking, high-pass, and high-peaking filters. The center frequency and slope of a filter is adjusted based on the client's error(s) while he listens and feels speech.

For example, Figure 19–1 in Essay 19 shows a parent using a body movement, a speech-vibrating board, and wrist-vibrator with her son. Figure 19–2 shows the first author using a body movement with three children, each wearing a speech-vibrator and a headset. These two figures demonstrate vibrotactile input and body movement.

Neurologic research supports that the vestibular-otoliths respond to sounds (i.e., vibrations) from 2 to 1000 Hz. As both the vestibule and the cochlea comprise the infant's inner ear, one may say that there is vestibular-cochlear listening. The perceptual frequency range of both organs overlaps from 20 to 1000 Hz, where the cochlea dominates above 1000 Hz, although the vestibule dominates

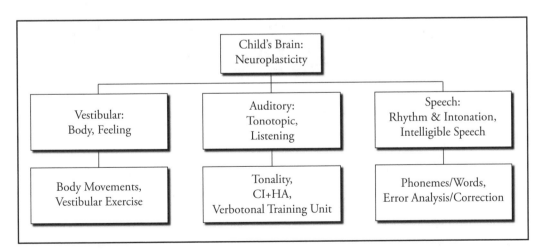

Figure 42–1. The child's brain receives simultaneous auditory, vestibular, and speech input, with propriocep-tive feedback from body movements. Used with permission from Asp (2006).

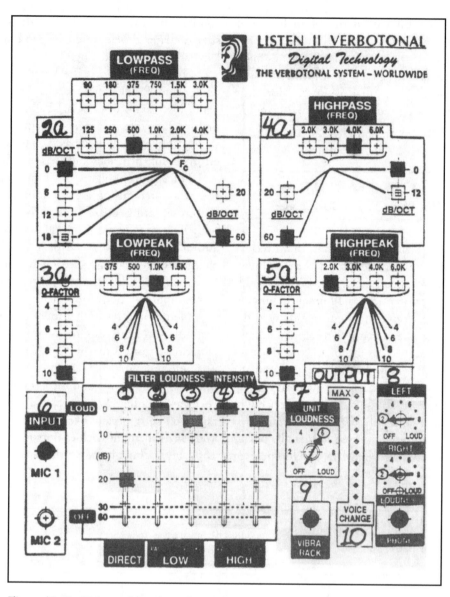

Figure 42–2. *Verbotonal five-channel control panel. Used with permission from Asp (2006).*

below 20 Hz (infrasonics) (Asp, 2006, revised, 2011).

In order to facilitate this vibrotactile phase of listening, a device called the Verbotonal speech vibrator responds from 2 Hz to 1000 Hz. It can be attached to the infant's wrist and/or a vibrating board that stimulates the infant's brain through the vibrotactile sense. Figure 19–1 in Essay 19 shows a picture of a parent using body movement while her two-year-old son feels/hears her speech through a speech vibrator on his wrist and one on a vibrating board against his lower body. With the use of the more dominant vibrotactile sense, it becomes easier and optimal for the infant even with profound hearing loss to become aware of sounds (vibrations). Furthermore, the infant feels his mother's speech rhythms, as he did in his mother's womb. This helps his babbling advance to rhythm and intonation patterns that become meaningful, as discussed in the next section. Table 19–1 in Essay 19 illustrates body movements and speech modification based on the seven perceptual parameters to correct errors.

LISTENING THROUGH RHYTHM AND INTONATION

Rhythm and intonation (suprasegmental or prosodic) is the foundation of both listening and spoken language. In a conversation, changes in rhythm and intonation and body language can affect the meaning of a phrase so that "no" may mean "yes" or "yes" may mean "no," depending on how the rhythm and intonation pattern of the word is altered. Natural vocal-pitch changes in conversation go an octave lower and higher than the mean vocal pitch. For example, when we say, "I cannot go out; it's raining" (Guberina, 1939), emotional vocal-pitch changes (intonation) alters the meaning (language) of this phrase (speech). The semicolon is a pause, created by the vocal pitch rising with tension to let the listener know there is more after the pause. Therefore, an upward inflection at the end of "go out" can mean "Yes, I dare go out," as if the child is questioning the authority of the mother. According to Mehrabian (1969), verbal components (lexicon and syntax) are only 7% of human communication, whereas 93% (38% and 55%, respectively) are from suprasegmental components (e.g., rhythm and intonation) and nonverbal components (e.g., facial expressions, eye contact, gestures, etc.). Verbotonal considers that it is important to incorporate this observation into actual habilitative and

rehabilitative therapies, emphasizing the development of good rhythm and intonation patterns in the early stage of spoken language.

In both adults and children, speech energy for rhythm and intonation typically lies below 300 Hz. Most children and adults with hearing impairment are observed to have hearing sensitivity below 300 Hz in the audiogram. Therefore, in order to ensure that children with profound deafness are able to perceive rhythm and intonation patterns, a Verbotonal training unit that can amplify the speech frequencies below 300 Hz effectively, with a wide frequency response bandwidth (2 to 20,000 Hz) that includes both extended lows (2 to 300 Hz) and extended highs (3000 to 20,000 Hz), has been designed and utilized for therapy. This is why most people who are deaf (90 dB) in the classical speech frequencies (300 to 3000 Hz), can learn to talk and listen with good rhythm and intonation and intelligible spoken language. Especially in the early stage of habilitation, Verbotonal training units may even include speech vibrators and headphones to create optimum listening to good rhythm and intonation, which ultimately helps to stimulate neural maturation in the brain. In this context, Verbotonal can be characterized as a multisensory strategy for rehabilitation of the brain.

In 1940, the AT&T Bell Research Lab determined an auditory memory span of eight syllables in 1.8 seconds, separated by a pause, was an essential part of a phone conversation. For example, a phone number 523 (pause) 0996 is easy for a normal listener to remember. The pause is an essential part of auditory memory. During a typical conversation, normal speech rate is five syllables per second. Each syllable has a vowel, with one or two consonants. The phoneme rate of a talker is 12 phonemes per second, 720 per minute, and 43,200 per hour. In a long conversation, the listener automatically "locks on" to the syllable stress and intonation patters of the talker, because the normal speech rate is too fast to "lock on" to all the phonemes. This is another reason why Verbotonal stresses listening through rhythm and intonation, that is, to enhance auditory memory to at least eight syllables.

ERROR ANALYSIS AND CORRECTION

American English has 25 consonants, and 15 vowels and diphthongs. Guberina (1972) proposed to use octave-band filters to determine what would be the most important frequency region for the perception of a particular phoneme (vowel or consonant). In his experiment, when he set the octave-band filter's center frequency at 200 Hz, the listener heard the recorded vowel /i/ as the vowel /u/. When the center frequency was changed to 1000 Hz, the vowel /i/ was heard as the vowel /a/, and so forth. Therefore, he concluded that all phonemes are contained in one phoneme, because the perception of different phonemes (e.g., the vowels /i/, /e/, /a/, /o/, /u/) was possible from the same phoneme (e.g., the vowel /i/) depending on which filter frequency in which the phoneme was passed. Guberina further defined each of these various filter settings as an *optimal octave* for each vowel or consonant. In practice, this principle is a helpful tool in analyzing errors, that is, why a certain error occurs with an individual with a certain audiometric pattern. For example, it would explain why a child with only low frequency hearing below 300 Hz, will say the vowel /u/ when the vowel /i/ is presented as a stimulus. The vowel /i/ is filtered through the child's hearing loss that is equivalent to a low pass filter, optimal for perceiving the vowel /u/.

Based on such research with optimal octaves, Guberina (1972) constructed a sequence of eight nonsense syllables, with their optimal octaves ranging from a low frequency to a high frequency continuum and defined them as *logatomes* (bru-bru, mu-mu, bu-bu, vo-vo, la-la, ke-ke, shi-shi, and si-si) (Asp, Guberina, & Pansini, 1981, p. 7). In practice, an abbreviated sequence of logatomes "mu-mu, la-la, si-si" has been used by Verbotonal clinicians to evaluate the detection and perception of these sounds through auditory training units, hearing aids, and cochlear implants.

Furthermore, in a paired-comparison experiment by Peterson and Asp (1971), normal-hearing listeners judged the unfiltered prevocalic consonant /s/ as higher in spectral pitch than /m/ and so forth. In 1979, Bessel and Asp, in a paired-comparison experiment, found that normal hearing listeners judged the unfiltered word "cease" as higher in pitch than the word "move." In 1980, Bessel and Asp acoustically analyzed 30 words judged to be different in spectral pitch. Both the consonant and the word results support a low to mid to high spectral-pitch continuum. At the syllabic and word level, this spectral pitch was defined as tonality.

Similarly, words were separated into low, mid, and high tonality categories (Asp, 2006, revised 2011). For example, low, mid, and high tonality words would be, "Moon-Hat-Cease." During diagnostic therapy, the appropriateness of a hearing aid's frequency response can be diagnosed by analyzing tonality errors. At the same time, possible adjustment may be made to the frequency response and/or gain of the hearing aid. For example, the clinician presents one tonality word, and each time the client says what is heard, without visual cues. It is commonly observed that when the client has a high frequency hearing loss above 2000 Hz, a high tonality word such as "cease" can be mistakenly perceived as words from the lower tonality category, for example, "use" or "ooze." Analysis of errors enables the clinician to provide further auditory therapy with use of the Verbotonal training unit that has adjustable acoustic filters and slopes to enhance the correct perception of the test words and/or to adjust the settings of the hearing aid to optimize the perception of high tonality sounds.

One of the unique treatment tools Verbotonal uses in the correction of speech errors, either at the suprasegmental level (rhythm and intonation) or at the segmental level (phoneme, word, and sentence), is body movements. A detailed explanation of why and how body movements are utilized is available in Essay 19.

within various contextual cues. Progression of teaching various phonemic utterances also follows the developmental progression of normal hearing children (e.g., the acquisition of words like "mama" and "baby" occurs earlier than words like "sister" and "scissors") (Asp, 2006, pp. 152–153). Interestingly, low tonality words are generally developed earlier than high tonality words. Just as slides and DVD are used in the teaching of foreign language courses (e.g., SGAV), the use of situational teaching with audiovisual materials is frequently incorporated into therapy sessions with hearing-impaired children.

LISTENING THROUGH SPOKEN LANGUAGE

The ultimate goal of Verbotonal is to develop good, intelligible spoken language among children and adults with hearing impairment, so that they can communicate and be educated among normal hearing peers. As described above, Verbotonal initially utilizes multisensory input (vibrotactile, vision, audition, and proprioception in the form of body movements) for rehabilitation of the brain. In the process, however, audition (listening) must be established as the primary sensory input in learning spoken language.

Verbotonal evolved from Guberina's observation of how people learn a foreign language. The process of teaching children with hearing impairment is almost analogous to how hearing children learn their native language. Infants begin with a babbling stage, where they begin to imitate the mother's utterances, feel affectionate changes in rhythm and intonation, and see facial expressions and gestures. As they mature, they begin to form wordlike utterances, where the meaning of spoken language begins to be defined

SUMMARY

The five Verbotonal areas and five principles above comprise the Theory. Essay 19 describes the Treatment Tools, with emphasis on Verbotonal Body Movements.

Acknowledgments. The authors appreciate the editing by Mary Koike, Wayne Kline, and Jan Asp.

REFERENCES

Asp, C. W. (1967). *The effectiveness of low-frequency amplification and filtered-speech testing for preschool deaf children.* University of Tennessee, Knoxville, TN. U.S. Department of Health, Education & Welfare, Grant No. OED-0-9-522113-3339 (032).

Asp, C. W., (2006, rev. 2011) (casp@utk.edu). *Verbotonal speech treatment.* San Diego, CA: Plural.

Asp, C. W., Guberina P., & Pansini, M. (1981, rev. 2011) (casp@utk.edu). *The verbotonal method for rehabilitating people with communication problems.* New York, NY: World Rehabilitation Fund.

Bessel, C. S. (1979). *Pitch difference among 30 English monosyllabic words.* Unpublished master's thesis, University of Tennessee, Knoxville, TN.

Bessel, C. S., & Asp, C. W. (1980). Acoustic analysis of 30 English monosyllabic words judged to be different in spectral pitch, *Journal of the Acoustical Society of America, 67*(Suppl. 1).

Black, J. W. (1963). *Perception of altered acoustic stimuli by the deaf.* Ohio State University Research Foundation, Columbus, OH. U.S. Department of Health, Education & Welfare: Social & Rehabilitation Services Grant No. RD-1226-S-68-C4.

Guberina, P. (1939). *Speech intonation and language.* Unpublished PhD dissertation, Sorbonne University, Paris.

Guberina, P. (1972). *Case studies in restricted bands of frequencies in auditory rehabilitation of deaf.* U. S. Office of Vocational Rehabilitation, OVR-YUGO-2-63.

Mehrabian, A., (1969). Some referents and measures of nonverbal behavior. *Behavior Research Methods Instrumentation, 1,* 203–207.

Piaget, J. (1973). *The child and reality.* New York, NY: Grossman.

Peterson, N. M, & Asp, C. W. (1972). The perceived pitch of 23 English consonants. *Journal of the Acoustical Society of America, 59*(Suppl. 1).

Renard, R., & Van Vlasselaer, J. J. (1976). *Foreign language teaching with an integrated methodology: The SGAV (structuro-global audio-visual) methodology.* Paris, France: Didier.

Roberge, C. (1973). [In Japanese]. What is the verbotonal system? In C. Roberge (Ed.), *Zagreb language education: Theory and application* (Chapter 1). Tokyo, Japan: Gakushobo.

ESSAY 43

❧ Timing Is Everything ❧

At Least for MCI

Kathryn Bayles

Sadanand Singh knew the truth of this axiom and were he with us, he would likely have a book about MCI in the pipeline. Singh had a gift for seeing the clinical implications of basic science and identifying clinical observations deserving of scientific investigation. He was equally gifted in the art of persuasion and routinely convinced overcommitted professors to add the challenge of writing a book to their busy schedules. Singh used his talents to make profound contributions to speech-language pathology and audiology. Although the publications he brought to life could be counted, we could never take the full measure of their influence on clinicians, researchers and individuals with communication disorders. Singh changed the course of my career as he likely did for all the essayists in this commemorative text. His passion for science and its translation to clinical practice was infectious and his timing impeccable.

INTRODUCTION

What Is MCI?

MCI is the acronym for the psychogeriatric disorder of mild cognitive impairment.

Many characterize MCI as a transitional zone between normal cognitive function and dementia (Winblad et al., 2004), although not all individuals with MCI develop dementia. MCI is associated with many etiologies but Alzheimer disease (AD) is by far the most common. Increasingly, attention has been given to identifying individuals with MCI and the effectiveness of treatments for slowing or stopping progression to dementia. Whereas pharmacologic interventions, approved for individuals with AD, are being tested on individuals with MCI, none has emerged as capable of preventing dementia. What has emerged, however, is evidence of the benefit of cognitive stimulation for sustaining and improving function and quality of life in individuals with MCI.

Cognitive stimulation is noninvasive, cost effective, generally enjoyed by recipients, and free of the negative side effects of drugs. The thesis of this essay is that speech-language pathologists, who are expert in identifying cognitive-communication disorders and providing cognitive stimulation, have an important role in identifying and treating individuals with MCI. Supporting this thesis is a growing body of evidence that changes in language signal early stage MCI when intervention through cognitive stimulation would be most beneficial.

CRITERIA FOR DIAGNOSING MCI

In 2003 an international conference was convened in Stockholm to consider the clinical characteristics of MCI. The consensus of participants was that memory impairment is the signature characteristic (Winblad et al., 2004) and AD the most common cause. However, conference participants recognized the existence of other subtypes caused by vascular, metabolic, psychiatric, and other degenerative conditions.

Characterization of MCI subtypes has generated considerable debate that is likely to continue. When memory impairment is the prominent feature, the individual is said to have amnestic MCI; when multiple cognitive domains are affected, the individual is said to have multiple domain MCI; when memory is not affected, a diagnosis of non-amnestic MCI is given (Winblad et al., 2004). A challenge to characterizing the cognitive profiles associated with subtypes is a lack of consensus about what cognitive functions are tested by the neuropsychological tests used to detect MCI. For example, is a poor performance on the widely used category naming/verbal fluency tests best characterized as a memory problem, executive function problem, language deficit, or the result of multiple cognitive problems?

Criteria for diagnosing amnestic MCI, the most common type, include: self-report of memory problems, or report by a qualified informant; a Mini-Mental State Examination score ≥24; objective evidence of deficit; and generally intact cognitive functions, with no significant difficulties with instrumental activities of daily living (Petersen, 2004). The performance of individuals with MCI on cog-

nitive tests typically falls 1.5 standard deviations below the mean for age and education (Petersen et al., 1999).

Rate of Conversion to Dementia

Numerous investigators have evaluated rate of conversion to dementia (Gauthier et al., 2006), with varying results ranging between 12% and 20% after 30 months and approximately 48% thereafter. Petersen and Negash (2008) reported rate of progression to AD to be 10% to 15% per year. German investigators reported progression rates of 7.2 to 10.2% per year. Notably all of these progression rates exceed the population incidence figures for AD of 1 to 2% per year (Busse, Hensel, Guhne, Angermeyer, & Riedel-Heller, 2006).

Hodges, Erzinçlioğlu, and Patterson (2006) conducted a careful long-term follow-up study of ten individuals with MCI who were given extensive neuropsychological testing annually. All ultimately developed dementia (defined as <24 on the MMSE and/or a significant problem with activities of daily living), though onset ranged from 1 to 8 years. Those presenting with multiple cognitive deficits early converted faster.

EARLY CHANGES IN LANGUAGE

The first report that early language performance may be a harbinger of late life dementia came in 1996 from the now famous Nun Study (Riley, Snowdon, Desrosiers, & Markesbery, 2005; Snowdon et al., 1996). Investigators had access to the autobiographies of almost 200 American Roman Catholic sisters who are members of the School Sisters of Notre Dame. Although the nun study began when the sisters were between 75 and 103 years old, the autobiographies were written decades earlier as novices. Linguistic analyses of these autobiographies revealed that sisters whose text had lower idea density and grammatical complexity were more likely to develop AD later in life. Making this finding more compelling was that all the nuns had a similar existence by virtue of being in the same order, living under similar conditions, and 85% were teachers. Since the report of Snowdon and colleagues, others have found a relation between cognitive performance early in life and vulnerability to late life dementia (McGurn, Deary, & Starr, 2008; Whalley et al., 2000).

In 2002, Chapman and colleagues reported that individuals with MCI are impaired in processing discourse and deriving the gist of a story (Chapman et al., 2002). Sixty-nine individuals (20 with MCI, 24 with mild AD, and 25 cognitively normal elders) listened to a 578-word biographical narrative and were later asked to recount the story, including the gist. Additionally, they answered questions about story details. Analysis of performance data revealed that both MCI and AD subjects were impaired in recounting story details and producing *gist-level* responses. Their performance was interpreted as reflecting memory impairment for details and difficulty drawing inferences about the core meaning of the story that were not explicitly stated.

In 2005 the effects of early AD on the characteristics of the writings of a well-known author were published. Garrard, Maloney, Hodges, and Patterson (2005) analyzed the text of three of Iris Mudoch's novels, one written early in her career in her 30s, a second written during her prime, and her final novel written a few years before her death from AD. Comparisons were made of the degree of lexical diversity in the three works. In her last and least highly regarded work, vocabulary was more restricted, and there were fewer unique word types relative to overall word count.

Harris, Kiran, Marquardt, and Fleming (2008) reported subtle changes in the discourse of 10 adults with MCI, compared to 30 neurologically healthy young adults and 22 neurologically healthy older adults. A variety of discourse analyses were conducted: calculation of MLU, proportion of definite nouns, indefinite nouns, verbs and modifiers, and pronouns and mazed words (repetitions, false starts, reformulations, and self-corrections). Count was also made of the number of core concepts recounted that were related to the story theme. Subjects were instructed to describe, in detail, activities associated with preparing for and taking a trip to New York City. They were told to think about preparation, packing, and activities while there. Data analyses revealed that individuals with MCI provided less thematic information, more irrelevant comments, and were more verbose than normal subjects. Significantly, performance on the discourse task was associated with performance on cognitive measures including the MMSE.

In a related study, Fleming and Harris (2008) sought to determine whether performance on the Trip to New York discourse task differentiated normal elders from eight physician-diagnosed individuals with MCI in terms of discourse length, complexity, and quality using SALT analysis (Miller & Inglesias, 2006). Other analyses included counting the number of words and core elements of the 26 possible, plus calculating the average number of morphemes per T-units. MCI subjects produced significantly fewer words and core elements than control subjects, though the groups did not differ in average length of T-unit.

In 2009, an intriguing report of the sensitivity of language test scores for detecting MCI was published. Oulhaj, Wilcock, Smith, and de Jager (2009) followed a cohort of 241 normal healthy individuals for up to 20 years. The purpose of the study was to identify early markers of the later development of MCI. Subjects were periodically administered the Cambridge Cognitive Examination (CAMCOG), a widely used comprehensive neuropsychological battery comprising subtests of orientation, comprehension, expression, recent memory, remote memory, learning, abstract thinking, perception, praxis, attention, and calculation, as well as a derived Mini-Mental State Examination score. Only the subscores for language expression and learning/memory were predictors of time to conversion to MCI.

The CAMCOG expression subtest includes verbal fluency, spoken language descriptions, definitions, and comprehension. For each point lower on the composite expression score, the time to conversion was 17% shorter; for each point lower on the learning score, the time to conversion was 15% shorter; and for every 5 years of age, time to conversion was 14% shorter. The investigators emphasized that although memory impairment is the signature criterion for amnestic MCI and the recommended type of measure for assessing predementia AD, "expression" or language ability was a stronger predictor of duration to conversion than either "learning" or memory. It must be noted, however, that some would characterize verbal fluency as more a memory test than a language test. Nonetheless, it was just one of several language measures that formed the composite expression score.

In sum, one of the earliest and most telling manifestations of MCI is in language performance. Results of studies of language performance in young and older individuals strongly suggest that language changes occur very early, perhaps decades before a clinical diagnosis is made at a time when intervention would likely be most beneficial.

BENEFITS OF COGNITIVE STIMULATION FOR INDIVIDUALS WITH MCI

Advances in neuroscience have demonstrated the plasticity of the human brain throughout life. Abundant research supports the validity of the saying, "Use it or lose it." Rich environments, cognitive stimulation, and new experiences all increase synaptogenesis and neurogenesis. Animals placed in rich environments have greater neuron density, dendritic branching, increased brain weight, and cortical thickness than those in simple environments (Anderson, Eckburg, & Relucio, 2002; Biones, Suh, Jozsa, & Woods, 2006; Patoine, 2011). Humans with greater education and cognitively challenging careers have better cognitive reserves that reduce their risk of dementia (Katzman, 1993; Stern, 2002; Valenzuela & Sachdev, 2005; Zhang et al., 2004).

The science supporting plasticity of the human brain has given hope to individuals with brain injury and disease, including those with MCI. So also have reports of the benefit of cognitive stimulation programs (Jean, Bergeron, Thivierge, & Simard, 2010). Jean and colleagues reported that of the 15 cognitive intervention programs tested in patients with amnestic MCI, significant improvements were apparent at the end of training on 44% of objective measures of memory and 12% of other measures of cognition. Additionally, statistically significant post-treatment improvements were routinely observed on subjective measures of quality of life, mood, and memory.

ROLE OF SPEECH-LANGUAGE PATHOLOGISTS

As specialists in cognitive-communication disorders, speech-language pathologists can play an important role in educating people about MCI and identifying and treating those affected. The challenge is creating opportunities for education and screening. Some worth considering are screening seniors who visit clinics for hearing tests, are admitted to hospitals, reside in housing designed for elders, and are spouses of elders with communication problems. In a large study of 794 nondemented hospitalized patients aged 65 to 85, the prevalence of MCI was found to be 36% (Bicker, Mösch, Seigerschmidt, Siemen, & Förstl, 2006). Furthermore, the positive predictive value for cognitive impairment 3.5 months later was 61%. Particular attention should be paid to those with diabetes, high blood sugar, or depression, because these conditions appear to increase the risk of MCI evolving to AD (Palmer et al., 2010). Fortunately, seniors are increasingly seeking screenings for high cholesterol, osteoporosis, and cardiovascular disease, and these visits are another opportunity for MCI education. With greater awareness of MCI and the benefit of early detection, the demand for MCI screening will likely rise.

Screening and Treatment

What procedures are recommended for screening? A simple approach is a questionnaire about changes in language and memory. For those reporting awareness of change, in-depth testing can be scheduled. Verbal fluency (also called generative or category naming) is easily administered, takes little time and is sensitive to MCI (Hodges et al., 2006; Nutter-Upham et al., 2008). Two types of verbal fluency tests are widely used, those requiring the naming of words that begin with a particular letter, and those requiring the naming of items in a category. Nutter-Upham and colleagues gave both types to individuals with amnestic MCI, and reported statistically significant performance differences for both relative to cognitively intact age-matched older adults. Because verbal fluency tests are open-ended with no highest possible score, identification of MCI can be enhanced by pairing them with a test of episodic memory, such as story-retelling in an immediate and delayed condition.

As to treatment, cognitive stimulation helps individuals maintain function. Although an in-depth review of the literature on cognitive stimulation is beyond the scope of this essay, many researchers report improvement in memory and other cognitive functions (Jean et al., 2010). Particularly promising are cognitive stimulation programs designed to strengthen the processing of incoming sensory information (Smith et al., 2009). This approach is supported by a wealth of compelling evidence that age-related changes in the processing of sensory information contribute significantly to reports of age-related cognitive decline (Schneider & Pichora-Fuller, 2000; Wingfield & Stine-Morrow, 2000).

SUMMARY AND FUTURE DIRECTIONS

Awareness of MCI and its prevalence is growing and with it interest in interventions that can slow evolution to dementia. Many drugs are under study as are types of cognitive stimulation programs. To date, no drug has been approved for use, but researchers have demonstrated that cognitive stimulation can improve and sustain function. Of significance to speech-language pathologists are findings that indicate language change is a very early symptom of MCI. Were these findings shared with Dr. Singh, I have no doubt that he would recognize their significance to clinicians and individuals with MCI. Likely, he would ask the key questions needing future research. What language and other measures are most sensitive to the various subtypes of MCI? What cognitive stimulation programs are most effective for improving and sustaining function? Is cognitive stimulation more effective if paired with pharmacologic treatment? What variables predict those individuals with MCI who will develop dementia? What is the best way for speech-language pathologists to counsel individuals with MCI? With continued effort and additional research, we may soon find the answers to these questions.

REFERENCES

Anderson, B. J., Eckburg, P. B., & Relucio, K. I. (2002). Alterations in the thickness of motor cortical subregions after motor-skill learning and exercise. *Learning Memory*, *9*, 1–9.

Bickel, H., Mösch, E., Seigerschmidt, E., Siemen, M., & Förstl, H. (2006). Prevalence and persistence of mild cognitive impairment among elderly patients in general hospitals. *Dementia and Geriatric Disorders*, *21*(4), 242–250.

Biones, T. L., Suh, E., Jozsa, L., & Woods, J. (2006). *Experimental Neurology*, *198*(2), 530–538.

Busse, A., Hensel, A., Guhne, U., Angermeyer, M. C., & Riedel-Heller, S. G. (2006). Mild cognitive impairment: Long-term course of four clinical subtypes. *Neurology*, *67*, 2176–2185.

Chapman, S. B., Zientz, J., Weiner, M., Rosenberg, R., Frawley, W., & Burns, M. H. (2002). Discourse changes in early Alzheimer disease, mild cognitive impairment, and normal aging. *Alzheimer Disease and Associated Disorders*, *16*(3), 177–186.

Fleming, V. B., & Harris, J. L. (2008). Complex discourse production in mild cognitive impairment: Detecting subtle changes. *Aphasiology*, *22*(7–8), 729–740.

Garrard, P., Maloney, L. M., Hodges, J. R., & Patterson, K. (2005). The effects of very early Alzheimer's disease on the characteristics of writing by a renowned author. *Brain*, *128*(2), 250–260.

Gauthier, S., Reisberg, B., Zaudig, M., Petersen, R. C., Ritchie, K., & Brioch, K., . . . Windblad, B. (2006). Mild cognitive impairment. *Lancet*, *367*, 1262–1270.

Harris, J. L., Kiran, S., Marquardt, T., & Fleming, V. B. (2008). Communication Wellness Check-Up©: Age-related changes in communicative abilities. *Aphasiology*, *22*(7–8), 813–825.

Hodges, J. R., Erzinçlioğlu, S., & Patterson, K. (2006). Evolution of cognitive deficits and conversion to dementia in patients with mild cognitive impairment: A very-long-term follow-up study. *Dementia and Geriatric Cognitive Disorders*, *21*, 380–391.

Jean, L., Bergeron, M. E., Thivierge, S., & Simard, M. (2010). Cognitive intervention programs for individuals with mild cognitive impairment: Systematic review of the literature. *American Journal of Geriatric Psychiatry*, *18*(4), 281–296.

Katzman, R. (1993). Education and the prevalence of dementia and Alzheimer's disease. *Neurology*, *43*(1), 13–20.

McGurn, B., Deary, I. J., & Starr, J. M. (2008). Childhood cognitive ability and risk of late-onset Alzheimer and vascular dementia. *Neurology*, *71*, 1051–1056.

Miller, J., & Inglesias, A. (2006). *Systematic Analysis of Language Transcripts (SALT)*, English and Spanish (Version 9) [Computer software]. Language Analysis Lab, University of Wisconsin-Madison.

Nutter-Upham, K. E., Saykin, A. J., Rabin, L. A., Roth, R. M., Wishart, H. A., Pare, N., & Flashman, L. A. (2008). Verbal fluency performance in amnestic MCI and older adults with cognitive complaints. *Archives of Clinical Neuropsychology*, *23*(3), 229–241.

Oulahaj, A., Wilcock, G., Smith, A. D., & de Jager, C. A. (2009). Predicting the time of conversion to MCI in the elderly: Role of verbal expression and learning. *Neurology*, *73*(18), 1436–1442.

Palmer, K., Iulio, F. D., Gianni, W., Sancesario, G., Caltagirone, C., & Spalletta, G. (2010). Neuropsychiatric predictors of progression from amnestic-mild cognitive impairment to Alzheimer's disease: The role of depression and apathy. *Journal of Alzheimer's Disease*, *20*(1), 175–183.

Patoine, B. (2011). *Evidence grows for brain benefits of enriched environments in normal aging and disease*. The Dana Foundation. Retrieved from http://www.dana.org/media/detail.aspx?id=7142

Petersen, R. C. (2004). Mild cognitive impairment as a diagnostic entity. *Journal of Internal Medicine*, *256*, 183–194.

Petersen, R. C., & Negash, S. (2008). Mild cognitive impairment: An overview. *CNS Spectrums*, *13*(1), 48–53.

Petersen, R. C., Smith, G. E., Waring, S. C., Ivnik, R. J., Tangalos, E. G., & Kokmen, E. (1999). Mild cognitive impairment: Clinical characterization and outcome. *Archives of Neurology, 56*(3), 303–308.

Riley, K. P., Snowdon, D. A., Desrosiers, M. F., & Markesbery, W. R. (2005). Early life linguistic ability, late life cognitive function, and neuropathology: Findings from the Nun Study. *Neurobiology of Aging, 26,* 341–347.

Schneider, B. A., & Pichora-Fuller, M. K. (2000). Implications of perceptual deterioration for cognitive aging research. In F. I. M. Craik & T. A. Salthouse (Eds.), *The handbook of aging and cognition* (pp. 155–219). Mahwah, NJ: Lawrence Erlbaum.

Smith, G. E., Housen, P., Yaffe, K., Ruff, R., Kennison, R. F., Mahncke, H. W., & Zelinski, E. M. (2009). A cognitive training program based on principles of brain plasticity: Results from the improvement in memory with plasticity-based adaptive cognitive training (IMPACT) study. *Journal of the American Geriatrics Society, 57,* 594–603.

Snowdon, D. A., Kemper, S. J., Mortimer, J. A., Greiner, L. H., Wekstein, D. R., & Markesbery W. R. (1996). Linguistic ability in early life and cognitive function and Alzheimer's disease in late life: Findings from the Nun Study. *Journal of the American Medical Association, 275,* 528–532.

Stern, Y. (2002). What is cognitive reserve? Theory and research application of the reserve concept. *Journal of the International Neuropsychological Society, 8,* 448–460.

Valenzuela, M. J., & Sachdev, P. (2005). Brain reserve and dementia: A systematic review. *Psychological Medicine, 35,* 1–14.

Whalley, L. J., Starr, J. M., Athawes, R., Hunter, D., Pattie, A., & Deary, I. J. (2000). Childhood mental ability and dementia. *Neurology, 55,* 1455–1459.

Winblad, B., Palmer, K., Kivipelto, M., Jelic, V., Fratiglioni, L., Wahlund, L. O., . . . Petersen, R. C. (2004). Mild cognitive impairment —beyond controversies, towards a consensus: Report of the International Working Group on Mild Cognitive Impairment. *Journal of Internal Medicine, 256,* 240–246.

Wingfield, A., & Stine-Morrow, E. A. L. (2000). Language and speech. In F. I. M. Craik & T. A. Salthouse (Eds.), *The handbook of aging and cognition* (pp. 359–416). Mahwah, NJ: Lawrence Erlbaum.

Zhang, M., Katzman, R., Salmon, D., Jin, H., Cai, G., Wang, Z., . . . Liu, W. (2004). The prevalence of dementia and Alzheimer disease in Shanghai, China: Impact of age, gender, and education. *Annals of Neurology, 27*(4), 428–437.

ESSAY 44

Exploiting Eye-Mind Connections for Translation to Clinical Applications in Language Assessment

Brooke Hallowell

The zeal of my precious friend Dr. Sadanand Singh is unforgettable. Whether we were conferring about the best way to select grant reviewers, evaluate the promise of potential textbook authors, choose wine, grow vegetables, or raise children, he had the same degree of passionate responsiveness, dynamic facial expressions, delightful intonation, and profound joy. His influence on me was tremendous. He encouraged me in my forays into becoming as Indian as a Caucasian North American can be. He remained loyally connected to his roots and our Ohio University community in Athens, where he previously served on our faculty. He encouraged my career development when I was a whippersnapper and instilled in me his passion for fostering successes in others. He emanated profound inspiration by repeatedly emerging from tremendous hardships, always with that brilliant smile and continued vigor and success. His love of, and dedication to, our profession was spectacular, and he lived that love and dedication every day, through his publishing, philanthropy, teaching, writing, mentoring, and fostering of lasting connections amongst us. He also blessed our profession through his introduction of his wife, Anju, to our professional

world; Anju herself rose quickly to become a vibrant innovator and leader in our field and, thankfully, a gracious personal friend to so many of us. It is a great comfort that she and her vibrant family continue to give life to the Singh mission and legacy.

Where people look as they are looking at just about anything tends to tell us something about what they are thinking. This has been coined the *eye-mind assumption* (Just & Carpenter, 1980), the strongest form of which includes the suppositions that time spent fixating an item in a visual display is proportional to the time spent processing that item and that fixation sequences reflect sequences of visual items processed during a given task. As anyone who has ever daydreamed or anyone who is blind knows, the assumption may be invalidated. To be able to interpret data about eye fixation patterns in a way that reflects underlying cognitive and linguistic processing, we must ensure that any assumptions about the relationship between eye fixations and concurrent processing are valid in the context in which those data were collected.

It is important to note that eye fixations in this context are spontaneous (natural, unintentional or unprogrammed), not like those used purposefully in augmentative communication and computer and environmental control, although the latter uses have tremendous benefits for many people with motor speech difficulties. This is an important distinction in that one of the important strengths of methods for comprehension assessment described here is that people are not required to intentionally use eye movements to communicate; this helps control for potential ocular motor programming confounds that may affect an individual's intentional use of the eyes to convey propositional (intentional, meaningful) content.

Many scholars across a vast array of disciplines have developed clever ways to ensure close eye-mind relationships in a vast array of populations. There is tremendous potential in exploiting those relationships for translation of eyetracking methods into clinical use. Here we focus on applications for assessment of language comprehension in adults with neurological disorders, although additional clinical applications abound.

HARNESSING THE POWER OF THE EYE-MIND RELATIONSHIP

Although eyetracking research methods have been in use for over 100 years, eyetracking studies have grown in popularity over the past 30 years, because of the growing awareness of their value in studying cognitive activities, enhanced accuracy, improved ease of use, and decreasing costs. Eyetracking enables us to monitor where viewers' foveas (the highest-resolution portion of retinas) are fixated as they take in visual information. The technology used most commonly now entails video-based pupil-center corneal reflection systems, which come in myriad forms with diverse levels of accuracy, varied configurations (e.g.,

head-mounted, remote, and goggle-based, and entailing diverse ways of controlling or accounting for head movement), and a wide range of costs (Hallowell & Lansing, 2004).

Eyetracking methods have the advantage of allowing online measures, i.e., tracking of responsiveness during the actual task under study. They do not have the drawbacks associated with successive measures (e.g., recall, recognition, question answering) that require inferences about individuals' cognitive processes and allow for testing responses only after a studied task, leaving obscure the locus of the effect of manipulated variables.

Although other simultaneous measures exist, such as reaction times to prespecified stimuli, or shadowing (the repeating of verbal stimuli as they are heard), such measures are often so unnatural that they may alter normal processes. In contrast, eye-tracking provides a continuous record, and allows people to perform under relatively natural conditions. Numerous studies have demonstrated how eyetracking methods enable continuous mapping of responses during a variety of spoken language processing tasks (Altmann & Kamide, 1999; Anderson, Chlu, & Spivey, 2010; Blumenfeld & Marian, 2010; Eberhard, Spivey-Knowlton, Sedivy, & Tanenhaus, 1995; Mirman & Magnuson, 2009; Rayner, 1998; Sedivy, Tanenhaus, Chambers, & Carlson, 1999; Spivey, Tanenhaus, Eberhard, & Sedivy, 2002; Tanenhaus, Magnusan, Dahan, & Chambers, 2000; Tanenhaus, Spivey-Knowlton, Eberhard, & Sedivy, 1995).

EXPLOITING THE EYE-MIND RELATIONSHIP FOR IMPROVED TRANSLATION FOR THEORY AND PRACTICE

Many eye-tracking methods have been considered successful in their attempts to reveal underlying processes, because they have led to models that are compatible with, and/or predictive of, other eye-tracking results as well as the outcomes of experiments based on different response measures. Such successes would not occur if the eye-mind assumption were false; however, in a given context, the assumption may be violated. How? Cognitive tasks are not the only drivers of how we look at the visual world before us, including computer displays designed for research or clinical purposes. Our viewing patterns are also heavily influenced by physical stimulus characteristics (Heuer & Hallowell, 2007, 2009).

Given that there are open- (top-down) and closed-loop (bottom-up) influences on fixation sequences, it is important that we recognize that eye fixations do not *necessarily* reflect cognitive processes. For example, there are frequent cases of participants responding correctly to the informational content yielded by certain elements or features of pictures (e.g., to the presence of a particular object or characteristic of an object in a scene) and of text (e.g., one content word as opposed to another, or the disambiguating word in an otherwise ambiguous sentence) when these elements were never fixated. How can clinical and research methods be designed so that experimenters may be most confident of harnessing true eye-mind relationships? In addition to controlling for myriad participant characteristics and ensuring appropriate eye-tracker calibration and accuracy, it is critical that we adhere to a few key guidelines.

1. Control for possible peripheral viewing of elements of a visual display while different elements are being fixated.
2. Consider possible disparities between foveal and attentional fixation; recognize that there may be processing extraneous to any task under study. Set reasonable time limits tasks, taking into account task complexity and recognizing that speeded tasks may discourage extraneous processing.

3. Ensure that task instructions are well specified and understood, and reduce reliance on overt verbal instructions. Poor comprehension or hearing of task instructions can directly invalidate results.
4. Consider and control for the effects of contextual constraints on information processing. If visual stimuli used are simple or highly familiar, or if they contain much redundant information, it is not likely that viewers will fixate on all of their features.
5. Design visual stimuli carefully to control for properties of images that may extraneously influence scanning patterns. See Heuer and Hallowell (2007, 2009) for descriptions of specific visual stimulus and semantic content factors that may lead to confounds of bottom-up or closed-loop processes on eye-tracking results.
6. Have a clear rationale for the use of certain units of fixation-related analysis. The measures one adopts for particular eye-tracking applications has a direct impact on the interpretation of findings. Unfortunately, the eye-tracking literature is replete with studies in which dependent measures are ill conceived or poorly described such that interpretations of results are questionable. Also unfortunately, the publication of such work leads others to believe that they should follow suit and repeat erroneous uses of measures.
7. Have a clear rationale for the use of statistical methods used for eye-tracking analysis.

EXPLOITING THE EYE-MIND RELATIONSHIP TO STUDY COMPREHENSION

It is vital that people understand when listening to others speak or when reading, especially in cases of acquired neurologic disorders.

Knowing a person's comprehension abilities is vital to accurately diagnosing problems with cognition and communication, and to making appropriate decisions about treatment planning and life decisions. Despite the sheer number of test batteries we have for assessing comprehension and related cognitive abilities, we are still at a loss when it comes to knowing the true comprehension abilities of many of the patients and clients that we serve. After all, how do we really know what a person understands? Our assessments rely on *inferring* comprehension ability, based on overt responses. This is a problem because most people who have had a stroke or brain injury have motor, perceptual, and other deficits that may impair their ability to respond, or to respond correctly, when traditional comprehension tests are administered. Consequently, there is a high likelihood of inaccuracy when the existence and severity of comprehension deficits in such individuals are estimated through traditional test results, experimental data, and clinical judgment, as well as by the impressions of patients' caregivers and significant others (Hallowell, Wertz, & Kruse, 2002; Rosenbek, Kent, & LaPointe, 1984; Ross & Wertz, 2003, 2004). An important way to address this problem is by exploiting the eye-mind relationship for online assessment of comprehension via eye-tracking.

Excluding the work on Eye-tracking Comprehension Assessment System (ECAS) described below, only a few published studies address the use of eye-tracking in acquired neurogenic language disorders (Choy & Thompson, 2010; Dickey, Choy, & Thompson, 2007; Thompson, Dickey, & Choy, 2004; Thompson, Dickey, Choy, Lee, & Griffin, 2007; Yee, Blumstein, & Sedivy, 2004). The purpose of those studies was not to develop clinical assessment methods but rather to study grammatical and lexical processing from a theoretical perspective.

The focus of ECAS, now in progress in the Neurolinguistics Laboratory at Ohio University, is the translation of research-based eye-tracking methods for clinical comprehension assessment. This includes work toward a clinically applicable standardized method, verbal and visual testing stimuli, clinical norms, and instrumentation for assessing comprehension in any clinical population (see Hallowell, 1999; Hallowell, Wertz, & Kruse, 2002).

It is important that we *exploit* the eye-mind relationship, inducing viewing patterns that expose a person's underlying comprehension abilities to allow clinicians to gain information about comprehension that is currently unavailable for severely inexpressive patients and other patients who are difficult to diagnose. During an eye-tracking comprehension evaluation, a patient sits comfortably in front of a computer screen. The person is presented a series of test trials. In each trial, an auditory or written stimulus is presented along with a set of visual images. Within a trial, the image that best matches the content of the verbal stimulus is the target; the others are nontarget foils that have controlled degrees of semantic relationship with the verbal stimulus. Patients are not required to explicitly choose an answer or perform any intentional response, for example, speaking or pointing. Rather, they are asked just to look in whatever way is natural to them. Patients' eye fixations are tracked using a remote pupil-center corneal-reflection system.

Nothing is attached to the patient, who is able to move the head freely. Eye fixation data pertaining to the location, sequence, and duration of eye fixations on the image displays are analyzed through custom software.

To date, two different eye-tracking-based comprehension tests have been developed: The Multiple-Choice Test of Auditory Comprehension (MCTAC) and the Eye-tracking Picture Test of Comprehension (EPTAC). To evaluate their effectiveness with respect to traditional types of assessments, both tests have been developed in two forms: a computer-projected form where the eye-tracker tracks the patient's gaze on a computer monitor, and a printed paper form where the patient manually points to the choice. Both tests enable study of degrees of comprehension ability rather than simple correct/incorrect scoring; through systematic control of nontarget stimuli within visual displays, the influence of the degree of semantic relatedness of nontarget foils on eye-tracking and pointing responses can taken into account. Each of these tests has important strengths. A strength of the MCTAC is that its test items (varying in shape, color, size, prepositional and directional terms) are considered relatively culture free (McNeil & Prescott, 1978), because they do not require participants to understand culturally specific or unfamiliar words, or to interpret images of objects or action with which participants may not be familiar. A major strength of EPTAC is that its verbal stimuli represent common terms in everyday communication and were carefully developed to control for familiarity and frequency in English language usage. Also, EPTAC stimuli represent a broad array of linguistic structures, from short to long and simple to complex. Furthermore, EPTAC images include multicultural and multigenerational representation across all human characters depicted.

The psychometric properties of the eye-tracking tests bode well for clinical applications. For control participants (adults with no history of neurologic disorders, age 21 to 89, recruited for equal distribution across 10-year age ranges), the proportion of fixation duration on target images is consistently significantly greater than on any of the nontarget foil items. For each item and subtest and for overall tests, the proportion of fixation duration allocated to target images significantly exceeds chance expectations, whereas the proportion of fixation duration for each of the foil images is significantly lower than chance. The correlations between pointing scores and eyetracking scores for both tests are high for adults with no neurologic disorder. These results confirm previous findings (Hallowell, 1999; Hallowell,

Wertz, & Kruse, 2002; Heuer & Hallowell, 2009), again supporting ECAS and MCTAC validity and feasibility.

For people with aphasia, as expected, results indicate greater comprehension deficits, as indexed by reduced proportions of fixation durations allocated to target images. Also as expected, results have much greater variability than do those of control participants. With the more complex and longer stimuli, variability in performance among participants with aphasia increases. People with aphasia who achieve lower auditory comprehension scores on the *Western Aphasia Battery-Revised* (WAB-R, Kertesz, 2007) and on the pointing versions of the MCTAC and EPTAC tend to allocate smaller proportions of total fixation durations to target images on the eyetracking versions of those tests. It is important to consider differences among individuals with aphasia in terms of the degree of concordance among standardized behavioral test (WAB-R), pointing, and eye-tracking results.

Linear trend contrasts demonstrate that as the length of the verbal stimuli increases in the number of semantic elements to be understood, the proportion of fixation duration on the target declines. This indicates that the longer or more complex the verbal stimulus is, the more difficult it is for the individual with aphasia to identify the target image. Importantly, and consistent with results of control participants, results from the pointing version of the MCTAC and EPTAC are significantly correlated with eye-tracking version results.

The primary focus of ECAS research and development to date has focused on control participants to ensure methodological effectiveness and individuals with aphasia to ensure clinical feasibility and validity. The eye-tracking form of the MCTAC has been normed in American English, Russian, and Kannada, and is in development in Hindi, Mandarin Chinese, Bahasa Malaysia, and Korean. In addition to people with aphasia, the method is likely to benefit other individuals with any form of neurogenic disorder for whom comprehension assessment is challenging. This includes individuals with diffuse and focal traumatic brain injury (including blast injuries), locked-in syndrome, Alzheimer disease and other forms of dementia, multiple sclerosis, and amyotrophic lateral sclerosis. Current progress is encouraging in terms of future applications with additional conditions, including those in children, such as autism.

THE JOY OF SYMBIOSIS ACROSS DIVERSE AREAS OF EXPERTISE

A key to translational eye-tracking advances is the synergy of knowledge from diverse disciplines. For example, we seek interdisciplinary input on research design, clinical concerns, and attention to convergent validity through diverse eye-tracking applications by continuously tapping into the literature in psycholinguistics, cognitive science, neuroscience, neurology, speech-language pathology, marketing, human factors, computer science, and education (to name a few); this is vital to making sure that we do not reinvent solutions to problems already confronted by others and that we remain mindful of the relevance of our work. Also, for direct work on actual technological development, we benefit tremendously from the important work of graphic artists (development of carefully controlled visual stimuli); mechanical, systems, and biomedical engineering professionals (work on ergonomic and manufacturing considerations and hardware and software development); psychologists (consultation on assessment and scoring methods); and statisticians (data analysis). Furthermore, a key to making years of research in our laboratories translatable to clinical practice is engaging collaborators with diverse areas of expertise in health care, research commercialization, and business

development. This degree of interdisciplinary interdependence is a source of great joy for those of us who love the privilege of multifaceted exchange and knowledge sharing that is so fundamental to research and clinical practice in communication sciences and disorders.

Acknowledgments. The author thanks the numerous collaborators who have helped to advance the development of methods described here, including Hans Kruse, YoonSoo Lee, Vanessa Shaw, Sabine Heuer, Maria Ivanova, Dixon Cleveland, and Pete Norloff, and the clever graduate students in the Ohio University Neurolinguistics Laboratory. This work was supported by the National Institutes of Health/National Institute on Deafness and Other Communication Disorders (grants 5R43DC010079 and 5K23DC000153).

REFERENCES

Altmann, G. T. M., & Kamide, Y. (1999). Incremental interpretation at verbs: Restricting the domain of subsequent reference. *Cognition, 73*, 247–264.

Anderson, S. E., Chlu, E., & Spivey, M. J. (2010). On the temporal dynamics of language-mediated vision and vision-mediated language. *Acta Psychologica, 137*(2), 1–9.

Blumenfeld, H. K., & Marian, V. (2010). Bilingualism influences inhibitory control in auditory comprehension. *Cognition, 118*(2), 245–257. Retrieved from http://journals.ohiolink.edu/ejc/pdf.cgi/Blumenfeld_Henrike_K.pdf?issn=00100277&issue=v118i0002&article=245_biiciac

Choy, J., & Thompson, C. K. (2010). Binding in agrammatic aphasia: Processing of comprehension. *Aphasiology, 24*(5), 551–579.

Dickey, M. W., Choy, J. J., & Thompson, C. K. (2007). Real-time comprehension of wh-movement in aphasia: Evidence from eyetracking while listening. *Brain and Language, 100*, 1–22.

Eberhard, K. M., Spivey-Knowlton, M., Sedivy, J., & Tanenhaus, M. K. (1995). Eye movements as a window into real-time spoken language comprehension in natural contexts. *Journal of Psycholinguistic Research, 24,* 409–436.

Hallowell, B. (1999). A new way of looking at auditory linguistic comprehension. In W. Becker, H. Deubel, & T. Mergner (Eds.), *Current oculomotor research: Physiological and psychological aspects* (pp. 292–299). New York, NY: Plenum.

Hallowell, B., & Lansing, C. (2004). Tracking eye movements to study cognition and communication. *ASHA Leader, 9*(21), 1, 4–5, 22–25.

Hallowell, B., Wertz, R. T., & Kruse, H. (2002). Using eye movement responses to index auditory comprehension: An adaptation of the Revised Token Test. *Aphasiology, 16*(4/5/6), 587–594.

Heuer, S. & Hallowell, B. (2007). An evaluation of test images for multiple-choice comprehension assessment in aphasia. *Aphasiology, 21*(9), 883–900.

Heuer, S., & Hallowell, B. (2009). Visual attention in a multiple-choice task: Influences of image characteristics with and without presentation of a verbal stimulus. *Aphasiology, 23*(3), 351–363.

Just, M., & Carpenter, P. A. (1980). A theory of reading: From eye fixations to comprehension. *Psychological Review, 87,* 329–354.

Kertesz, A. (2007). *Western Aphasia Battery-Revised.* San Antonio, TX: Harcourt Assessment.

McNeil, M. R., & Prescott, T. E. (1978). *Revised Token Test.* Austin, TX: Pro-Ed.

Mirman, D., & Magnuson, J. S. (2009). Dynamics of activation of semantically similar concepts during spoken word recognition. *Memory and Cognition, 37*(7), 1026–1039.

Rayner, K. (1998). Eye movements in reading and information processing: 20 years of research. *Psychological Bulletin, 124,* 372–422.

Rosenbek, J. C., Kent, R. D., & LaPointe, L. L. (1984). Apraxia of speech: An overview and some perspectives. In J. C. Rosenbek, M. R. McNeil, & A. E. Aronson (Eds.), *Apraxia of Speech* (pp. 1–72). San Diego, CA: College-Hill Press.

Ross, K. B., & Wertz, R. T. (2003). Discriminative validity of selected measures for differentiating normal from aphasic performance. *American Journal of Speech-Language Pathology, 12,* 312–319.

Ross, K. B., & Wertz, R. T. (2004). Accuracy of formal tests for diagnosing mild aphasia: An application of evidence-based medicine. *Aphasiology, 18,* 337–355.

Sedivy, J. C., Tanenhaus, M. K., Chambers, C. G., & Carlson, G. N. (1999). Achieving incremental semantic interpretation through contextual representation. *Cognition, 71,* 109–147.

Spivey, M. J., Tanenhaus, M. K., Eberhard, K. M., & Sedivy, J. C. (2002). Eye movements and spoken language comprehension: Effects of visual context on syntactic ambiguity resolution. *Cognitive Psychology, 45,* 447–481.

Tanenhaus, M. K., Magnusan, J. S., Dahan, D., & Chambers, C. (2000). Eye movements and lexical access in spoken-language comprehension: Evaluating a linking hypothesis between fixations and linguistic processing. *Journal of Psycholinguistic Research, 29,* 557–580.

Tanenhaus, M. K., Spivey-Knowlton, M. J., Eberhard, K. M., & Sedivy, J. C. (1995). Integration of visual and linguistic information in spoken language comprehension. *Science, 268,* 1632–1634.

Thompson, C. K., Dickey, M. W., & Choy, J. J. (2004). Complexity in the comprehension of wh-movement structures in agrammatic Broca's aphasia: Evidence from eye-tracking. *Brain and Language, 91,* 124–125.

Thompson, C. K., Dickey, M. W., Lee, J., Cho, S., & Griffin, Z. M. (2007). Verb argument structure encoding during sentence production in agrammatic aphasic speakers: An eye-tracking study. *Brain and Language, 103,* 24–26.

Yee, E., Blumstein, S. E., & Sedivy, J. (2004). The time course of lexical activation in Broca's and Wernicke's aphasia: Evidence from eye-movements. *Brain and Language, 91,* 62–63.

ESSAY 45

Counseling Around the Edges of Traditional Treatment

Audrey L. Holland

I had the pleasure of knowing and working with Sadanand Singh, and his lovely staff and family, since his adventures in publishing began with his creation of College-Hill Press in 1980. His presses have published all of my books, all of them with good editing, good advice and fairness. More importantly, Sadanand Singh and all of his family have been my constant, warm, and caring friends. I always knew that when life got too complicated or boring or busy, I could find respite at their home in the hills above La Jolla. And I took great advantage of this—I even went to visit them when my first golden retriever died, so that their lovely dog could crawl into my bed to be petted and to help me mourn.

I am honored to be asked to contribute to this volume and, in fact, would have been heartbroken if I had not been.

INTRODUCTION

I have written extensively, as well as given a number of workshops on the role and the processes of counseling and coaching in speech-language pathology and audiology. Although my ideas have been well received, there is also a fairly constant undercurrent of concern voiced by readers and audiences. This concern results from a persistent professional paradox; although most speech-language pathologists and audiologists recognize the value and need for counseling for children and adult clients and their families, it is extremely difficult, if not impossible, to find time to provide it. Under these circumstance, it also seems ironic that the American Speech-Language-Hearing Association includes counseling in its Scope of Practice (2004, 2007), yet provides no mandate for counseling to be taught in our graduate programs nor provides guidelines for how to incorporate counseling time into evidence-based practice.

Both of these issues demand attention and change, ideally as soon as possible. In the meantime, however, the counseling needs of the populations we serve currently also demand at least our cursory consideration. In this paper, I outline a stopgap way to meet counseling needs around the edges of our required interventions. I begin with a rationale for the approach I will then describe. I use poststroke aphasia as my example, although I mean it as a more general metaphor for the practice of both speech-language pathology and audiology.

WHY COUNSELING? A RATIONALE FOR THE TREATMENT OF HUMAN COMMUNICATION AND ITS DISORDERS

The basic science of human communication and its disorders appears to be alive and well, attested to by the professions' own journals and by those of related fields such as linguistics, acoustics, neuroimaging, and so forth. The applied science of human communication, and indeed the art of applying it fares not nearly as well. There are a number of reasons for this, including the rather interesting article of professional faith that the basic science somehow outweighs the human side of things, and research and writing on those issues are somehow less important. It is beyond the scope of this work to explain, or even to consider in detail, the various societal forces that influence this neglect. Nevertheless, most readers will agree that acknowledgment of personhood, that is, learning to know the child or adult or family on whom a communication disorder has been inflicted, is not the high priority it should be.

Diane Ackerman's (2011) account of her spouse Paul West's aphasia is quite instructive, and probably should be required reading across master's training programs. Although she is charitable to the SLPs who worked with him, it is clear that that they did not know who he really was, and failed to consider the person to whom this devastating problem occurred. That is, they failed to acknowledge Dr. West's (and Dr. Ackerman's) personhood. Things improved remarkably in his recovery when she took over, putting her lifelong experience with him centermost in helping with his recovery.

Communication is an interpersonal act, not a scientific one. Language is merely the playing field on which the game of communication occurs, and of course it demands care and nurturance, for without it the communi-cation game cannot be very well played. Nevertheless, the game itself is even more critical. Identifying the players is central, acknowledging who they are, and what positions they play, and so forth, are all relevant for playing the communication game.

Good clinical intervention demands genuine acknowledgment of the person or family with the problem. Communication problems exist in people and their interactions. This is particularly important in today's health care climate. Because we professionals cannot fix problems, only provide help in solving them, it is necessary that we enlist and nourish the involvement of significant others. This is a counseling issue. Clinicians can work most effectively in their limited time if they can get both the family, and the adult or child with the problem to buy into the therapeutic process itself. This means incorporating them into the rehabilitation team as partners and experts; family, for information concerning what it is like to live with the problem, client for what it is like to live in the problem. Clinicians are, of course, the technical experts. These three sources of expertise should serve as a viable rehabilitation team.

There appear to me to be two attitudinal issues that determine how effectively family and clients buy in to the clinical process, and both require counseling skills. In what follows, I discuss these two pervasive counseling attitudes first. I then discuss a few much more specific counseling tools and how and when to apply them.

PERVASIVE COUNSELING ATTITUDES

The Thou Attitude

The key to making clinical alliances with family and client, in my experience, is the clinician's attitude. At heart, approaching persons and families with communication problems should be no different from the way in which we approach friends and loved ones, an attitude for which Martin Buber (1958, 2003) coined the terms "I-Thou." As opposed to "I-It" relationships, when one approaches others as I-Thou, others are fully respected and valued, based not on facts one knows about others, but on their personhood. To be sure, many aspects in our clinical field require I-It, in which facts are crucially important. For example, what is the nature and severity of the person's language or speech disorder, and what are appropriate clinical techniques for its management. But as the disorder exists in the person, the direct techniques of treatment cannot be applied well if the person with the disorder is not taken into account. This is a basic, even overarching counseling issue, and without it few long-term effects of intervention will result.

The good news is that learning and applying what I am going to call the "Thou Attitude" is solely within the control of individual clinicians. We SLPs choose this profession because we are intrinsically helpers. Rigorous training in the science of the discipline, as in almost every other health-related profession, focuses on the disorders. In accord with highly motivated medical students, SLP students are taught to shift their attention to the relevant science. But just as truly dedicated physicians (Jerome Groopman, Abraham Verghese, and Atul Gawande come to mind) return to the importance of recognizing personhood, so can we. And this shift is a major, pervasive, and most important part of "counseling around the edges."

Practicing clinical respectfulness is not difficult. For some, simply reading Martin Buber's short book on I-Thou (1958) or Kramer's practical interpretation of his work (2003), or some other volume, such as Davis (2011) that focuses on how to develop and maintain

respect for others could be the answer. For others, even the very simple practice of remembering to whisper the Thou pronoun (better not to do this aloud!) before entering a clinic room might do the trick. In a nutshell, learning to respect one's clients, regardless of their differences from ours in beliefs, lifestyles, politics, issues of importance, and so on, is the counseling foundation of our work. It leads naturally to finding out how our clients perceive their lives, who they communicate with, and what they talk about. For example, if an aphasic person's central interest is in his grandkids, then helping him with the language that addresses this interest is where the intervention should be centered. If his world revolves around the Pittsburgh Steelers, the wise clinician will try to get a grasp of NFL football allegiances' rather fascinating subcultures, possibly using the client's expertise as as the treatment focus. For example, my colleague Margaret Forbes describes a program of successful language therapy for a fan that was largely built around videotapes of the Steelers' glory years of the 1970s. She knows little about football and could care less, but she knows how to plan engaging and effective treatment. Whatever it is, an individual's passions are where the word retrieval activities and the relevant grammar reside.

Reading and writing provide other examples. How much clinical emphasis is to be placed on these modalities should depend on the client's preaphasic reading and writing needs and habits. Attempting to retrain skills that were used minimally beforehand rather ignores the client's personhood, or at least that what it is likely to be motivated to relearn. Thus, one of the two aspects of counseling that permeates the entire treatment scene is the clinician's attitude of respect for the client and the honoring of his or her unique personhood. The other is the clinician's understanding of his or her role in the treatment process, the next topic.

Metaphors for Clinicians

In his workshops on collaborative brain injury intervention (Ylvisaker & Feeney, 1998), Ylvisaker urged clinicians to develop a metaphor that addressed how they see themselves as clinicians. He maintained that having a metaphor in the first place was more important than what the metaphor actually was. He believed that we all have a personal metric against which we judge our professional work and how we do it, even if we don't recognize the metaphor without a bit of soul searching. Finding the best-fit metaphor reveals our personal professional standards. These metaphors could be anywhere along a spectrum ranging from coach to advocate to fairy godmother to movie director, to animal trainer, with many stops in between. When you find the metaphor you are comfortable with, it will resonate with how you go about your clinical job. It will reflect your own values and principles. This is an easy way to develop a sense of one's clinical persona. In my counseling classes and workshops, I routinely ask the participants to work this out to their satisfaction.

I agree with Ylvisaker on the importance of developing insight into ourselves as clinicians, but I question whether all of those metaphors are appropriate for those who aspire to be respectful and honoring of their clients. Does any clinician really believe that human communication is similar to how our family pets are trained? (If treatment consists solely of stimuli used to elicit single word responses, then this format has a lot in common with teaching Fang to "sit.") Nor can clinicians can improve communication by a simple whoosh of a clinical wand. (Not likely. Not a useful metaphor.) The bottom line is to look for the consistencies in one's own clinical behavior, and realize your metaphor. It is always possible that if it isn't what one intends, then find a better one and organize your interactions accordingly.

A final comment on counseling attitude. In no way is it to be implied that counseling attitudes are to kept in one's clinical back pocket, and only brought out when clinicians actually talk to their clients, as opposed to when they get to work on language. My belief is that talking to clients is the most important part of our clinical work. However, even the drills and the practices that center on the language part of communication are enhanced by the attitudes of respect and consistent application of a well-conceived, internally consistent rationale (metaphor) for our undertakings. The next section of this essay abandons these generalities, and describes more specific ways of providing counseling around the edges of our client interactions. It emphasizes some core counseling skills, followed by a detailed discussion of the concept of counseling moments. Finally, it briefly describes other client-oriented venues for meeting client's and family's counseling needs.

TRAINING IN COMMUNICATION COUNSELING

There is no substitute for formal training in counseling, where hands-on practice and role playing have a prominent role. However, a number of counseling workshops, geared to SLPs are available annually. As a former university instructor involved in teaching counseling to graduate students, and as a current provider of 1- and 2-day workshops to professionals in the field, I feel comfortable in saying that that their prior experience (and the self-selection process that gets them to the workshops) makes them very effective learners and participants. There are also useful texts in communication counseling (Flasher & Fogle, 2011; Holland, 2007; Luterman, 2008) that work well. A useful adjunct to texts is Simple Counseling (Chial & Flahive, 2011) a "self-contained Web site on CD-ROM" (authors' description). The goal is to provide examples, hands-on exercises and practice material that focuses on principles and method of counseling with people with aphasia (PWA). Regardless of one's professional area of specialization, clinicians can learn from them. As is true of this paper, generalization to other speech and language disorders across the life span is really pretty straightforward. Finally, alternatives to improving counseling skills involve finding a role model, or journaling.

Many counseling techniques are variants on a few underlying themes. Because the goal of this paper is to assist clinicians in seeing counseling opportunities around the edges of their more straightforward treatment approaches, only the most important are described here. Once you feel confident and comfortable with a few of them, try them out in appropriate interpersonal situations, such as when a friend or family member seeks your opinion on an important matter. It is likely to be useful for the people who seek either your ear or your advice, or both. And you get relevant practice!

THE QUIET TECHNIQUES

Focus on Listening

Clarifying, disclosing, and affirming are important quiet skills that reflect empathy to the person being counseled, but they are secondary in importance to listening. If one has the time and energy to improve only one direct counseling skill, it probably should be the skill of listening, for it is the most basic. Listening is an active process. Webster (1977) reminds us that listening is the primary tool to help us understand how the world looks to the person that is being counseled, not how closely it mirrors how we see the world. This is essential to the Thou, of course.

Buddhists consider the concept of using the space between our two eyes as an extra-sensitive space for deepening our awareness of what we see, that is, the Third Eye. The counselor in us should supplement it with developing a Third Ear. Listening effectively, that is really listening, takes concentration and effort, time, and constant underlying attention to Webster's definition. It is the client's world we seek to understand through listening (and looking), and we need those conceptual extra eyes and ears to do it.

What Is Heard Versus What Is Meant

Sometimes, messages have at least one more level of meaning. To Freud, manifest content was the actual plot of a dream, whereas its latent content was its hidden meaning. But the manifest/latent distinction can be noted in more mundane interchanges. One of my own personal favorites was when an acquaintance, commenting on an outfit I was wearing, said "I like your dress. I wish I could wear things designed for younger people!" Was this a compliment? Is the latent content really that hard to detect?

Usually, latent content is more subtle, and requires the combination of our real and our extra eyes and ears to detect it. For example, the spouse of a severely aphasic man buys him a computer with all the bells and whistles, and complains that the clinical staff is not taking the time to teach him how to use it. (A third ear hears that she is failing to accept the severity of her spouse's disorder; a counseling issue, probably for both of them.)

Practice with Listening

Our ability to apply those other aspects of counseling: explaining, advising, helping clients and families to understand the process of change, depends on these listening skills, what Luterman (2008) calls "deep listening." Deep listening is hard work, and although it is tempting to say it should be employed in all interpersonal interactions, it is not appropriate for many of them. However, if friends often remind you that you are "not listening" (a circumstance not unfamiliar to many husbands), it might be wise to sharpen up your listening skills a bit for all-around everyday use as well. But in counseling, deep, active listening is indispensable. Here are some practical tips for the counseling art of listening.

Practice applying a 3- to 5-second delay between the end of a friend's comments and your response when you are involved in a meaningful and important conversation. Use the time to consider a few alternative responses and choose the one you consider best for your reply. (This is the 5-second rule.)

In such conversations, make an effort to understand your partner's point of view before offering your own.

If you are not sure that you have it right, ask for clarification before responding (and repeat the 5-second rule then.)

Remember that many messages have both manifest and latent content. Make sure you try to hear both.

Involve your body in the act of listening. Look, lean in, and don't assume a confrontational posture. The more you look like you are listening, the more likely you are to be listening!

Remember the power of silence. There is no such thing as "just listening." Sometimes silence is its own therapy, permitting the speaker to hear him or herself. A pat on the hand here doesn't hurt either.

THE LOUD TECHNIQUES

The loud techniques include informing and explaining, teaching, advising, and helping others to change. Robert Shum, a noted clinical psychologist with lots of experience with language disordered children and their families, once commented that SLPs are masters at informing and explaining, but often at the expense of other counseling skills. I agree. We frequently equate providing information and explanation to counseling. Although they are certainly squarely within our professional counseling responsibilities, they are secondary to communicating our empathy, which relates to our attitudes and our listening skills. Finally, the loud skills require some acknowledgment of the persons we are informing and advising, as well as some modulating by our own experience. For example, I readily acknowledge my years of experience to clients, for it increases my credibility. But I also readily acknowledge that these years of experience have done little to guarantee that I am right. My mantra goes something like, "In my experience . . . but . . ." This does not mean that less experienced clinicians lack credibility. What it means is that they should acknowledge their experience, reassure the questioner that they know how to get answers to the questions they might not be able to answer, and will get back to them asap, etc. The bottom line is that none of us really knows, and that we all have to show the questioner that our skills include seeking out the answers. It also keeps us honest.

Among the loud skills, I believe that helping others to change is the most valuable. First, it involves a bit of all of the others, but it also holds the key for successful intervention. Again, the issue of time is paramount. We do not have enough time to effect change in our clients, and frankly, communication is so ubiquitous that if PWA and their families do not provide extra support, as well as understand and provide practice outside the clinical environment, long-lasting effects are probably not going to be forthcoming. There are self-help books available on methods for effecting change, and responsible clinicians should review this literature and either rely on them for some helpful suggestions, or even better, suggest that they be read by family members and discussed in treatment with clients. Two strong suggestions are books by Heath and Heath (2010) and Seligman (2007). Both are readable, theoretically sound, and provide very useful plans and suggestions.

SUMMARY OF COUNSELING TECHNIQUES

This was a brief tour of counseling skills. They were selected for their salience, but there are plenty of other skills that fall within the purview of counseling. Readers are encouraged to read, study as many of them as possible, and then to use them judiciously. Be alert to instances in which others can be seen doing effective counseling, that is, find and study role models. Practice them, and when they seem relevant, begin to apply them as well to clients and personal interactions.

COUNSELING MOMENTS

"Counseling moments" is a term I have adapted from my training as a life coach. The life coach has to be alert for little nuances and comments that suggest the need for direct interaction, questioning, reminders that you are really listening, from the coach. (Most of my coaching has been done over the telephone, which, incidentally, has greatly increased my ability to listen actively.) I have borrowed the term to apply to counseling in communication disorders.

There are predictable places in the dance we call intervention where counseling moments are most likely to occur. They are when a session is just starting up, or when it is drawing to a close. Unfortunately, dealing with those that happen near the end of the session can disrupt a session scheduled to follow it. But comments like, "We'll talk about it next week" are totally unsatisfactory, and I prefer to take the consequences of possibly annoying the next client. But apologizing is within most of our skill sets, and seems the lesser demon.

Although clinicians need to be particularly alert for them at beginnings and ends, counseling moments can occur any time in a clinical session. This means maintaining counseling attitudes during the more traditional parts of our interactions as well.

Here are a few counseling moments. Take 5 seconds (or longer) to organize your answer before you say it, then let your imagination guide you to the next step.

Counseling Moments for PWA

"I know what's wrong . . . but my kids — no way."

"I know why . . . speech here . . . you listen . . . but home? no good. 'Do your homework' . . . yes. But listen . . . no."

"Talking . . . talking . . . I get so . . ." (pounds table with hand).

Counseling Moments with Caregiver

"We have no social life anymore."

"I'm not getting any help from his children, and I am just overwhelmed."

"I'm afraid to leave her alone. What if she had another stroke?"

Simmons-Mackie and Damico (2011) provide a number of actual interchanges that exemplify what they call missed opportunities to help persons with aphasia to deal more adequately with the raft of problems that surround them. They are all good examples of unfulfilled counseling moments. Here is one of them, from near the end of a diagnostic evaluation:

CLIN: So his scores show that he has . . . uh . . . pretty severe aphasia and something called apraxia of speech

That . . . that has to do with the motor movements . . . moving your lips, and . . .

WIFE: He can move his lips.

CLIN: Yes . . . he does, but he has trouble making movements for speech. At least making movements that are the right ones . . . um . . . for speaking.

WIFE: Oh mmmmm.

CLIN: He has a lot of trouble with word finding, See here the score is only 20% on naming pictures.

PWA: (Eyes are starting to get tears.)

CLIN: The stroke damaged your language area in the brain (points to head). And here are the comprehension scores . . . these look a bit better.

WIFE: Okay (reaches over to PWA and puts her hand on top of his).

CLIN: Do you have any questions?

WIFE: He has gotten a lot better. He couldn't talk at all . . . nothing. I mean, what (XX) expect?

CLIN: He probably will improve, but we can't really predict how . . . how much. If I could do that I could make a fortune (short laugh). (Closes folder and pushes back in chair.)

(Wife and PWA stand)

CLIN: So I'll call you, and we'll get started soon.

The client and his wife are not treated as Thou. Instead, test scores are the focus, and the session becomes an I-It as a result. The person with aphasia is depersonalized, with all conversation directed to the spouse. Simmons-Mackie and Damico (2011) note that by strictly cataloging the facts, as she sees it, this relatively experienced clinician provides information at the expense of dealing with the emotionality that is apparent even by reading the text. Probably, the clinician is uncomfortable with direct personal contact, and one has to wonder what her clinical metaphor might be. Regardless, she has also missed the opportunity to engage this man and his wife in helping them to understand their own predicament, and I suspect, undermining future successful treatment by failing to make them members of the team. The clinician appears also to have set herself up for an unsuccessful future clinical experience with this couple, should they decide to return for treatment.

Note the manifest/latent contradiction not in the aphasic couple, but in the clinician's behavior, when she says, "Do you have any questions?" and, when the wife appears about to ask one, dismisses it with a (failed) attempt at humor, closes the folder, and stands up. Is it likely that this family will respond favorably to the clinician's promised call? Certainly, it is a missed opportunity to help people in obvious need. And it provides an excellent example of failing to provide counseling around the edges of a clinical session.

How would a counseling-oriented clinician handle the situation? Admittedly, what follows is a crass breaking of the 5-second rule. (I thought about it more carefully.) But below are some modifications that, hypothetically, could turn this into a counseling moment instead of a missed opportunity. I have changed none of the wife's questions.

CLIN: I'm sorry this took so long, and was so difficult for you, Mr. Z. And I know this news is not going to make either of you happy. But John, your scores show that you have . . . uh . . . pretty severe aphasia and something called apraxia of speech. That . . . that has to do with the motor movements . . . moving your lips, and . . .

WIFE: He can move his lips.

CLIN: Mrs. Z, you are right! And I kind of misspoke . . . It has more to do with your husband's brain not being able to tell any of his speech muscles how to move. It is a very frustrating situation for you, right, Mr. Z? I know this word "apraxia" is a new one for you, but as we work on it, it will get clearer, and probably less severe.

WIFE: Oh mmmmm.

CLIN: And Mr. Z, we both know that you have a lot of trouble with names of stuff.

PWA: (Eyes are starting to get tears.)

CLIN: (reaching over and taking his hand) I know this is hard for you, but the stroke damaged some of the brain parts involved in talking. But, Mr. Z, we also did some tests that were about how well you were understanding. You did much better on those, and that is a very good thing! It makes it so much easier to work on the stuff that is hard.

WIFE: Okay (reaches over to PWA and puts her hand on top of his).

CLIN: (puts her hand on top of theirs as well) I want to help you work out some ways to improve your communication, and if you want to, we will work on some. But meanwhile, do you have any questions?

WIFE: He has gotten a lot better. He couldn't talk at all . . . nothing. I mean, what (XX) expect?

CLIN: Both of you, I expect, with a lot of work from all of us, and a lot of patience, you should improve, Mr. Z. And as you said, Mrs. Z, he has already improved some. I wish I could predict better, but frankly, I can't. I do know that there are a lot of things we can try, and I assure you that I will do my best. Mr. Z, are you okay? In this stroke business, the only thing we can be sure of is that if all goes well medically, it won't get worse. (Closes folder and pushes back in chair)

(Wife and PWA stand)

CLIN: Is it okay if I call you? We will try to get started as soon as possible. Meanwhile, you have my card . . . if you think of other questions, please call me. I'm truly sorry that this has happened to you, but I will do the best I can to help.

My chattiness has probably added no more than 2 to 5 minutes, including unanticipated responses from the PWA and his wife. So it is probably not all that time consuming. Regardless, it should increase the likelihood of buy-in into the therapeutic process for this couple. There are many other ways to do this, of course. We all have the privilege of working within the constraints of our own metaphors, and I suspect mine would have dictated a somewhat different approach.

OTHER VENUES

Speech-language pathologists seldom consider developing other venues for providing counseling to their clients and families. A very satisfactory way to approach it is to go far beyond the edges, by creating "short courses" to families and PWA for dealing with the personal counseling issues surrounding an individual's language disorders. In my book (2007), I outline some ways to help families and PWA (not necessarily at the same time) deal with issues such as developing resilience. Such workshops and short courses are outside the purview of the current healthcare system, but with minimal financial investment from the sponsoring hospital or rehab center, and perhaps a small charge for participants, they can at least cover costs and become a viable adjunct to the problems of providing badly needed counseling to our clients.

CONCLUSIONS

The goal of this essay has been to support clinicians in their efforts to be of service to their clients and their families, not just by providing the services mandated by our flawed healthcare system, but by taking the step of reaching beyond it. This means recognizing and reaching out to forge relationships with the person who has a communication disorder and his or her significant others. Although the focus here was on aphasia, these comments apply to the broader spectrum of speech, language, and hearing disorders across the life span.

REFERENCES

Ackerman, D. (2011). *One hundred names for love.* New York, NY: W. W. Norton.

American Speech-Language-Hearing Association. (2004). *Scope of practice in audiology.* Available at http://asha.org

American Speech-Language-Hearing Association. (2007). *Scope of practice in speech-language pathology.* Available at http://asha.org

Buber, M. (1958). *I and thou* (2nd ed.). (R. Smith, Trans.) New York, NY: Charles Scribner.

Chial, M., & Flahive, M. (2011). *Simple counseling.* San Diego, CA: Plural.

Davis, C. (2011). *Patient practitioner interaction: An experiental manual for developing the art of healthcare* (rev. ed.). Thornton, NJ: Slack.

Flasher, L., & Fogle, P. (2011). *Counseling skills for speech pathologists and audiologists* (2nd ed.). Clifton Park, NY: Delmar.

Heath, C., & Heath, D. (2010). *Switch: How to change things when change is hard.* New York, NY: Broadway Books.

Holland, A. (2007). *Counseling in communication disorders: A wellness approach.* San Diego, CA: Plural.

Kramer, P. (2003). *Martin Buber's I and thou: Practicing living dialogue.* Mahwah, NJ: Paulist Press.

Luterman, D. (2008). *Counseling persons with communication disorders and their families* (5th ed.). Austin, TX: Pro-Ed.

Luterman, D. (2008). *Sharpening counseling skills.* DVD produced by The Stuttering Foundation of America, Memphis, TN.

Seligman M. E. P (2007). *What you can change and what you can't: The complete guide to successful self-improvement.* New York, NY: Vintage Press.

Shrum, R. (2004). *Remarks made at the annual Van Riper Conference*, Western Michigan University, Kalamazoo, MI.

Simmons-Mackie, N., & Damico, J. (2011) Counseling and aphasia treatment. *Topics in Language Disorders, 31,* 1–16.

Webster, E. (1977). *Counseling parents of handicapped children: Guidelines for improving communication.* New York, NY: Grune & Stratton.

Ylvisaker, M., & Feeney T. (1998). *Collaborative brain injury intervention: Positive everyday routines.* San Diego, CA: Singular.

✌ Index ✌

A

AAA (American Academy of Audiology), 109
AAC (Augmentative and Alternative Communication), 307–310
Academia, nurturing clinical expertise in, 78
Acceptance Based Therapy, 165
Ackerman, Diane, 344
Acoustical Society of America, 10
Acoustic analysis, of amusia, 277–280
Acute Otitis Media (AOM), 226–227
Adaptability, aphasia, 302–303
ADHD (Attention Deficit/Hyperactivity Disorder), 157
Adults
  with hearing loss, 220–222
  with normal hearing, 218–220
AERP (Auditory event-related potential), 215
  simple experiment, 217–218
African Americans, diagnosis of cancer and, 70
Air-conduction audiogram, 220
Alcohol, cancer and, 71
Alzheimer disease, Mild cognitive impairment (MCI) and, 327
American Academy of Audiology (AAA), 109
American Academy of Audiology Task Force on the Quality of Life Benefits of Amplification in Adults, 227–228
American Sign Language (ASL), 201
American Speech-Language-Hearing Association (ASHA), 72, 107, 109, 343
Amusia, acoustic analysis of, 277–280
ANSD (Auditory neuropathy spectrum disorder), 172
AOM (Acute Otitis Media), 226–227

APDs (Auditory Processing Disorders), 179–183
  defined, 180
Aphasia
  coping with
    external threats, 303–304
    internal threats, 304–305
    mechanisms unavailable to patients with, 305
  defense mechanisms/adaptability, 302–303
  psychological reaction determinants, 301
Applied behavior analysis, 152
ASHA (American Speech-Language-Hearing Association), 107, 109, 343
  examinations for cancer by, 72–73
ASHA Leader, 33
ASHA Working Group on Auditory Processing Disorders, 187
ASL (American Sign Language), 201
Asp, Carl, 319
Asperger disorder, 150
Attention Deficit/Hyperactivity Disorder (ADHD), yoga and, 157
Attitudes, counseling, 344–346
Audiograms, 100–101, 323
  air-conduction, 220
  overuse of, 103–104
  pure-tone, 172
Audiology, evidence-based practices (EBP) in, 225–229
Auditory event-related potential (AERP), 215
  simple experiment, 217–218
Auditory evoked potentials, evoked by words, 215–216
Auditory nerve (AN), dysfunction, inner hair cell (IHC) and, 171–175